# PHYSICIAN SERVICE PATTERNS
# AND ILLNESS RATES

# *Physician Service Patterns and Illness Rates*

Helen Hershfield Avnet

A Research Report
on Medical Data
Retrieved from
Insurance Records

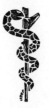

Group Health Insurance, Inc.

© 1967 by Group Health Insurance, Inc.
Library of Congress Catalog Card Number: 67-31143
Printed in the United States of America

 60

# ACKNOWLEDGMENTS

The research presently reported was translated from a series of proposed studies to an operating demonstration project as a result of the interest of Winslow Carlton, Chairman of the Board, and the late Arthur H. Harlow, Jr., then President, of GHI. The latter's successor, George W. Melcher, Jr., M.D., was responsible for the decision to continue the organization's policy of publishing and disseminating research results pertinent to current problems of medical care planning and distribution.

GHI's purpose was to demonstrate, by examples, the wealth of not-otherwise-available medical data which could be regularly retrieved from medical insurance records. Implementation involved procurement of data through data-processing, claims, membership, and medical department personnel. Assurance of cooperation from all these departments permitted the demonstration to proceed.

The project was conducted by the GHI Research Department, headed by the author, who is grateful to Joseph Krinsky, staff statistician, Lawrence Ort, research assistant, Florence Freed, chartist; to members of the office staff who assisted, for varying intervals of time, in various phases of production of the Report—Helen Ackenheil, Lucille Ball, Mary Lutz, Frances Reilly, Ruth Young; and, for his efforts in expediting publication, to Walter Perry, GHI public relations staff.

# PREFACE

This study was undertaken by Group Health Insurance (GHI) to demonstrate the wealth of medically relevant data which can be produced as a by-product of medical insurance administration.

The flow of original source data presented in "Physician Service Patterns" contains much of substantive value; equally important is the demonstration of what can be done.

It is our belief that every type of data examined for this exploratory project bears directly or indirectly on the work of medical care analysts and planners, epidemiologists, sociologists, physicians, hospital administrators, insurers, welfare fund trustees and research fund allocators.

Without repeating what is already in the body of the Report, the unprecedented variety of subjects treated specifically or by implication is illustrated in this selection of questions based on the contents:

What proportion of people will seek private medical care when given access to all types of physician service through their medical insurance? To what extent does this vary according to age, sex, marital status, family size, social class, area?

How many services does the average insuree receive in a year? How many different doctors does a family visit in a year? Where are people most likely to find doctors willing to make home calls? Which are the busiest months for surgery? for office care? for home calls? for preventive visits? for births?

How are the practicing physicians distributed—geographically, by age, by type of practice, by qualifications? Has the disappearance of the general practitioner been exaggerated? What proportions of physicians have voluntary hospital staff appointments? Are there significant local variations?

How does our emphasis on specialization compare with that in other countries? How do specialists in the different fields vary as to proportion of services rendered in office, home or hospital? What role does the general surgeon play as compared with surgical subspecialists? How does this vary in different types of hospitals? How extensive is the role of the nonspecialist? Does the rate of specialist consultations appear to be associated with higher proportions of specialists or of general practitioners practicing in a given area?

Are hospital admission rates lower among insurees covered for out-of-hospital services? What proportion of physician services is received out of the hospital?

How are hospital admissions distributed among medical school affiliates, other voluntaries and proprietaries? In what areas are proprietary admissions concentrated? Why do physicians and patients continue to use proprietary hospitals?

What differences are found in utilization rates of various x-ray and laboratory procedures? What proportions of office x-rays are accounted for by radiologists? by other specialists?

Instead of fragmented reports, is it feasible to develop serial data on illness trends via an integrated index of the incidence of treated illness, by diagnosis, including acute, chronic, hospitalized and non-hospitalized disorders?

How would reporting of annual incidence rates of each diagnosis, surgical or diagnostic procedure and other correlated treatment data for age-sex subgroups, provide a more equitable base for comparing and evaluating care under different systems of medical care distribution?

How can quantitative studies of insurance records suggest promising leads to studies of medical care quality, adequacy, standards?

The above questions come no closer to encompassing the material in the book which follows than the book comes to exhausting the possible types of analysis permitted by available data. But even if only a fraction of such data were regularly available on populations insured under various systems of distribution and residing in different areas (abroad as well as in the United States), the base for scientific evaluation and planning efforts would be vastly strengthened.

This volume is the third original research report to be published by GHI-GHDI in five years. Like its predecessors ("Psychiatric Insurance" and "Insured Dental Care") it is distributed as a community service. We hope that by showing what can be done as a first step by one organization, we shall be helping to stimulate further action in this sphere, by those in strategically appropriate positions, toward our common ultimate goal of improved medical care distribution.

GEORGE W. MELCHER, JR., M.D.
*President, Group Health Insurance, Inc.*

# CONTENTS

Chapter 18 *(Cont'd)*

# TABLES

xxiii / Tables

## xxiv / Tables

# GRAPHS

# PHYSICIAN SERVICE PATTERNS
# AND ILLNESS RATES

# Chapter 1

# INTRODUCTION AND HIGHLIGHTS

Medical insurance systems in the United States and abroad have generally neglected their opportunities to retrieve and report medical information accumulating as a by-product of the insurance. The neglect has persisted over the years despite the well-recognized need for medical care—morbidity statistics and the increasing capabilities of data-processing machinery. With occasional exceptions, mainly involving hospitalization data, references to medical insurance experience usually concern costs or coverage.

At the level of individual plans or associations of plans in the United States, failure to explore and develop potentially useful medical data can be ascribed to many factors—indifference, unwillingness to disclose information, absence of suitable personnel, or, probably most consistently, pressures to minimize expenditures not contributing obviously and directly to growth or operating efficiency. (The latter explanation would suffice also for the frequent inadequacy of basic population records required for interpretation of experience.)

At the national level of research leadership, there has been a tendency to emphasize insurance data limitations rather than to encourage exploration for positive contributions.

Whatever the causes, the situation calls for thoughtful review in the light of two factors: admitted shortcomings of currently available medical care and morbidity indices; and the increasing medical data potential of insurance records as comprehensive coverage broadens its membership base.

## The Household Interview as a Source of Medical Data

Medical care and sickness rates, however narrowly or elastically conceived, must by definition relate to a population at risk: within a stated time interval, $x$ persons are treated with $y$ units of specified service for $z$ cases of specified illness—all described in relation to the total population of which these persons are a part.

The requirement of a known population at risk rules out the use of most medical records as sources for computation of rates and description of trends. As a result, heavy reliance has been placed on household interviews by means of which questions on health, disability, medical care and illness pertaining to all members of households are addressed to one of its members.

Most national health and medical care statistics for the United States are based on this approach, applied through the Health Interview Survey. The latter is one of three types of surveys comprising the National Health Survey, an ongoing activity of the Federal Government since 1957; the others are the Health Examination Survey, which seeks data on health defects by means of actual health examinations of representative population samples, and the Health Records Survey, consisting of miscellaneous studies of facilities or special population groups such as hospital patients.

The household interview has long been regarded by many as the only practical method of collecting population-based information in this field. Among its advantages, the following are outstanding:

Stratified sampling procedures permit the drawing of population samples from any desired universe of study—e.g. the nation, a region, a city, children, civilians, etc.

The interview method permits more "one-stop" questions than any other possible source. All questions as to health and medical care of families can be asked at the one interview, including topics such as days of disability, and untreated illness, on which only the interviewee would have information.

Standardized questionnaires ensure uniformity of records from place to place and over the years.

The opportunity to bring the intrinsic advantages of the interview technique to full fruition is assured when government agencies adopt it, as in the case of the Health Interview Survey, automatically adding the blessings of adequate time to experiment and ample funds to implement research plans. This combination of advantages cannot be approached by any alternative data source.

On the other hand, a serious limitation is also inherent in the household interview approach: reliance on the capacity of the householder to understand, remember, and relay health and medical information.

Criticisms of the Health Interview Survey, voiced in its own reports and in publications of allied agencies, stem mainly from uncertainties as to accuracy of medical reporting by household respondents. Most confidence seems to be placed in respondents' ability to recall major events such as hospitalization or disability, and to list medical expenditures. Special studies which might have been reassuring on other counts, however, have had the opposite effect.[1]

One project designed to check interview responses against data recorded by physicians found "that the survey information does not conform even moderately well to the universe of conditions inferred from physician reporting." This was based on findings, for example, that of all persons for whom physicians noted a service during the two weeks prior to interview, only

---

[1] For example see Sanders, Barkev S., *"Have Morbidity Surveys Been Oversold?,"* American Journal of Public Health, Volume 52, Number 10, October 1962.

about 60 per cent were reported on interview to have seen a physician, while, on the other hand, 60 per cent of chronic conditions reported by respondents could not be matched with any entries on medical records. The same study called attention to the difficulty of disease identification by laymen:

> "A wide variety of orthopedic conditions—characterized by physicians as osteomyelitis, Paget's disease, sacroiliac sprain, degenerative disc syndrome . . . —are matched in the household interview with a respondent report of arthritis. Many specific dermatological diagnoses made by physicians (eczema, seborrheic dermatitis, contact dermatitis, psoriasis, neurodermatitis, lichen simplex, alopecia) were matched on survey by a respondent report of a skin disorder stated to be due to allergy. An appreciable number of cases of arteriosclerotic and/or hypertensive heart disease were matched on interview by respondent reports, simply, of high blood pressure." [1]

Such disquieting findings have led to frank statements, by responsible officials, as to the need for reevaluation of interview limitations:

> "There is an enormous field here for methodological research work. We visualize this as perhaps a crisis in social science. More people are taking surveys of more things, . . . asking people questions without any commensurate amount of work in trying to test the accuracy with which these questions can be answered or are answered."

> "The National Health Survey, and particularly the Health Interview Survey, seems to be discussed as a perfected instrument, and it is by no means such . . . We are in the midst of a program of reappraisal of the whole survey to try to bring to bear the methodological research that has been carried out over the past 5 or 6 years and make such

---

[1] *Health Interview Responses Compared with Medical Records,* report by Eve Balamuth, Division of Research and Statistics, Health Insurance Plan of Greater New York, published by U.S. Department of Health, Education and Welfare, Public Health Service Publication Number 1000–Series 2–Number 7, 1965.

improvements as we can, and perhaps cut back on the objectives at points where we think that it is pretty evident that we are not accomplishing the job and don't yet know how to accomplish the job." [1]

Dissatisfaction has also been expressed as to the inability of the National Center for Health Statistics to relate data on physician visits to diagnosis.[2] This is only one manifestation of the type of criticism generated by the Center's piecemeal approach to morbidity and medical care analysis, as well as by the absence of detailed data on sources of service and on services received, all of which suggests that interviews with laymen regarding their medical experiences need to be supplemented by data from other sources.

## Growth of Private Medical Insurance

It has been estimated that the proportion of consumer expenditures for physicians' services met by private insurance in the United States rose from 12 per cent in 1950 to 38.4 per cent by 1964.[3]

The number of people privately insured for at least a portion of physician expenses was estimated as of 1965 at 146 million for surgery, 113 million for "regular medical" (mainly in-hospital), and 52 million for "major medical" insurance.[4]

From these figures, it may be inferred that the great majority of the non-military, non-welfare, non-Medicare popula-

---

[1] Dr. Forrest Linder and Theodore D. Woolsey, Director and Deputy Director, National Center for Health Statistics, speaking before the Fifteenth Anniversary Conference of the U.S. National Committee on Vital and Health Statistics. Public Health Service Publication Number 1000–Series 4–Number 4, U.S. Department of Health, Education and Welfare, June 1966.

[2] *Economic Costs of Cardiovascular Diseases and Cancer*, by Dorothy P. Rice, Health Economics Series Number 5, p. 537, U.S. Department of Health, Education and Welfare, 1965.

[3] Reed, Louis S. and Hanft, Ruth S., *National Health Expenditures, 1950–64*, Social Security Bulletin, U.S. Department of Health, Education and Welfare, January 1966.

[4] *1966 Source Book of Health, Insurance Data*, Health Insurance Institute, New York, 1966.

tion has some degree of private insurance coverage for physician services. It is also clear that the tendency has been toward "catastrophic" rather than comprehensive coverage (the latter usually being defined to include office, home, diagnostic and preventive care); but that with the dramatic growth of "major medical" coverage—from 100,000 in 1951 to 52 million in 1965— a large number of people incidentally acquired partial protection for office-home expenditures.

The influence of Medicare, together with the near-saturation of the voluntary medical insurance market in terms of numbers of persons reached, is expected to result in increasing pressure from both buyers and sellers toward broader ambulatory benefits.[1] The voluntary portion of Medicare provides a more inclusive level of coverage to those past 65 than that held by most employed groups. It is anticipated that the difference will be a popular subject in collective bargaining sessions, while for their part the insurers, particularly in the non-profit plans, will be more responsive than in the past to suggestions that they broaden their benefits.

## Insurance as a Source of Medical Data

The health interview method is one way of obtaining population-based data. Insurance experience is also based on a known universe, a population at risk.

As the volume and scope of medical insurance increase, the volume of medical records in the files of insurers becomes a problem—in most instances a problem of whether or when to throw them out.

The term "medical records" as used here distinguishes the insured population's medical services, sources of service, and reported diagnoses from the financial aspects of insurance (premium income and benefits paid) usually reported. These medically relevant aspects of insurance records could, with

---

[1] *"Sees Medicare Affecting All Health Cover,"* Journal of Commerce, October 18, 1966.

proper attention to necessary preparatory steps, permit calculation of use rates and treated morbidity rates based on matching records of the population at risk to the physician or hospital rendering service, the type and amount of services rendered, and the diagnosis reported by the physician. The last three variables can also be matched to describe patient care in relation to diagnosis, independently of rate calculations.

Continuing neglect of insurance records may be regarded with varying degrees of indifference or indignation. The need for quantitative medical data in connection with planning and evaluation is not disputed. Difficulties appear when decisions center on which sources of data are worth the considerable effort required for their development.

Those deprecating the potential usefulness of medical insurance data have in the past offered a variety of reasons—that there is "self-selection" of the insured, that records are of no value unless they represent the national population, that morbidity statistics which exclude untreated morbidity are useless, that plans offering limited benefits or excluding any population segments are not likely to accumulate worthwhile data.

The objection that insurees are "self-selected", thus unrepresentative, has been negated by the emergence of group insurance as the mechanism for blanketing in the vast majority of insurees. Insurees today are representative of the non-institutionalized, non-government-subsidized population; their medical care reflects the level prevailing in the country.

The notion that all statistics must be based on nationwide samples has been modified by practical demands for local information; but in any case, the growth and distribution of coverage have removed geographic limits of individual plans as an automatic disqualifier.

The validity attached to the other arguments against insurance as a source of medical data depends on research objectives and on available alternatives.

Is it necessary that morbidity statistics, to be useful, include untreated illness? It would seem not always, as for example when the purpose is to determine the reasons for the medical care being received, or to plan resources needed to meet demands. In fact, in some respects, the mixture of untreated and treated morbidity rates in one index could create confusion for planners, particularly if it were not known why the untreated illnesses were untreated, or whether they required any professional care.

Must an insurance plan cover all services before retrieval of medical data on any type of service becomes worthwhile? This appears to be an unreasonable prerequisite to the recovery of data on insured segments. There is no really good reason, for example, why surgical data of the type retrieved for the present studies could not have been forthcoming regularly by now for the nearly 150 million people with such coverage, and analyzed by procedure, by type of treating physician, by type of medical organization system, and by area, to help answer the ultimate questions as to what is "normal", which procedures are overutilized, which may be underutilized in which situations.

As for the necessity of including all population segments, it seems self-evident that the exclusion of welfare, military and institutionalized populations from the insurance universe need not circumscribe the usefulness of insurance data. Separate studies of various population categories receiving care under different systems could in fact be helpful if presented in comparable form.

Insurance data can definitely be discounted where the objective is to measure the totality of health or health care, or define health status in terms of prevalence of disease or defects including unknown or untreated conditions, or devise similarly inclusive morbidity indices, or measure days of disability, or determine consumer expenditures for various medical purposes. All such information is obviously beyond the scope of medical insurance records.

The chief advantage of medical insurance records over records based on household interviews is access to data reported by physicians.

Each source has its drawbacks; each can complement the other. No single approach can satisfy all data needs.

In evaluating alternative objectives and sources, it is necessary to distinguish between the somewhat vague concept, health, and the measurable concept, medical care. Medical care is only one aspect of health care, frequently a negligible aspect as compared with environmental health influences such as fresh air, plumbing and garbage-disposal facilities, rat-free domiciles, and so on; but it is the only aspect reflected in medical records of whatever origin. Similarly, "need" for medical care, when it includes unrecognized need, is an ill-defined concept which is difficult to relate to current realities of the medical market; expressed demand for care is the measure of medical liability as of any given time.

None of the limitations on scope of insurance data need detract from their potential capacity to depict major aspects of the private medical care complex as it exists and changes. The private sector still delivers most of the service; it is still the recourse of the great majority of the population for the great majority of services. Little is systematically measured and reported as to what goes on in this sector. Private insurance experience holds one key. The scope of possible studies enlarges with the scope of the insurance. Data from comprehensive plans can answer the most questions, but worthwhile data can also be produced by limited plans, given adequate incentive to engage in the necessary preliminaries of planning and data preparation.

Potential and realization are far apart. The prepayment group practice or capitation plans which service members through salaried physicians have received financial encouragement to provide data in some depth on their experience.[1] Since the great majority of services to the noninstitutionalized civilian population is still rendered by private practitioners on a fee-for-service basis, however, it would seem prudent to study medical care in such settings as well, irrespective of preferences for one setting or the other.

---

[1] *Group Health and Welfare News,* November 1965.

## Group Health Insurance, Inc.

GHI is the largest independent non-profit community fee-for-service plan for insuring physician services in the United States. As such it usually creates classification problems for medical insurance analysts: it is too large to ignore, it cannot be categorized as medical-society-sponsored, but it is equally out of place among consumer-sponsored prepayment group practice plans.

Consumers and physicians each comprise half of its Board of Directors.

The "group" in its name refers to enrollment methods, not to manner of providing service; the plan operates within the established system of medical care distribution. Subscribers have freedom of choice of physician. Those choosing partici-pating physicians, who accept GHI fees as full payment, are promised paid-in-full service benefits. Fees for services of non-participating physicians equal those paid to participants, but the subscriber in this case has no protection against out-of-pocket expense.

A medical insurance innovator since 1938, when it began as Group Health Cooperative, Inc., GHI offered in-hospital med-ical-surgical coverage of physician services in the 'Forties; added first-visit, unlimited office, home, preventive and ambulatory diagnostic coverage in the 'Fifties; was first with a community dental insurance plan (its sister organization, Group Health Dental Insurance, Inc.); pioneered with short-term psychiatric insurance experimentation in the 'Sixties; plans to add hospitali-zation to give subscribers the opportunity for medical-hospital-dental coverage under one administrative roof.

GHI now protects over a million people, most of them in the New York-New Jersey metropolitan area and covered under the comprehensive "Family Doctor Plan" of physician coverage in office, home, hospital.

It was the addition of this coverage, around the mid-'Fifties, which triggered GHI's greatest growth. Up to then, the choice of medical coverage in the area had been between limited coverage under the prevailing system of medical care distribution, and comprehensive coverage under closed panel salaried or capitation arrangements, with or without group practice. The offer of comprehensive benefits under the prevailing free-choice, fee-for-service system combined in one plan what were regarded by many potential buyers as the advantages of the two other choices.

The timing of the new plan was also opportune, coinciding with increasing interest in medical care as an area for broadened fringe benefits to union members and permitting fringe-benefit shoppers to purchase the coverage they wanted without disturbing their members' patterns of seeking care. Consumer preference for this type of plan, initially exhibited by many welfare fund advisors and managers, was subsequently verified when individuals within groups were allowed "dual choice".

With the launching and enthusiastic reception of the broadened coverage plan, GHI's administrative focus turned from hospital to ambulatory services. The number of claims skyrocketed as a result of increased membership and increased claims per member. This in turn dictated acquisition of computers to expedite claims-processing.

The developing situation offered undeniable research opportunities: a "goldmine" of accumulating records on members, patients, physicians, services, illnesses; and generous assertions, during negotiations for computer equipment, of its incidental potential for medical data retrieval and analysis.

The opportunity was accepted by GHI as a challenge. Its leaders, never satisfied with running an ordinary insurance operation, were proud of GHI's long history of innovating successful experiments in the voluntary medical insurance field, and were also concerned that its original purpose of social usefulness to the community at large be maintained. They thought of the "Patterns Project", as it came to be called, in these terms. Their support promised the necessary cooperation between

GHI Claims Processing and Research Departments, and their personal integrity ensured continuation of the policy of unbiased research and reporting previously established.

## The GHI "Patterns Project"

The thesis behind the present effort holds that a number of sources should be tapped to produce needed data; that as long as the fee-for-service free-choice system of distributing care remains as the dominant method, what happens under that system needs to be studied and reported with some precision and without prejudice as to whether or not it is a good system, this being irrelevant to the need for facts; that private medical insurance is, increasingly, a potential source of such data; and that GHI, because of its broad coverage and broad range of "matchable" records on membership, physicians, services, and diagnoses, provides a logical base for a demonstration project.

The general purpose of the project was to investigate and illustrate the range of medical care and morbidity data which is potentially available to administrators of comprehensive medical insurance and which could be produced at regular intervals by the application of currently feasible electronic data processing techniques.

The phrase "potentially available" admittedly describes varying degrees of data availability in different plans. At GHI, preparations for medical data retrieval involved special attention to "input" information on the study population, physician characteristics, diagnosis entry and coding, x-ray and laboratory procedure coding, and hospitalization information. Except for physician records, such efforts at special preparation were generally designed to minimize the number of incomplete or uncoded records on types of information routinely collected, rather than to add other items.

The entire project was devoted to planning, preparation, retrieval, analysis and presentation of quantitative measurements. Inferences drawn from the quantitative findings as to quality of care received by the GHI population would require further data, mainly of a type not found in insurance records, for verification. Similarly, there may well be implications of an epidemiological nature in the data; here again, the experience presented may serve as a source of pointed questions for further investigation.

Except for Chapter 2, a necessary antecedent to an understanding of objectives and of data limits applicable to all aspects of the work, the report on this experiment consists largely of substantive results, presented as a series of interrelated but not necessarily interdependent studies, each illustrating a different facet of the retrieval program.

Most of the studies are based on the reported illnesses and medical care of the membership insured with comprehensive physician coverage; but data on service utilization are shown in terms of service components, with tabulations in separate chapters arranged to suggest, or for comparison with, segmented studies feasible under limited coverage plans.

The book by its nature achieves a range of topics unprecedented in medical insurance literature.

## HIGHLIGHTS

In the scant field of medical care and morbidity reporting, the significance of GHI's initial explorations comes less from their substantive content than from the fact of their development.

Aside from studies based on interviews with household respondents, whose medical reporting abilities have been seriously challenged, most of the limited research effort in this field has been directed either toward a relatively infrequent medical care segment (hospitalization), toward minority (disadvantaged) population segments not covered by voluntary insurance, or toward prepaid group practice plans affecting only a small fraction of the population.

*What happens to the self-supporting privately-insured great majority who obtain medical care under the traditional system of medical care distribution could be systematically reported by insurers, at least in part, but is not. This is the message of the present report.*

At a time when more and more emphasis is being placed on the need for planning and on "health services research," corresponding emphasis is suggested on the feasibility of converting a wasted information resource into a planning tool. The message assumes the more cogency as the growing demand for more comprehensive medical insurance broadens the potential scope of population-based, physician-reported medical data accumulating in insurance files; medical facts are increasingly at the disposal of insurers, but thus far little has been done to rescue and coordinate them.

Most of the data in this book (except for the study of available physicians) apply to the study population's experience of the year 1964, were retrieved in 1965 and 1966. Once past the struggle of initiation, with "bugs" removed and with adequate financing, regular production of any analyses deemed desirable on a serial basis could be scheduled within a few months of the experience studied. Continuous studies offer the opportunity for trend analysis, one of the most valuable aspects of this type of data, which unfortunately could not be incorporated into plans for the present experiment.

Aside from the sections describing source data and some of the problems faced in translation, this book is a series of illustrations of data retrieval possibilities and of simple analytic approaches to interpretation.

Data describing population composition are generally not produced on insured groups, but could be; and are a prerequisite to comparison of experience under different plans, or for projection of findings to other populations.

Data on physician resources help to restore perspective in an area where reporting and recommendations are sometimes distorted by limited viewpoints or unrealistic objectives. Information must be available in some detail and on a continuing basis if there is to be intelligent discussion of what is practically feasible as of any given point in time.

Data on ambulatory care, employed in the development of

both service and illness rates, recall what is often ignored—that *out-of-hospital care still constitutes the bulk of medical service, represents the average person's contact with the medical profession.*

On the other hand, the project's hospitalization studies provide information in a medical care sphere where comparable data could be most readily and regularly available to researchers seeking explanations of wide variations in utilization.

Similarly, the type of detailed analysis provided on surgery contains the seeds for a better understanding of frequency differences found for specific procedures under different systems of distributing medical care—another area characterized by more heat than light.

Data on proportions of membership subgroups using medical service reflect demand unencumbered by financial restraints.

Data on volume and types of service received from different types of physicians by different population segments in different areas, or for various conditions, are of interest in themselves, as well as a helpful preliminary to estimates of future demand and, conceivably, to ultimate plans for the setting of standards.

Integrated data on treated illness rates for age-sex subgroups suggest how medical insurers could eventually provide a much-needed supplement to mortality statistics as a measure of medical problems and progress.

In direct contrast to statistics on incidence of treated disease are the charts listing types and sources of treatment accorded individual patients during the study period. By integrating the data at the patient level, this approach demonstrates how insurance records may illuminate two generally inaccessible areas: the clusters of illnesses suffered, and the series and types of physicians visited, by individual patients.

If the GHI medical data retrieval program were to be repeated, some analyses would be expanded, others omitted; the selection process is initially difficult, improves with hindsight.

It is also difficult to select highlights from the mass of

substantive findings presented; varying disciplines or fields of interest of possible readers preclude agreement as to areas of greatest concern. The points made below are therefore chosen arbitrarily, with no attempt at inclusiveness, but with the same general focus as the book itself on illustrating applications of the project's basic thesis.

### Physician Supply

The supply of privately practicing physicians in the eight-county New York metropolitan area where most GHI members reside totals nearly 23,000 (of whom 17,000-plus are credited to the five counties of New York City proper), provides an overall ratio of one physician to 490 residents. The ratio ranges from 1:240 in Manhattan to 1:800 in Suffolk County.

Of the total, 55 per cent are listed as specialists; this compares with 61 per cent claimed nationally. When the definition of specialist is limited to Diplomates of various American Specialty Boards, about one of three practicing physicians qualifies —a ratio much closer to the proportions of specialists listed for countries in Western Europe.

Wide variations were found as to proportions and qualifications of specialists in different areas and age groups. The highest proportions of practicing Diplomates, 35 per cent or more, are in Manhattan, Westchester and Nassau, while about one in four practicing physicians were thus classified in Bronx, Brooklyn, Queens, Richmond, and Suffolk. The highest proportions with only the State Workmen's Compensation specialist designation were found in areas with lowest overall physician ratios, Richmond and Suffolk, raising the question as to differing standards in different areas and the possible effect of such practices on attempts to set nationwide criteria.

Despite the continuing downward trend in ratios of general practitioners, they still remain the single largest source of physician care. The notion of replacing them with internists and pediatricians is dispelled on realistic examination of resources.

Psychiatry now ranks third among specialty fields in the

eight-county area as a whole. This largely reflects its strong position in Manhattan, however, where it ranks second only to internal medicine, outranks general surgery. In the other areas of New York City and in Nassau County, psychiatrists are still outnumbered by internists, general surgeons, obstetricians, and pediatricians. This is also the order at the national level.

In general, the inclusion of Manhattan's resources in descriptions of the eight-county area masks the situation in the other seven counties. Manhattan has 271 specialists per 100,000 population, as against 64 to 128 in the other counties; and 148 general practitioners as against 62 to 88. The same type of disparity affects descriptions of hospital bed resources.

The study of physicians' status with respect to hospital staff appointments indicated over half the physicians with no appointment to a voluntary hospital staff. The situation is most acute in Queens, Nassau, Bronx, Brooklyn—where two thirds of the population in the eight-county area reside.

## Hospital Bed Supply

Throughout much of the eight-county New York metropolitan area, the number of general voluntary or proprietary hospital beds available for private patients, in proportion to population, is well below national averages. The true situation is frequently disguised by the inclusion of municipal hospital beds, or by averaging Manhattan's extraordinary resources with the relatively meager resources of other counties. Outside of Manhattan, the only counties that appear to have adequate facilities as compared with national averages (which are lowered by the southern states) are Westchester and Richmond.

## Free Access

Comprehensive insurance lacking financial deterrents such as "deductibles" and coinsurance requirements, offered without limiting stipulations as to physician or place of service, presents optimal inducements for initiation of medical service by insurees. The resulting index, user rates, probably comes closest to reflecting insuree awareness of need for medical care, along with awareness of insurance rights. Other indices, involving volume and types of services received, are complicated by the role of the physician and the extent of hospital facilities.

Study results demonstrated high user rates generally and among almost all major population subgroups in the sample.

The overall proportion of users among those with comprehensive coverage was 80 per cent. (The proportion of user families was even higher—86 per cent—connoting almost universal awareness of coverage.)

85 per cent of the children and 77 per cent of the adults used one or more services. Highest proportions of users (over 90 per cent) were found among women aged 20 to 24, boys aged 15 to 19, boys and girls under age 10, and women policyholders. Lowest proportions of users occurred among spouseless male categories; only 46 per cent of widowed, divorced or separated men, and 52 per cent of single men, were users during the study year.

At all ages past 19, women were likelier users than men, regardless of marital status or relationship. 86 per cent of the women vs. 68 per cent of the men used some service.

Relative availability of physicians in different areas does not appear to have affected the proportions seeking medical service. Except for Manhattan and New Jersey, the percentage of users in each area varied only within a small range, from 79 to 88 per cent of the resident membership, and the highest percentage occurred in Suffolk County, where the physician ratio was found to be the lowest in the eight-county New York metropolitan area.

Although significant class differences were found in use of certain types of service, there was no evidence of reluctance to visit physicians on the part of any class. The difference in proportions who became patients was considerably greater among the various white-collar segments than between blue-collar and white-collar groups as a whole, indicating awareness and willingness to use medical service irrespective of social levels.

*Comprehensive vs. Limited Coverage*

In contrast to the high proportion of users among those with comprehensive coverage of physician services, only one of four persons with limited coverage used it, reflecting the exclusion of most ambulatory services.

A more meaningful comparison of experience under the two types of coverage involved hospital utilization. Both groups had equivalent coverage of physicians' hospital services and equivalent access to medical care resources. It was found, after adjustment for differences in age composition of the two groups, that extent of physician coverage was not a factor in admission rates—contrary to the hypothesis sometimes offered in explanation of large utilization differences between comprehensive group practice and limited community fee-for-service prepayment plans. Those with limited coverage did, however, tend toward longer stays, once admitted, thereby incurring an annual hospital day rate 57 days higher, per thousand eligible members, than the group with comprehensive insurance.

*Free Choice*

The operation of the free-choice-of-physician principle was evident in the use of 13,203 different physicians by the study sample of 42,611 persons insured with comprehensive coverage.

Many of these physicians were part of a multiple-choice option exercised by the members. One of every three families using any service used four or more physicians, one of seven used six or more. Half the families used at least three different physicians.

*Insurance Principle in Action*

One out of ten members accounted for 39 per cent of all claims; 27 per cent accounted for 67 per cent of claims.

*Service Locale*

85 per cent of the services were rendered out of the hospital (73 per cent in physicians' offices, 12 per cent at patients' homes).

Significant variations were associated with age and area of residence. Eight per cent of services to children were in hospital, 21 per cent were home visits. After age 19, 18 per cent were in hospital, 8 per cent at home. Males aged 65 or over had 27 per cent of services in hospital, vs. the overall average of 15 per cent.

In Westchester and Richmond Counties, 21 and 23 per cent, respectively, of all services were in hospital as against 13 to 16 per cent in other New York counties. The comparatively generous supply of private hospital beds in these two counties is cited as a possible explanation.

## Timing

The most popular months for starting service were January, followed by March, April, October. The lightest volume was recorded in July, followed by August and December.

These overall findings are heavily weighted by the most frequent type of service, general office visits. Variations were found for other types. Preventive visits were most frequent in June, September and October. Obstetrical deliveries were highest in four consecutive months, October through January. Home calls were relatively least frequent in June, July and August, most frequent from December through April. Hospital surgical admissions peaked in April, May and June, were lowest in August. For medical admissions, the busiest times were January and the fall months from September through November.

## Specialist Use

Three out of five hospital services of private physicians were performed by specialists, as against 35 per cent of office and 19 per cent of home services.

Highest proportions of specialist service occurred in connection with hospital surgery and office x-rays. This was true in every area.

Specialists performed 78 per cent of hospital surgery (ranging from 68 per cent for children under age 10 to 89 per cent for the 65-plus group).

Of the hospital surgery performed by specialists, general

surgeons performed less than half (44 per cent); the five leading surgical subspecialties accounted for 46 per cent (otolaryngology, gynecology, urology, orthopedic surgery, ophthalmology).

The proportion of hospital surgery performed by specialists other than general surgeons rose with a rise in hospital status: 27 per cent in unaccredited proprietaries, 45 per cent in voluntary hospitals approved for training residents or interns, 53 per cent in medical-school-connected hospitals. As these proportions rose, the proportion attended by non-specialists decreased from 41 per cent to 9 per cent, while general surgeons accounted for a relatively constant proportion, 38 to 32 per cent.

Non-specialists had more freedom to hospitalize their medical cases. They were responsible for a third of the GHI medical admissions to medical-school-affiliated hospitals, half or more of the admissions to other voluntaries, and over three out of four to proprietaries.

65 per cent of out-of-hospital diagnostic x-rays were performed by specialists, but of these fewer than half, 47 per cent, were by radiologists (who were thus responsible for only 30 per cent of all out-of-hospital x-rays). 31 per cent of specialists' x-rays were by internists, 6 per cent by orthopedic surgeons, and 2 to 3 per cent each by pediatricians, general surgeons, gastroenterologists, urologists, cardiologists.

Of the general office visits to specialists, 65 per cent were to internists, general surgeons, pediatricians and obstetricians. This contrasts with office consultations, where ophthalmology, internal medicine and otolaryngology were the fields most in demand.

Use of specialists was related not only to type of service and age but to social class and area. Contrast between the professional class and blue-collar groups was in evidence for all types of service, was particularly pronounced with respect to medical services in hospital, where 69 per cent of professional class vs. 40 per cent of blue-collar admissions were by specialists.

The greatest geographic variation in use of specialists occurred with respect to hospital medical admissions, where the inter-area range in proportions under specialist supervision was from 29 per cent to 57 per cent; and office surgery, ranging from 41 per cent to 65 per cent performed by specialists for members residing in different areas.

## Volume of Service

An average total of 6.7 insured physician and out-of-hospital laboratory services accrued per eligible member during the study year. Those using service averaged 8.4 services each.

Aside from retired members, the greatest variation in total service volume was shown for age-sex subgroups. The lowest utilizers were girls aged 10 to 14, with 3.55 services each; the highest were women aged 65 or more, with 11.247 services each.

Boys used more service than girls, especially in the teen years, but a marked reversal occurred at age 20.

Women were not only more likely to become users; they also used more services once they started. Men of 20 to 34 averaged less than half the number of services used by women of corresponding ages. At each subsequent age level the differential was reduced but still marked. Maternity services were only partially responsible for the differential; except after age 65, all types of service, especially surgery, were characteristically utilized at substantially higher rates by women than by men.

Women generally used more service than men at all ages, whether single or married, and regardless of whether they were policyholders or spouses of policyholders. Single women used nearly 60 per cent more services than single men.

Except for hospital medical care, married people of both sexes generally used more services than the single or widowed-divorced-separated groups.

The larger the family, the fewer the services per person. The additional children in large families and the lower average utilization of children as compared with adults fail to account for this finding; per capita utilization in large families including parents was lower than average rates shown for children.

The longer the period of coverage, the higher the service utilization rate. There was a steady rise in services per capita from the second through the seventh years. Much of this trend, however, is known to be attributable to differences in age composition of members enrolled for varying periods of time.

Service utilization rates ranged from 5.00 services per member in New Jersey to 7.41 in Brooklyn. In other areas, however, the range was much smaller—between 6.15 and 7.26 per capita. No conjectures are made as to reasons for the relatively low New Jersey rates, which applied both to proportions using any service and to number of services per patient.

As with proportion of members using any service, total service volume revealed no pattern ascribable to social class; members of blue-collar families and professional-executive families used precisely the same total number of services per person.

Of all employed categories, the sales category was outstanding, showing a service utilization rate 16 per cent higher than the average for the membership as a whole. These members had a higher proportion of users, and more services per user, than any group except retirees.

The latter group used over two services per capita for every one incurred by the membership as a whole (14.18 vs. 6.73) and also incurred service rates a third higher than the age group 65-plus, presumably reflecting a better state of health among the elderly working than among the elderly retired.

### Component Services

Of the 6.7 services per eligible member, one represented an in-hospital physician service. The majority of the 5.0 out-of-hospital physician services per person were general office visits (3.5). Consultations and out-of-hospital diagnostic tests accounted for one service per member. The ratio of all office services to reported home calls was about six to one. The number of preventive visits listed as such was 230 per 1000 members. The surgical procedure rate of 218 per 1000 persons included 157 out-of-hospital procedures, of which 21 per cent were diagnostic (mainly sigmoidoscopy). In-hospital surgery involved 370 different procedures for the study population, but the 25 leading procedures accounted for over half the total volume.

Analyses of utilization of component services by population subgroups showed age, sex, social class and area as primary variables associated with use of one or more types of service. Marital status also seems to have shown an independent association. Variables such as relationship to subscriber, and family size, would be chiefly useful in the absence of age-sex data or for comparison with other experience measured in these terms. Age and sex presumably reflect physiological sources of demand, while variations among marital subgroups, social classes and in different local areas are more likely to reflect environmental or professional influences. Such influences were more in evidence with respect to the less frequent component services.

The tendency for volume of service to rise with age was apparent for most types of service, but much less pronounced for ambulatory care components than for hospitalization. Members aged 65 or more used over two-and-one-half times as much hospital care, but only 40 per cent more ambulatory services than the rest of the population. Men past 65 used more hospitalization, particularly surgery, than did women of that age, who had more office and home services than the men. Older groups in general registered few preventive visits as such, but had relatively high rates of consultations and diagnostic tests as well as general office visits. Their home call rates were the highest of any adult group.

As expected, young children had highest rates of preventive visits and home calls; nevertheless, large families used less of each of these as well as most other types of service.

Spouseless adults generally used fewer office services of all kinds than the married—preventive, diagnostic x-ray and laboratory tests, consultations, ambulatory surgery—as well as home calls. Only in their use of hospitalization did subgroups of the unattached outdo the married. Both men and women, but especially the men, of the widowed-divorced-separated class, had far higher medical admission rates than the married. Once admitted, these members also stayed longer, for both surgical and medical admissions. On the latter index, length of stay per medical admission, they were joined by the single men and women in outdoing the married contingent by a significant margin, averaging two to four days longer per stay. It is hypothesized that the absence of a spouse may have influenced both the lower use of ambulatory service and the longer medical stays, independently of medical need.

Surgery rates in and out of the hospital showed varying age-sex patterns. The greatest frequency of office surgery was found for females aged 20 to 24 and past 64, males 15 to 19 and past 64. Boys of 15 to 19 underwent ambulatory procedures at rates nearly 90 per cent higher than girls of corresponding ages (much of the difference being attributable to treatment of injuries and nosebleeds), whereas the rates of hospitalized procedures were the same for both sexes, at that age. Women's rates of hospital surgery spurted ahead rapidly after the teen years, reaching a level of one procedure for every ten women aged 35 to 54. Gynecological and breast surgery accounted for more than half the procedures at ages 35 to 44. Married women underwent hospital procedures at rates 60 per cent higher than married males, 48 per cent higher than single women, whose rate in turn was 27 per cent higher than that of single men.

Use of hospitalization was found to be related to practically every variable tested. The largest range of use during the study year occurred among age-sex subgroups—from 171 days per 1000 girls aged 5 to 9, to 2,678 for men past 64 (2,742 for the retired). Such differences are assumed to have been related to need, in contrast to local variations, at least a part of which appear to have stemmed from varying facilities.

Admission rates and length of stay were both lower than national averages reported for the same period, resulting in an annual day rate of 897 for the GHI sample populations vs. 1,119 nationally. It is hypothesized that age composition and type of hospital included in the index, as well as bed availability, were all contributory factors. With the comparison limited to insured populations and to the days-per-stay index, GHI experience conformed rather closely to that of Blue Cross in Northeastern United States for the same period.

Exclusive of government hospitals, rank in the hospital

hierarchy was directly related to average length of stay; the higher the hospital's rank, the longer the average stay, for both medical and surgical admissions. The range was from 13.4 to 8.9 days per medical stay and 8.8 to 5.6 per surgical admission.

The 25 per cent of all admissions remaining 10 days or more accounted for 58 per cent of all hospital days. The 55 per cent remaining 5 days or less accounted for 22 per cent of the total days.

Two categories of diagnosis, circulatory and digestive disorders, contributed 42 per cent of the total days listed for medical stays. Surgery of the digestive system and of neoplasms accounted for 46.5 per cent of the days listed for surgical stays.

Although neither the proportion of members using any service, nor the total number of services used, varied significantly among occupation subgroups, *social class* may have been an important factor in the use of specialists, diagnostic aids, and preventive services. For office consultations this variable demonstrated a broader range of use rates than any other (including age and sex). The clerical and blue-collar classes were very close here, with rates of 70 to 78 office consultations per 1000 members, as contrasted with rates of 106 for professional-executive classes and 185 for the sales group. (Higher use rates of all types of office services were typical of the sales class, with differences particularly marked for consultations, x-rays and laboratory tests.)

In the use of diagnostic x-rays, the blue-collar class topped the clerical class by a wide margin, but the professional-executive class rate was 25 per cent higher. Professional-executive class males had 19 per cent more chest x-rays and abdominal x-rays than blue-collar class males. Similar class differences were found for laboratory tests, the blue-collar class showing a much higher rate than the clerical because of more tests per user, and the professional-executive group incurring a higher rate than either. The sales class exceeded all groups, with every fourth member tested, and 1,073 tests per 1000 persons as compared with the average of 693.

The pattern as to preventive visits was different. There

were higher proportions of users in all white-collar categories than in the blue-collar class. On this index the sales class was 56 per cent higher, the clerical class 37 per cent higher, and the professional-executive class 19 per cent higher, than the blue-collar group.

Class differences in rates of what might be termed preventive surgery may also have been of significance. The rate of treatment for local tumors and cysts, including benign neoplasms, was double among males and more than double among females of professional-executive families as compared with corresponding categories of blue-collar groups.

There appears to have been no class pattern in the use of hospitalization or general office visits (although the sales class was lowest on one index, highest on the other).

*Local variations* in utilization of various types of service are of particular interest as a possible reflection of varying professional attitudes or facilities.

Overall service volume per capita was fairly consistent in most areas. But geographic analysis of other indices of use (user rates, services per user), and breakdown of service volume into its components, showed this variable to be one of the most productive as a generator of further research queries. While the total area is not large, the variety of population densities and of medical resources to be found in its subdivisions (bed supply, physician supply and characteristics, presence or absence of medical schools) may represent a cross section of the major types of variations encountered over much of the country.

Area differences in frequency (or infrequency) of home visits provided clear-cut evidence of local differences in physician customs. In four of the five counties of New York City, members were more likely to have had home calls than in any of the areas outside the City. In Brooklyn, 39 per cent of the resident members were recorded as recipients of home calls, as compared with 21 per cent in Suffolk County, despite the relatively high proportion of children in the latter county. The lowest proportion of home call users in any area was recorded for "other New York," i.e., outside the eight-county New York metropolitan area. It was also observed that the number of home calls per recipient was lowest in the areas with fewest recipients. The combination of the two indices resulted in a utilization rate of 390 home calls per 1000 members in the lowest area, as against 1,277 in the highest. The average rate of home calls in New York City for its five counties combined was 40 per cent higher than the highest rate outside New York City.

Large area variations also characterized the incidence of preventive visits, office consultations, diagnostic x-rays and laboratory tests. Part of the variations are attributable to local differences in age composition of the membership, but additional unmeasured factors were clearly involved. The frequency of office consultations in the area with the highest rate more than tripled that in the area with the lowest.

Laboratory and x-ray tests and office consultations generally were less frequent in the outlying areas. Manhattan members were less likely than residents of other areas to use any service; but once they did become patients, these members averaged more services than others and were most likely to have x-ray and laboratory tests, as well as office consultations.

Local variations in surgical rates were among the most challenging findings. Incidence was highest in outlying areas whose relatively high percentage of children would have been expected to lower the overall surgical rate. The apparent conflict calls for further analysis of surgical incidence by type of procedure within area and age-sex subgroups.

A related topic concerns choice of office or hospital for surgical performance. Two areas, Richmond and Westchester, showed abnormally high rates of surgical procedures performed in the hospital. Both of these areas have more private voluntary or proprietary hospital beds in proportion to their population than most of the other areas. In one, Richmond, the ambulatory surgical rate was significantly lower than the overall average, raising the possibility of freer choice open to physicians practicing there. (The same theory is offered in explanation of lower rates of ambulatory diagnostic tests in Richmond.) In Westchester, however, both ambulatory and hospital surgical rates were higher than average.

In New Jersey, which was found to be far below average on utilization indices of all ambulatory services, the rate of hospitalized surgery slightly exceeded that for the five counties of New York City.

Hospital admission rates also varied strongly by area. Evidence of the tendency for hospital use to rise with the level of bed availability came in comparison of local admission rates, which for the GHI study populations were 50 per cent higher in the two suburban areas having higher-than-average ratios of general private beds to population. In one of these areas, length of stay of medical admissions was lower than average, raising questions as to possible differences in diagnostic criteria for admissions.

As to type of hospital used, a direct relationship was found in all areas between voluntary bed scarcity and use of proprietary hospitals (the higher the private voluntary bed ratio to population, the lower the proportion of proprietary admissions)—indicating the fallacy of assuming that patients en masse can exercise a significant degree of control as to their use of proprietaries.

### Illness Rates

Morbidity rates were calculated for all reported illness, whether treated in or out of hospital and whether acute or chronic.

Respiratory illness was by far the leading category, being recorded during the study year for 40 per cent of the population; the most frequent form of illnesses thus classified were pharyngitis, bronchitis, tonsillitis. The next most frequent categories were diseases of the digestive system (listed for 12 per cent of the population), infective diseases (10 per cent), skin diseases (10 per cent), allergic or metabolic conditions (9 per cent), circulatory diseases (8 per cent), disorders of bones or joints (excluding injuries, 7 per cent), ear disorders (7 per cent), eye conditions (5 per cent). Many persons had disorders in more than one category.

Differences in total treated illness rates between males and females were minor to age 14, substantial at ages 15 to 19, with boys 16 per cent higher, major from ages 25 to 64, with women's rates always much higher, and minor after age 65.

Disorders for which male rates were significantly higher included many of the more serious conditions—e.g. most types of heart disease, malignant neoplasms of digestive, respiratory, urinary systems, ulcers and hernias, lung and liver disorders. This finding, together with the lower proportions of medical service users found among middle-aged men, raised the question of neglect or postponement of care as a possible factor in shorter life expectancy of men.

Females were treated more frequently for multiple sclerosis, arthritis, thyroid disorders, and especially for gall bladder disorders; and for obesity, anemia, migraine, headaches in general, varicose veins, gastroenteritis and colitis, nasopharyngitis, sinusitis, cystitis.

Male and female rates coincided or were close for treatment of appendicitis, disorders of pancreas, muscular dystrophy, chicken pox, measles and mumps, mononucleosis, tonsillitis, pneumonia, benign skin neoplasms, asthma and hay fever, epilepsy, conjunctivitis, cataract, glaucoma, deafness, skin disorders, hemorrhoids, general arteriosclerosis, infective myositis, osteomyelitis.

The highest rate of treatment for respiratory conditions, intestinal complaints, and ear disorders occurred in the preschool group, those under age 5. Skin treatment rates reached their highest point for boys aged 15 to 19. The same group had the highest injury rate—274 boys with 331 reported injuries, per 1000 in this class—and this accounted for most of the difference in total treatment rates of boys and girls aged 15 to 19.

At ages 20 to 24, the total female incidence rate of treated disorders nearly doubled the male rate, attesting to dramatic decreases of male rates in almost all previously high categories and large increases of female rates—not only of pregnancy and disorders of female organs but in most other categories as well.

For both sexes, age trends showed the expected pattern of increasing morbidity rates in certain categories—malignancies, diseases of nervous system, eye disorders, diseases of bones and joints, circulatory disorders. At ages 55 to 64, the treated malignancy rate doubled that found for the previous age interval.

Among male adults, those past 65 generally recorded highest treatment rates for most conditions, whereas women aged 35 to 44 often had highest rates.

Analysis of treated illness rates by class revealed instances of apparently significant differences—for example, the rate of treatment of malignancies and of glaucoma among males of the professional-executive-sales class was double the rate found for males of the blue-collar class.

## Quality and Adequacy

Although no attempts were made to evaluate adequacy of care, quantitative findings of various types may be interpreted as having qualitative connotations.

The most detailed source would be the type of data available on individual patients, illustrated in the samples of treatment histories on members with selected diagnoses. But variations in average numbers and types of services received by different population or patient subgroups may also generate tentative observations or further queries concerning adequacy of care received. Questions for follow-up might relate to:

why, despite free access, women of the study population were apparently not observing cancer prevention program recommendations with respect to Pap smear tests, while men past 45 were not having routine chest x-rays and electrocardiograms;

whether the children were undergoing too many tonsillectomies;

adequacy of referrals for specialist consultations;

variations in treatment patterns (or diagnosis patterns) associated with physician type and field of practice,

qualifications, age, location, hospital appointment
status;

reasons for local variations in proportions of patients having diagnostic tests, preventive visits, home calls, surgery, medical hospitalization;

the significance of apparent social class differences in rates
of preventive visits, diagnostic procedures, specialist
services, preventive surgery, elective surgery, and
treatment of such conditions as malignancies and glaucoma;

the relative roles of members, physicians, hospital facilities,
in generating significant local and class differences.

Some of these and other queries could be partially satisfied
by fuller examination of entries in the insurance records, but in
general, supplementary data would be required. It is felt that
while record studies skirt the ultimate question—how to evaluate not only treatment, but results of treatment—they can be of
value, particularly if they encompass the area of ambulatory
diagnosis and care where so little is reported. Current medical
practice is presumably based on experience with previous suc-
cesses and failures. Studies of records which reflect changing
practices over time, as well as varying practices as of any one
time among population and physician subgroups, can become
useful references for the definition of "norms" and the development of standards.

# Chapter 2

# PROJECT SCOPE, DESIGN, PROBLEMS

The problem of how to develop medical data accruing as a by-product of an insurance operation, using the same type of data-processing machinery as in processing claims, was approached with a modest budget, supplied by GHI, sufficient to experiment with a sample of one year's data.

An initial experiment was designed, modified for reasons of economy, delayed for higher priorities, finally programmed, and developed in 1965–6, using 1964 data as input to IBM 1401 and 1410 computers.

The opportunity for the research project had been promised in the original sales messages accompanying GHI's initiation into the computer world. It was a long interval between promise and realization, during which a succession of computer models seemed always to be under consideration, ordered, awaited, and, by the time of installation, outgrown or obsolescent or both.

The period of upheaval and delays netted certain research benefits, however, permitting introduction of innovations which improved the scope and quality of "input" data and which as it turned out also proved helpful to GHI program and policy planners.

The physician file was expanded to include data on nonparticipants as well as participants. The numbering system which had previously identified hospitals by name was amended to provide a simple classification code. Characteristics of the membership, never before studied, were obtained for a 10 per cent sample and thereafter regularly updated for additions and dropouts. In addition, claims coding practices were reviewed and instructions to coders were revised where necessary to improve specificity and completeness. Diagnosis, previously omitted from punched cards, was gradually added to the list of items required and coded for all claims, including surgical claims.

These and other steps, while considerably enhancing the value of "input" data, by no means achieved the perfect source. Perfection was regarded as an impossible prerequisite, insistence upon which would have indefinitely postponed all action.

## Purposes

The purposes of the experiment were:

to investigate the range of medical data acquirable as a by-product of administering comprehensive medical insurance under the prevailing system of medical care distribution;

to test the application of computer techniques to the retrieval of such data;

to devise an expandable system for deriving periodic population-based indices on treated morbidity and on utilization of specific service components;

to illustrate, with one year's findings, various types of substantive medical analyses permitted by the program;

to publicize results, in the hope of calling attention to this neglected resource and furthering the development of medical statistics from insurance data.

In the present series of studies, no attempt was made to ascertain whether the population studied was receiving appropriate care. Objectives did not include evaluation of medical care adequacy or effectiveness. Effectiveness, or results, can never be judged on the basis of insurance records. As for adequacy (or inadequacy or overadequacy), it may be possible to draw inferences with respect to certain services such as consultations, where the frequency seems low, or tonsillectomies, where it seems high; but generally, in the absence of standards or norms, it would be inappropriate to conclude that "high" utilizers overused their insurance or that "low" utilizers lacked needed care.

It was recognized from the start, however, that quantitative measurements of the type presented, particularly those relating services to diagnoses, might serve some useful function in connection with attempts to develop standards or evaluative procedures. In fact, one impetus to activation of the project was a series of conferences on the quality of ambulatory care, which led to the recommendation that extraction of quantitative data precede evaluative efforts.

Also excluded from consideration in the present studies were judgments as to appropriateness of subscriber choice of physician. Whether or not it may be the proper responsibility of medical insurers to influence such decisions, and if so, on the basis of what criteria for what types of services, is another facet of the quality debate. Here again the project demonstrated the feasibility of collecting facts pertinent to decisions of this nature—e.g. on available physicians and who performed various services.

Although the aims of the project seemed remote from day-to-day operating problems, the innovations introduced into the records system, as well as results of component studies, frequently provided useful information which would not otherwise have been available.

## Immediate Objectives

To implement its general purposes, the immediate objectives of the research project were, or became as plans progressed:

to draw plans, mainly in the form of dummy tables, indicating to computer systems and programming personnel the substantive data objectives proposed for an initial program;

to accommodate these plans to the physical proportions feasible within computer tabulating format limitations;

to select and describe the study population;

to describe physician resources;

to emphasize analyses involving ambulatory services but also

to include analyses of services most frequently insured elsewhere;

to employ varied analytical approaches to data interpretation;

to derive several types of indices from the same data;

to relate population data to service utilization, service utilization to physicians used, treatment to diagnosis, and diagnosis to population—thus indicating how regular periodic studies of medical data from insurance records could serve medical planners and epidemiologists.

## Selection of Study Sample

To serve the major purposes of the research project as economically as possible, it was necessary to minimize coverage and administrative differences affecting the study population, except where such differences contributed to the value of the research.

This requirement eliminated groups with "deductible" clauses applicable to the first one, two or three office visits, as well as groups which were "self-administered" and for which GHI therefore lacked detailed membership data.

The remaining subscribers and their dependents constituted the universe of study. Within this universe, the sampling unit was the subscriber (policyholder).

Sample specifications next called for easy identification of sample member claims by various GHI departments cooperating in retrieval efforts. The terminal-digit method of random selection, placing approximately every tenth subscriber and his dependents in the sample, satisfied this requirement while also providing a representative cross section of the GHI population (except for those excluded from the universe of study).

The latter characteristic of the sample, representativeness, was not essential to the purposes of the research project, but it was of importance when GHI administrators turned to the Research Department for information—e.g. as to membership characteristics by age and geographic distribution, or utilization of hospitalization or of specific types of procedures—relevant to practical management or planning problems.

As of 1964, the year of experience selected for study, the research project sample of subscribers and dependents chosen by the terminal-digit method numbered 59,308, of whom 49,618 were covered by the comprehensive "Family Doctor Plan" and 9,690 had only limited coverage, mainly physicians' services in hospital, under the "Semi-Private Plan."

To simplify rate calculations, utilization and morbidity analyses in the present series were usually based on the experience of full-year members only. Exclusion of part-year members reduced the sample population to 50,529, 42,611 with comprehensive and 7,918 with limited coverage.

Finally, since the nature of the analyses generally involved ambulatory services, directly or indirectly, most of the report refers to the experience of the full-year sample covered by the comprehensive plan—42,611 members.

Characteristics of the sample populations are shown in Chapter 3.

*The substantive data presented in this report relate to the experience of the study population during the study year. They have not been projected to any other population or year.*

## Sources and Scope of Available Data

### Computer-Stored Records

*Membership Data.* Members in the project sample had GHI certificate numbers with a common terminal digit which automatically selected them and their records for the study.

Demographic and other data on sample members were taken from application cards and punched onto IBM cards.

Information recorded for each member (subscriber or dependent) included date of birth, sex, marital status, relationship to subscriber, size of enrolled family, subscriber occupation, area of residence, date of enrollment, group through which enrolled, type of coverage. Marital status was entered as one of three categories—married, single, or widowed-divorced-separated; subdivisions of the latter category are not indicated on application cards.

Data on educational attainment and income levels of subscribers are unavailable. These two characteristics, which are generally sought and emphasized as social status indicators in studies based on interviews with consumers, are seldom available in insurance records. Like race and religion, education and income are regarded as personal information to which the insurer is not entitled. Accordingly, all such items are omitted from enrollment cards completed by applicants. The only way to obtain any of them is by special survey.

Occupation of subscriber has been used here as a rough indicator of social class. Aside from the misclassification that may result when the family of a married female subscriber is classified according to her occupation rather than that of her husband, occupation probably provides a fairly good class index of itself, as well as a likely indication of educational attainment. It is, in fact, preferred by some researchers:

> "The great significance of a person's occupation for all other aspects of his life makes occupational level one of the prin-

cipal indices for differentiating social classes. Although
some studies have also used such indices as education and
area of residence, as the sociologist Clausen has pointed
out, in modern industrial living class is linked most closely
with occupational status." [1]

*Physician Record.* Characteristics of participating and
non-participating physicians filing claims with GHI are recorded by the GHI Medical Department, using directories,
signed agreements, and correspondence as sources of data. Recorded information includes office location, year of graduation
from medical school, type of practice, field of practice, professional qualifications, hospital affiliation. Data are punched on
IBM cards, sent for electronic processing, taped and continually
updated by IBM computer machine number 1401, using a program specifically designed for this purpose by GHI program-
mers.

*Hospital Record.* All hospitals in New York State and the
surrounding metropolitan (commuter) areas have been assigned
a code number. This number designates location by county;
voluntary, proprietary or government sponsorship; accredita-
tion status; and whether attached to a medical school or ac-
credited for training residents or interns.

*Claim Record.* Computer systems personnel tape the following information for each claim:

> Type and place of service (office visit, home visit, annual
> examination or other preventive visit, in-hospital sur-
> gery, out-of-hospital surgery, obstetrical care, in-hos-
> pital medical care, consultation in or out of hospital,
> diagnostic x-ray, laboratory examination, anesthesia,
> visiting nurse service, radiation therapy, professional
> nursing, ambulance service, drugs, oxygen, appliances,

---

[1] Wolford, Jack A., M.D., "Mental Health and Occupation," *Public Health
Reports,* Volume 79, No. 11, November 1964, p. 979.

psychotherapy, electroshock therapy in or out of hospital, psychological testing)

First date of service, this claim (year, month, day)

Last date of service, this claim (year, month, day)

Number of services of each type

Diagnosis

Specific surgical, x-ray, or laboratory procedure

Fee paid

Fee charged by physician

Patient identifying data (to relate to membership analysis tape): Certificate number, first name, date of birth, sex, relationship

Physician identifying number (to relate to physician tape)

When service rendered in hospital:

> Type of accommodation, number of days, hospital code number.

*Composite Record.* For the present studies, all of the above sources of data on services, diagnoses, physicians, hospitals, patients, members were integrated by means of a series of computerized matching operations—claims tape matched with physician tape, claims-physician tape matched with hospital tape, claims-physician-hospital tape matched with membership analysis tape. The resulting composite record was the source of most service and morbidity tabulations planned for the initial experiment in medical data retrieval.

### Limitations on Scope of Available Service Utilization Data

The term service as used here refers to GHI insured services except where otherwise specified.

Service utilization data measure the expressed demand for covered physician and laboratory services as determined from claims prepared by treating physicians.

It was not within the scope of the research plan to investigate medical care received by GHI enrollees outside the GHI system. This applies to services not covered as well as to services covered and used but not charged to GHI. (It is felt that the latter category would not be of significance for GHI, which pays any physician, as it might be under a prepaid group practice or clinic arrangement whereby members must use group or panel physicians in order to qualify for benefits.)

Comprehensive services include office, home and hospital physician services; out-of-hospital x-ray and laboratory services and other auxiliary services such as visiting nurse, ambulance, radiotherapy. Optional riders are available for coverage of prescription drugs and appliances, full-time nursing, short-term psychotherapy.

Services specifically excluded from GHI coverage are the usual insurance exclusions—cosmetic surgery, routine eye refractions and routine podiatric care, services covered by Workmen's Compensation legislation or veterans' facilities or provided at subscriber's place of employment.

Diagnostic x-ray and laboratory procedures performed for hospital in-patients are billed to hospitalization insurers, not to GHI. Ambulatory tests are paid by GHI without limit except for the exclusion of routine urinalyses and hemoglobin tests, which are regarded as integral parts of general office care, thus included with the office fee and not reported separately.

Anesthesia administered by salaried hospital employees is not covered.

Psychiatric care in hospitals is covered only in general hospitals.

Telephone consultations are not covered.

## Scope of Analysis

The variety of available data, plus promised computer capacity to link component variables in any desired combination, presented researchers with a virtually unlimited potential for sheer volume of tabulations.

Practical considerations dictated a relatively modest retrieval design and curtailed multivariate analyses which would have been desirable from a substantive viewpoint; but it is believed that those included in the initial design served the purpose of illustrating feasible types of analysis.

The major portion of the analyses contributed in some way to the central question: *How much and what kinds of physician services did different classes of members receive from what types of physicians, where, when, why?*

In addition, hospitalization, which is not yet insured by GHI but on which information could be retrieved from claim forms involving physician in-hospital services, was the subject of a number of studies.

The research design set limitations on types of services to be analyzed for the initial program. Services covered by contract riders for only part of the membership, such as nursing, drugs, appliances, were excluded from retrieval plans. Services used comparatively infrequently such as radiotherapy, ambulance or visiting nurse were combined in retrieval plans and generally ignored in analysis. Anesthesia experience was tabulated separately but not analyzed because of the irregular pattern of insurance liability. The incidence of psychiatric hospitalization was also disregarded in analysis, for the same reason.

The emphasis throughout on medical data deliberately snubbed the financial aspects of insurance experience, to reverse the usual tendency. Proposed tabulations on costs were the first to be discarded when savings in computer time were required. Aside from the fact that the studies were not intended as cost studies, it is believed that utilization rates are a superior indicator of insurer risk, providing a more flexible method of estimating costs. Fees must be taken into account in deciphering the meaning of costs reported for a given situation at a given time. Utilization rates obviate the need for that step. If, despite these arguments, cost data were required, they could be retrieved from the same tape which produced the utilization tabulations.

Tabulations began with analysis of membership characteristics by age-sex, marital status-sex, relationship-sex, size of family, subscriber occupation, area of residence, and duration of enrollment in GHI. Once provisions for "input" data were assured, this study and the study of private practicing physician characteristics were each programmed for retrieval from separately-maintained tapes.

In the analysis of service utilization and illness data, most computations involved development of indices related to the population at risk; others presented findings in the form of percentage distributions, as is done elsewhere when population-at-risk data are lacking. Thus some analyses were based on the eligible population, some on the patient population. For many of the analyses involving ambulatory care and illness, there appears to be no precedent; for others, particularly those concerned with hospitalization, both usual and unusual indices were developed.

Patterns of service use were analyzed for combined services and for each type of service (office call, home call, hospital call, preventive care, consultation, office surgery, hospital surgery, maternity care, ambulatory laboratory and diagnostic x-ray procedures, hospitalization) in relation to each recorded characteristic of the population at risk, the type of practitioner rendering, and diagnosis.

Record matching (or linkage) permitted tabulation not only of number of *services* rendered each population subgroup but number of *members* using each or any type of service. Thus it was possible to calculate a variety of use indices for each population subgroup:

> Number of users per thousand exposure years, any service and each type of service
> Number of users of each type of service per thousand users of any type of service
> (e.g. What percentage of patients were x-rayed?)
> Number of services per thousand exposure years, all services and each type of service
> Number of services per thousand patients

In addition to overall incidence of surgical and diagnostic procedures, determined in connection with the above series, frequencies of individual procedures were analyzed by age, sex, and occupation class.

Patterns of physician use were analyzed in terms of impact of the free-choice principle on total sample use and on individual subscriber use; extent of use of general practitioner and each type of specialist; who used specialists, where, for what types of service; which specialty fields were called upon most frequently; and likely locale of service rendered by specialists in each field.

Indices of hospital use, developed within type of admission (medical, surgical, obstetrical), included number of annual admissions per thousand eligibles, number of patients per thousand eligibles, admissions per patient, days per stay, days per thousand eligibles, days per thousand patients—all by eight membership variables and by type of physician coverage (comprehensive or limited); and admissions of each diagnosis per thousand eligibles.

Hospital data were also analyzed independently of the population base; admissions were distributed in a series of analyses to show monthly variations, geographic spread, types of hospitals used in areas with varying facilities, length of stay in different types of hospitals.

Treated morbidity rates were obtained by diagnosis for age-sex subgroups and were also adjusted to the age-sex distribution of the general population in the study area. In analyses limited to patients, diagnosis was related to treatment using two different methods—one revealing average types and volume of each type of treatment per case of each diagnosis, the other serving as case-finder-treatment-recorder for individual cases of selected diagnoses drawn from the 10 per cent of the population registering 39 per cent of the claims.

## Problems of Data Conversion
## and Interpretation

*Converting Claims to Services*

The unit of measurement in insurance records is the claim. The unit of measurement in medical care reporting is the service (or contact or visit). In order to calculate the total number of units of care received, as well as to maximize comparability with other types of source data, it was necessary to adopt a common unit of measurement for conversion of insurance data to medical data.

This problem was partially solved by counting each physician-patient contact and each laboratory test as a unit of service, regardless of number of claims involved. In many instances, however, the number of physician contacts is unknown. One claim will suffice per surgical procedure, per maternity case, per hospital case; for insurance purposes these are considered and paid for as single services. But since they involve multiple physician contacts, they cannot be equated with, say, single office visits, in a count of total medical services. Assignment of more appropriate weights to these services requires assumptions, sometimes arbitrary, as to probable average numbers of physician services actually rendered.

Calculations of volume of physician and laboratory services were based on the following guidelines:

One physician service was counted for each office call or home call.

One physician service was counted for each day of hospitalization. (In this case, "hospital day" includes both entry and discharge dates, since GHI includes both in calculating physician payments for medical admissions. For purposes of hospitalization studies, however, data were adjusted to exclude the extra day, to conform with methods of hospitalization reimbursement.)

For each hospital surgical admission, two office visits were assumed to have been included for the surgical fee; office surgery was assumed to involve an average of one extra office visit; obstetrical cases were assumed to involve eleven pre- and postnatal office visits [1] except for abortions or miscarriages, where five such visits were assumed.

Diagnostic x-rays were classified as physician services on the assumption that interpretations were by physicians.

One laboratory service was counted for each procedure paid for by GHI, which means routine urinalyses and hemoglobin tests, as well as all hospital tests, were excluded.

### Converting Claims to People

Insurance use of claims as the unit of measurement permits calculation of number of claims per policyholder. It generally precludes ready identification of the proportion and characteristics of covered individuals who used services, or the combination of services used by one individual.

The computer matching or data linking operations previously mentioned facilitated conversion of services to a person basis where requested in the research design (e.g. proportion of eligibles using service, services per user). The same principle was involved in reporting diagnosis and treatment on a person, rather than claim, basis; it was necessary to combine all claims per diagnosis per person as a first step in arriving at morbidity rates and per case treatment rates.

---

[1] The latter figure was based on Health Information Foundation studies of maternity care trends. See *Maternity Care and Costs: A Ten-Year Trend*, Progress in Health Services, Volume XV, Number 2.

*Other Problems of Interpretation*

The problems discussed above were recognized in advance and taken into account in programming data retrieval. There were other troublesome aspects of the data, also known in advance, which were beyond computer remedy; and there were problems created on inspection of some of the emerging tabulations. A few examples:

The problem of missing data occurred most frequently in connection with surgical and obstetrical hospitalization, where despite preliminary precautions in the form of special instructions to coders of "Patterns" claims, the number of days hospitalized was sometimes omitted. The arbitrary decision here was to project the known experience of other similar cases to the unknown cases.

Previously established systems of data classification created some problems—as when a large proportion of surgery was found to have been performed by internists and other non-surgical physicians. This was explained by reference to the system which classifies many diagnostic procedures, and much of the work of dermatologists, as surgical procedures.

There were problems of interpretation caused by uncertainty as to extent of interaction of measured population variables; these could have been avoided by more elaborate plans for multivariate analysis and data adjustment than were possible in the initial program. An outstanding instance concerned the relationship between duration of enrollment and use of service, which was found to be too consistent, on some indices, for unblinking acceptance. On further analysis, a correlation not attributable to length of time in GHI was also found between duration of enrollment and age—a finding which there was no reason to suspect in advance but which, once unveiled, eliminated duration of coverage from consideration as an independent utilization variable.

Some problems of interpretation concerned questions of data credibility. These could not be resolved as part of the initial experiment because of the time and expense involved.

Further references to problems of data interpretation will be found under subject presentations.

## Computer Processing and the Analyst

As previously noted, one of the purposes of the present project was to test the application of computer techniques to the retrieval of medical data from insurance records. The test was successful; all the data presented were retrieved in this fashion.

It should be mentioned, however, that the blessings of computer processing were found to be not entirely unmixed. Once the research design is programmed, the possibilities for speedy massive data retrieval, record linkage, and machine computations are unquestionable computer advantages over any previous data processing system. But there are also drawbacks which can become sources of frustration for the researcher exploring new areas.

Aside from the apparently characteristic inability of computer systems personnel to set reasonably accurate time schedules for programming and delivery of planned tabulations, at least with respect to medical care data, there are difficulties associated with the comparative inflexibility of the system.

To the extent that research plans anticipate the findings they are designed to unearth, flexibility in retrieval methods is not important. It is the unanticipated which causes problems. Any revisions, any additional analyses suggested by unfolding results, require the writing of new programs and signal further delays and expense. Such revisions and additions would presumably be minimized in a mature program. During the experimental phase preceding the development of routine reporting, however, flexibility is an important analytic tool. It was more readily achieved when data processing relied on cards, counters, and sorters.

In a sense, the analyst is a prisoner of the computer.

# Chapter 3

# THE STUDY POPULATION

The GHI population of subscribers is representative of self-supporting, largely unionized, lower-middle—and—middle-class salaried workers and wage earners. In terms of white-collar—blue-collar distribution, it corresponds more closely to the employed national than the employed local population (but is not strictly comparable, in the absence of GHI data on spouse occupation). Professional, executive and sales classes are underrepresented as compared with either the national or local employed populations. Other underrepresented categories are age groups past 65 and 20 to 24, and widowed-divorced-separated adults.

The method of selecting the study populations, and limitations on available descriptive information, have already been outlined (Chapter 2).

The sample studied for most analyses consisted of 42,611 persons enrolled for the full study year under the comprehensive "Family Doctor Plan" (full coverage of physician services in office, home, hospital). The additional sample of 7,918 persons with the limited "Semi-Private Plan" was included for purposes of comparing utilization experience where possible. (In the present report, comparison is limited to hospitalization experience.)

Membership characteristics were transcribed from application cards to IBM cards, to tape, and tabulated by computer. First tabulations included all sample members, full-year and part-year. Following the decision to restrict the study base in most analyses to full-year members, it was found that the composition of the sample was not greatly altered by exclusion of part-year members. The primary tabulations presented below apply to full-year members as of 1964. A few cross-tabulations include part-year members as well.

### Age Distribution

The two GHI sample populations differed substantially as to age distribution (Table 1). The attraction of the comprehensive plan to families with children is demonstrated by the 40 per cent aged 19 and under in this group as compared with 27

TABLE 1. Number and Distribution of Study Population Members, by Age and Sex (Full-Year Members)

| AGE | COMBINED PLANS | | | COMPREHENSIVE PLAN | | | LIMITED PLAN | | |
|---|---|---|---|---|---|---|---|---|---|
| | *Total* | *Male* | *Female* | *Total* | *Male* | *Female* | *Total* | *Male* | *Female* |
| | NUMBER OF MEMBERS | | | | | | | | |
| Under 5 | 4,626 | 2,363 | 2,263 | 4,160 | 2,142 | 2,018 | 466 | 221 | 245 |
| 5–9 | 5,444 | 2,752 | 2,692 | 4,856 | 2,439 | 2,417 | 588 | 313 | 275 |
| 10–14 | 5,311 | 2,734 | 2,577 | 4,685 | 2,397 | 2,288 | 626 | 337 | 289 |
| 15–19 | 3,934 | 1,936 | 1,998 | 3,484 | 1,673 | 1,811 | 450 | 263 | 187 |
| 20–24 | 1,581 | 632 | 949 | 1,128 | 434 | 694 | 453 | 198 | 255 |
| 25–34 | 5,791 | 2,747 | 3,044 | 4,896 | 2,315 | 2,581 | 895 | 432 | 463 |
| 35–44 | 8,262 | 4,126 | 4,136 | 7,122 | 3,586 | 3,536 | 1,140 | 540 | 600 |
| 45–54 | 8,207 | 4,069 | 4,138 | 7,018 | 3,537 | 3,481 | 1,189 | 532 | 657 |
| 55–64 | 5,312 | 2,999 | 2,313 | 4,242 | 2,510 | 1,732 | 1,070 | 489 | 581 |
| 65 and Over | 2,061 | 1,232 | 829 | 1,020 | 676 | 344 | 1,041 | 556 | 485 |
| TOTAL | 50,529 | 25,590 | 24,939 | 42,611 | 21,709 | 20,902 | 7,918 | 3,881 | 4,037 |
| | PER CENT OF MEMBERS | | | | | | | | |
| Under 5 | 9.2 | 9.2 | 9.1 | 9.8 | 9.9 | 9.7 | 5.9 | 5.7 | 6.1 |
| 5–9 | 10.8 | 10.8 | 10.8 | 11.4 | 11.2 | 11.6 | 7.4 | 8.1 | 6.7 |
| 10–14 | 10.5 | 10.7 | 10.3 | 11.0 | 11.0 | 10.9 | 7.9 | 8.7 | 7.2 |
| 15–19 | 7.8 | 7.6 | 8.0 | 8.2 | 7.7 | 8.7 | 5.7 | 6.8 | 4.6 |
| 20–24 | 3.1 | 2.5 | 3.8 | 2.6 | 2.0 | 3.3 | 5.7 | 5.1 | 6.3 |
| 25–34 | 11.5 | 10.7 | 12.2 | 11.5 | 10.7 | 12.3 | 11.3 | 11.1 | 11.5 |
| 35–44 | 16.3 | 16.1 | 16.6 | 16.7 | 16.5 | 16.9 | 14.4 | 13.9 | 14.9 |
| 45–54 | 16.2 | 15.9 | 16.6 | 16.5 | 16.3 | 16.6 | 15.0 | 13.7 | 16.3 |
| 55–64 | 10.5 | 11.7 | 9.3 | 9.9 | 11.6 | 8.3 | 13.5 | 12.6 | 14.4 |
| 65 and Over | 4.1 | 4.8 | 3.3 | 2.4 | 3.1 | 1.7 | 13.2 | 14.3 | 12.0 |
| TOTAL | 100.0 | 100.0 | 100.0 | 100.0 | 100.0 | 100.0 | 100.0 | 100.0 | 100.0 |

per cent in the limited coverage group. At the other extreme, the latter group also had 27 per cent aged 55 and over, compared with only 12 per cent of those with comprehensive coverage. (It should be noted that the distributions are pre-Medicare.)

Comparison of the combined GHI samples with the United States and local area populations shows greatest proportionate differences at ages 20 to 24 and past 65, where GHI has relatively fewer people (Table 2).

TABLE 2.   Age Distribution of United States Population and of GHI Study Populations, 1964

| | | | GHI STUDY POPULATIONS 1964 | | |
| | | New York-Northeast | (FULL-YEAR MEMBERS) | | |
| AGE | United States 1964 [1] | New Jersey 1960 [2] | Combined Plans | Comprehensive Plan | Limited Plan |
|---|---|---|---|---|---|
| | % | % | % | % | % |
| Under 5 | 10.9 | 9.7 | 9.2 | 9.8 | 5.9 |
| 5–9 | 10.8 | 8.9 | 10.8 | 11.4 | 7.4 |
| 10–14 | 9.7 | 8.2 | 10.5 | 11.0 | 7.9 |
| 15–19 | 8.4 | 6.2 | 7.8 | 8.2 | 5.7 |
| 20–24 | 6.3 | 5.5 | 3.1 | 2.6 | 5.7 |
| 25–34 | 11.4 | 13.4 | 11.5 | 11.5 | 11.3 |
| 35–44 | 12.8 | 14.7 | 16.3 | 16.7 | 14.4 |
| 45–54 | 11.5 | 13.3 | 16.2 | 16.5 | 15.0 |
| 55–64 | 8.8 | 10.6 | 10.5 | 9.9 | 13.5 |
| 65 and Over | 9.4 | 9.5 | 4.1 | 2.4 | 13.2 |
| TOTAL | 100.0 | 100.0 | 100.0 | 100.0 | 100.0 |
| N = | 189,371 (in 000's) | 14,759 (in 000's) | 50,529 | 42,611 | 7,918 |

[1] Current Population Reports, Series P-25, No. 321, U.S. Department of Commerce, November 30, 1965.
[2] U.S. Census of Population, 1960 General Population Characteristics, New York, Final Report, PC (1)–34B, 1961.

## Sex Distribution

The proportion of males in the GHI study populations was somewhat higher than in the national population—50.6 vs. 48.6 per cent. This was almost entirely accounted for at ages past 55, where the increasing preponderance of males under the com-

TABLE 3. Sex Distribution of United States and GHI Populations, by Age, 1964

| | % MALE | | | | % FEMALE | | | |
| | UNITED STATES[1] | GHI STUDY POPULATIONS | | | UNITED STATES[1] | GHI STUDY POPULATIONS | | |
| AGE | | Combined Plans | Comprehensive Plan | Limited Plan | | Combined Plans | Comprehensive Plan | Limited Plan |
|---|---|---|---|---|---|---|---|---|
| Under 5 | 51.0 | 51.1 | 51.5 | 47.4 | 49.0 | 48.9 | 48.5 | 52.6 |
| 5–9 | 50.8 | 50.6 | 50.2 | 53.2 | 49.2 | 49.4 | 49.8 | 46.8 |
| 10–14 | 50.8 | 51.5 | 51.2 | 53.8 | 49.2 | 48.5 | 48.8 | 46.2 |
| 15–19 | 49.7 | 49.2 | 48.0 | 58.4 | 50.3 | 50.8 | 52.0 | 41.6 |
| 20–24 | 45.4 | 40.0 | 38.5 | 43.7 | 54.6 | 60.0 | 61.5 | 56.3 |
| 25–34 | 47.9 | 47.4 | 47.3 | 48.3 | 52.1 | 52.6 | 52.7 | 51.7 |
| 35–44 | 48.2 | 49.9 | 50.4 | 47.4 | 51.8 | 50.1 | 49.6 | 52.6 |
| 45–54 | 48.6 | 49.6 | 50.4 | 44.7 | 51.4 | 50.4 | 49.6 | 55.3 |
| 55–64 | 48.0 | 56.5 | 59.2 | 45.7 | 52.0 | 43.5 | 40.8 | 54.3 |
| 65 and Over | 44.0 | 59.8 | 66.3 | 53.4 | 56.0 | 40.2 | 33.7 | 46.6 |
| TOTAL | 48.6 | 50.6 | 50.9 | 49.0 | 51.4 | 49.4 | 49.1 | 51.0 |

1 Current Population Reports, Series P-25, No. 321, U.S. Department of Commerce, November 30, 1965

54

prehensive plan was in marked contrast to their declining proportions in the general population (Table 3).

### Relationship to Subscriber

As would be expected, dependents outnumbered subscribers (policyholders), 64 to 36 (Table 4). Over half the male population consisted of subscribers, while only 14 per cent of females were in this category. The distributions were markedly different in the two GHI samples, especially for females, of whom 31 per cent with limited coverage were subscribers as against 11 per cent of females under the "Family Doctor Plan."

TABLE 4.  Number and Distribution of Study Population
Members, by Relationship to Subscriber
(Full-Year Members)

| RELATIONSHIP | COMBINED PLANS | | | COMPREHENSIVE PLAN | | | LIMITED PLAN | | |
|---|---|---|---|---|---|---|---|---|---|
| | Total | Male | Female | Total | Male | Female | Total | Male | Female |
| | NUMBER OF MEMBERS | | | | | | | | |
| Self | 18,190 | 14,595 | 3,595 | 14,524 | 12,194 | 2,330 | 3,666 | 2,401 | 1,265 |
| Spouse | 13,069 | 1,213 | 11,856 | 10,993 | 888 | 10,105 | 2,076 | 325 | 1,751 |
| Child | 19,270 | 9,782 | 9,488 | 17,094 | 8,627 | 8,467 | 2,176 | 1,155 | 1,021 |
| TOTAL | 50,529 | 25,590 | 24,939 | 42,611 | 21,709 | 20,902 | 7,918 | 3,881 | 4,037 |
| | PER CENT OF MEMBERS | | | | | | | | |
| Self | 36.0 | 57.0 | 14.4 | 34.1 | 56.2 | 11.2 | 46.3 | 61.9 | 31.3 |
| Spouse | 25.9 | 4.8 | 47.5 | 25.8 | 4.1 | 48.3 | 26.2 | 8.4 | 43.4 |
| Child | 38.1 | 38.2 | 38.1 | 40.1 | 39.7 | 40.5 | 27.5 | 29.7 | 25.3 |
| TOTAL | 100.0 | 100.0 | 100.0 | 100.0 | 100.0 | 100.0 | 100.0 | 100.0 | 100.0 |

### Marital Status

Of those aged 20 or over, 88 per cent with comprehensive and 75 per cent with limited coverage were married, 10 per cent and 15 per cent respectively were single. One out of ten with limited coverage was widowed, divorced or separated, compared with only 2 per cent of those with the comprehensive plan, reflecting the higher concentration at older age levels characterizing the limited coverage sample (Table 5).

TABLE 5. Number and Distribution of Study Population
Members Aged 20 or Over, by Marital Status
(Full-Year Members)

| MARITAL STATUS | COMBINED PLANS | | | COMPREHENSIVE PLAN | | | LIMITED PLAN | | |
|---|---|---|---|---|---|---|---|---|---|
| | Total | Male | Female | Total | Male | Female | Total | Male | Female |
| | NUMBER OF MEMBERS | | | | | | | | |
| Married | 26,802 | 13,520 | 13,282 | 22,489 | 11,367 | 11,122 | 4,313 | 2,153 | 2,160 |
| Single | 3,298 | 1,899 | 1,399 | 2,452 | 1,471 | 981 | 846 | 428 | 418 |
| Widowed, Divorced, Separated | 1,159 | 389 | 770 | 576 | 244 | 332 | 583 | 145 | 438 |
| TOTAL | 31,259 | 15,808 | 15,451 | 25,517 | 13,082 | 12,435 | 5,742 | 2,726 | 3,016 |
| | PER CENT OF MEMBERS | | | | | | | | |
| Married | 85.7 | 85.5 | 86.0 | 88.1 | 86.9 | 89.4 | 75.1 | 79.0 | 71.6 |
| Single | 10.6 | 12.0 | 9.0 | 9.6 | 11.2 | 7.9 | 14.7 | 15.7 | 13.9 |
| Widowed, Divorced, Separated | 3.7 | 2.5 | 5.0 | 2.3 | 1.9 | 2.7 | 10.2 | 5.3 | 14.5 |
| TOTAL | 100.0 | 100.0 | 100.0 | 100.0 | 100.0 | 100.0 | 100.0 | 100.0 | 100.0 |

## Family Size

Nearly half (47 per cent) the limited plan members were
in families of one or two enrolled members, as against only a
fourth of the comprehensive members.

A third of the "Family Doctor Plan" membership was in
families of five or more, and another 25 per cent in families of
four. Each of these categories accounted for only 18 per cent
of the "Semi-Private Plan" members (Table 6).

As compared with the family population of the United
States, the average size of family in the GHI "Family Doctor
Plan" seems somewhat smaller—3.45 vs. 3.71; but the inference
is not justified because of a difference in definition.

Family size under GHI or other insurance contracts is not
comparable to available statistics on the general population,
which are stated in terms of all related household members, thus
can include offspring past age 19 as well as grandparents, aunts,
uncles, cousins. The average size of the GHI enrolled family
with comprehensive coverage appears to be larger than national

TABLE 6. Number and Distribution of Study
Population Members, by Size of Family
(Full-Year Members)

| SIZE OF FAMILY | Combined Plans | Comprehensive Plan | Limited Plan |
|---|---|---|---|
| | NUMBER OF MEMBERS | | |
| 1 Person | 4,572 | 3,075 | 1,497 |
| 2 Persons | 10,000 | 7,780 | 2,220 |
| 3 Persons | 8,529 | 7,209 | 1,320 |
| 4 Persons | 12,000 | 10,560 | 1,440 |
| 5 Persons | 7,750 | 7,060 | 690 |
| 6 or more Persons | 7,678 | 6,927 | 751 |
| TOTAL | 50,529 | 42,611 | 7,918 |
| | PER CENT OF MEMBERS | | |
| 1 Person | 9.0 | 7.2 | 18.9 |
| 2 Persons | 19.8 | 18.3 | 28.0 |
| 3 Persons | 16.9 | 16.9 | 16.7 |
| 4 Persons | 23.8 | 24.8 | 18.2 |
| 5 Persons | 15.3 | 16.6 | 8.7 |
| 6 or more Persons | 15.2 | 16.2 | 9.5 |
| TOTAL | 100.0 | 100.0 | 100.0 |

TABLE 7. Distribution of Families of Two or More Persons,
United States and New York-Northeast New Jersey
Population, and GHI Study Population,
by Family Size

| SIZE OF FAMILY | PER CENT OF FAMILY UNITS | | |
|---|---|---|---|
| | United States (1964)* | New York-Northeast New Jersey (1960)* | GHI Study Population: Comprehensive Plan (1964)† |
| 2 | 32.2 | 33.5 | 34.0 |
| 3 | 20.7 | 23.6 | 21.0 |
| 4 | 19.9 | 22.0 | 23.1 |
| 5 | 13.2 | 11.9 | 12.3 |
| 6 or more | 14.0 | 9.0 | 9.6 |
| TOTAL | 100.0 | 100.0 | 100.0 |
| N = | 47,436 (in 000's) | 3,883 (in 000's) | 11,449 |

* Family includes persons related by blood, marriage or adoption and residing together.
† Family includes subscriber, spouse, and natural or adopted children to age 19.
Sources: Current Population Reports, U.S. Department of Commerce, Series P-20, No. 139,
Table 6, June 11, 1965 and 1960 Census of Population, Volume 1, Part 34, Table 110.
New York, U.S. Department of Commerce, 1963.

or local averages when the GHI definition (parents and children to 19) is taken into account (Table 7).

### Subscriber Occupation Class

In Table 8, the sample populations, including dependents, are distributed according to occupation class of the subscriber.

It has been previously noted (p. 40) that occupation class, in the absence of data on educational attainment level or income category, provided the only indication of insuree social class.

The GHI comprehensive plan membership is dominated by blue-collar subscribers and their families (61 per cent). This reflects the tendency of large unions to purchase comprehensive benefits for their members. The composition of the limited plan membership contrasts markedly, with 23 per cent in professional, executive, or sales categories (as against 9 per cent of the comprehensive plan membership), 10 per cent in the retired category, and less than half in the blue-collar class.

TABLE 8.   Number and Distribution of Study Population
Members Including Dependents Classified by
Occupation Class of Subscriber
(Full-Year Members)

| OCCUPATION CLASS | Combined Plans | Comprehensive Plan | Limited Plan |
|---|---|---|---|
| | NUMBER OF MEMBERS | | |
| *White-Collar* | | | |
| Professional | 1,741 | 1,234 | 507 |
| Executive | 2,104 | 1,632 | 472 |
| Sales | 1,524 | 877 | 647 |
| Clerical and | | | |
| White-Collar Unspecified | 14,005 | 12,522 | 1,483 |
| | 19,374 | 16,265 | 3,109 |
| *Blue-Collar* | 29,153 | 25,890 | 3,263 |
| | 48,527 | 42,155 | 6,372 |
| *Retired* | 965 | 250 | 715 |
| *Student* | 82 | 34 | 48 |
| TOTAL * | 49,574 | 42,439 | 7,135 |

* Excluding Unknown.

| | PER CENT OF MEMBERS | | |
|---|---|---|---|
| *White-Collar* | | | |
| Professional | 3.5 | 2.9 | 7.1 |
| Executive | 4.2 | 3.8 | 6.6 |
| Sales | 3.1 | 2.1 | 9.1 |
| Clerical and | | | |
| White-Collar Unspecified | 28.2 | 29.5 | 20.8 |
| | 39.0 | 38.3 | 43.6 |
| *Blue-Collar* | 58.8 | 61.0 | 45.7 |
| | 97.8 | 99.3 | 89.3 |
| *Retired* | 2.0 | .6 | 10.0 |
| *Student* | .2 | .1 | .7 |
| TOTAL | 100.0 | 100.0 | 100.0 |

## Area of Residence

Half the study population (51 per cent) was concentrated
in three counties, with Brooklyn first, Queens second, and
Nassau third. This pattern was true of both samples.

The remainder of each sample was distributed somewhat
differently; New Jersey and Manhattan were more heavily rep-

resented among the limited membership, but were outranked by the Bronx and upstate New York among the comprehensive membership (Table 9).

TABLE 9.  Number and Distribution of Study Population
Members, by Area of Residence
(Full-Year Members)

| AREA OF RESIDENCE | Combined Plans | Comprehensive Plan | Limited Plan |
|---|---|---|---|
| | NUMBER OF MEMBERS | | |
| Manhattan | 4,039 | 3,279 | 760 |
| Bronx | 4,937 | 4,204 | 733 |
| Brooklyn | 11,306 | 9,578 | 1,728 |
| Queens | 7,639 | 6,339 | 1,300 |
| Richmond | 864 | 803 | 61 |
| Nassau | 6,496 | 5,533 | 963 |
| Suffolk | 3,528 | 3,139 | 389 |
| Westchester | 1,655 | 1,366 | 289 |
| Other New York | 4,182 | 3,940 | 242 |
| New Jersey | 4,397 | 3,530 | 867 |
| Other | 1,203 | 630 | 573 |
| TOTAL * | 50,246 | 42,341 | 7,905 |

* Excluding Unknown.

| | PER CENT OF MEMBERS | | |
|---|---|---|---|
| Manhattan | 8.0 | 7.8 | 9.6 |
| Bronx | 9.8 | 9.9 | 9.3 |
| Brooklyn | 22.5 | 22.6 | 21.9 |
| Queens | 15.2 | 15.0 | 16.4 |
| Richmond | 1.7 | 1.9 | .8 |
| Nassau | 13.0 | 13.1 | 12.2 |
| Suffolk | 7.0 | 7.4 | 4.9 |
| Westchester | 3.3 | 3.2 | 3.6 |
| Other New York | 8.3 | 9.3 | 3.1 |
| New Jersey | 8.8 | 8.3 | 11.0 |
| Other | 2.4 | 1.5 | 7.2 |
| TOTAL | 100.0 | 100.0 | 100.0 |

## Year of Enrollment

The "Family Doctor Plan" membership covered for the full study year had apparently been entering at a fairly steady rate during the preceding years, each year from 1959 through 1963 accounting for about 14 to 16 per cent of the 1964 full-year membership. In the limited plan the picture was entirely different; 38 per cent of these members had joined in 1957 or before, when the "Family Doctor Plan" was either nonexistent or a novelty (Table 10).

TABLE 10. Number and Distribution of Study Population Members, by Year of Enrollment (Full-Year Members)

| YEAR OF ENROLLMENT | Combined Plans | Comprehensive Plan | Limited Plan |
|---|---|---|---|
| | NUMBER OF MEMBERS | | |
| 1957 and before | 9,091 | 6,081 | 3,010 |
| 1958 | 4,988 | 4,445 | 543 |
| 1959 | 7,359 | 6,621 | 738 |
| 1960 | 6,454 | 5,872 | 582 |
| 1961 | 6,704 | 5,907 | 797 |
| 1962 | 7,886 | 6,883 | 1,003 |
| 1963 | 7,327 | 6,122 | 1,205 |
| 1964 | 720 | 680 | 40 |
| TOTAL | 50,529 | 42,611 | 7,918 |
| | PER CENT OF MEMBERS | | |
| 1957 and before | 18.0 | 14.3 | 38.0 |
| 1958 | 9.9 | 10.4 | 6.9 |
| 1959 | 14.6 | 15.5 | 9.3 |
| 1960 | 12.8 | 13.8 | 7.3 |
| 1961 | 13.3 | 13.9 | 10.1 |
| 1962 | 15.5 | 16.1 | 12.7 |
| 1963 | 14.5 | 14.4 | 15.2 |
| 1964 | 1.4 | 1.6 | .5 |
| TOTAL | 100.0 | 100.0 | 100.0 |

## Selected Cross-Tabulations

The remaining tabulations are based on the total GHI sample, including full-year and part-year members. It was economically unfeasible to plan multivariate demographic analysis of utilization data, and these cross-tabulations were useful as a rough gauge of variable interaction.

TABLE 11. Age Distribution of Study Population Members,
by Area of Residence
(Full-Year and Part-Year Members)

| AREA OF RESIDENCE | COMBINED PLANS | | | | | COMPREHENSIVE PLAN | | | | | LIMITED PLAN | | | | |
|---|---|---|---|---|---|---|---|---|---|---|---|---|---|---|---|
| | Total | 19 and Under | 20-44 | 45-54 | 55 and Over | Total | 19 and Under | 20-44 | 45-54 | 55 and Over | Total | 19 and Under | 20-44 | 45-54 | 55 and Over |
| | % | % | % | % | % | % | % | % | % | % | % | % | % | % | % |
| Manhattan | 100.0 | 28.2 | 36.9 | 17.3 | 17.6 | 100.0 | 30.4 | 36.7 | 17.5 | 15.4 | 100.0 | 18.5 | 38.1 | 16.5 | 26.9 |
| Bronx | 100.0 | 33.6 | 33.2 | 16.0 | 17.2 | 100.0 | 35.3 | 32.7 | 16.6 | 15.4 | 100.0 | 24.4 | 36.3 | 12.1 | 27.2 |
| Brooklyn | 100.0 | 35.0 | 34.1 | 15.8 | 15.1 | 100.0 | 36.9 | 34.2 | 16.0 | 12.9 | 100.0 | 24.6 | 33.6 | 14.6 | 27.2 |
| Queens | 100.0 | 33.9 | 31.5 | 17.4 | 17.2 | 100.0 | 35.8 | 31.8 | 17.7 | 14.7 | 100.0 | 24.1 | 30.1 | 16.3 | 29.5 |
| Richmond | 100.0 | 38.4 | 29.5 | 17.6 | 14.5 | 100.0 | 39.8 | 30.3 | 17.5 | 12.4 | 100.0 | 21.1 | 20.0 | 18.9 | 40.0 |
| Nassau | 100.0 | 42.5 | 32.2 | 15.2 | 10.1 | 100.0 | 43.6 | 32.5 | 15.3 | 8.6 | 100.0 | 36.8 | 30.8 | 14.7 | 17.7 |
| Suffolk | 100.0 | 45.2 | 34.5 | 12.6 | 7.7 | 100.0 | 46.1 | 34.4 | 12.8 | 6.7 | 100.0 | 39.9 | 34.9 | 11.0 | 14.2 |
| Westchester | 100.0 | 37.3 | 32.4 | 17.6 | 12.7 | 100.0 | 39.3 | 32.9 | 17.6 | 10.2 | 100.0 | 26.8 | 29.5 | 17.5 | 26.2 |
| New Jersey | 100.0 | 37.7 | 32.0 | 16.5 | 13.8 | 100.0 | 40.0 | 32.6 | 16.8 | 10.6 | 100.0 | 29.4 | 29.8 | 15.6 | 25.2 |
| Other New York | 100.0 | 41.9 | 34.5 | 12.7 | 10.9 | 100.0 | 42.6 | 34.5 | 12.8 | 10.1 | 100.0 | 31.8 | 35.1 | 10.4 | 22.7 |
| TOTAL | 100.0 | 36.7 | 33.4 | 15.7 | 14.2 | 100.0 | 38.5 | 33.5 | 15.9 | 12.1 | 100.0 | 27.7 | 32.8 | 14.5 | 25.0 |

**TABLE 12.** Distribution by Residence Area, White-Collar–Blue-Collar–Retired Segments of Study Populations, Including Dependents Classified According to Subscriber Status (Full-Year and Part-Year Members)

| AREA OF RESIDENCE | COMBINED PLANS | | | | COMPREHENSIVE PLAN | | | | LIMITED PLAN | | | |
|---|---|---|---|---|---|---|---|---|---|---|---|---|
| | Total | White Collar | Blue Collar | Retired | Total | White Collar | Blue Collar | Retired | Total | White Collar | Blue Collar | Retired |
| | % | % | % | % | % | % | % | % | % | % | % | % |
| Manhattan | 8.0 | 7.7 | 8.2 | 8.5 | 7.8 | 7.0 | 8.4 | 7.2 | 9.3 | 11.4 | 7.4 | 9.1 |
| Bronx | 9.6 | 6.6 | 11.4 | 10.5 | 9.6 | 6.4 | 11.6 | 6.9 | 9.1 | 7.8 | 9.7 | 12.2 |
| Brooklyn | 22.5 | 14.1 | 28.0 | 20.5 | 22.6 | 13.1 | 28.4 | 20.1 | 22.1 | 18.7 | 25.3 | 20.6 |
| Queens | 15.9 | 11.7 | 18.6 | 18.2 | 15.9 | 11.0 | 18.8 | 19.3 | 16.2 | 15.3 | 16.8 | 17.7 |
| Richmond | 2.1 | 1.3 | 2.4 | 1.3 | 2.2 | 1.3 | 2.7 | 1.1 | .9 | 1.3 | .5 | 1.4 |
| Nassau | 12.5 | 15.6 | 10.6 | 8.5 | 12.4 | 16.1 | 10.2 | 7.8 | 12.9 | 13.5 | 13.0 | 8.8 |
| Suffolk | 7.4 | 10.7 | 5.3 | 5.7 | 7.8 | 11.9 | 5.3 | 10.0 | 5.3 | 5.0 | 6.0 | 3.7 |
| Westchester | 3.6 | 4.5 | 3.1 | 2.3 | 3.7 | 4.8 | 3.0 | .9 | 3.3 | 2.9 | 3.8 | 3.0 |
| Oher New York | 7.8 | 16.0 | 2.7 | 8.4 | 8.7 | 18.5 | 2.7 | 19.3 | 2.8 | 3.0 | 2.4 | 3.6 |
| New Jersey | 8.3 | 7.7 | 8.7 | 8.2 | 7.8 | 7.4 | 8.1 | 3.7 | 11.1 | 9.5 | 12.7 | 10.2 |
| Other | 2.3 | 4.1 | 1.0 | 7.9 | 1.5 | 2.5 | .8 | 3.7 | 7.0 | 11.6 | 2.4 | 9.7 |
| **TOTAL** | 100.0 | 100.0 | 100.0 | 100.0 | 100.0 | 100.0 | 100.0 | 100.0 | 100.0 | 100.0 | 100.0 | 100.0 |

## TABLE 13. Age Distribution of Adults in Study Populations, by Marital Status (Full-Year and Part-Year Members)

| | COMBINED PLANS | | | | COMPREHENSIVE PLAN | | | | LIMITED PLAN | | | |
|---|---|---|---|---|---|---|---|---|---|---|---|---|
| AGE | Total | Married | Widowed, Divorced, Separated | Single | Total | Married | Widowed, Divorced, Separated | Single | Total | Married | Widowed, Divorced, Separated | Single |
| | % | % | % | % | % | % | % | % | % | % | % | % |
| Under 20 | .7 | .3 | .2 | 3.8 | .6 | .3 | .4 | 3.2 | .9 | .1 | – | 5.4 |
| 20–24 | 6.6 | 4.2 | 2.1 | 25.9 | 6.1 | 4.3 | 2.8 | 22.3 | 8.9 | 4.0 | 1.3 | 36.1 |
| 25–34 | 19.9 | 19.9 | 7.7 | 23.6 | 20.7 | 20.3 | 12.6 | 25.1 | 16.4 | 17.6 | 2.6 | 19.4 |
| 35–44 | 25.8 | 27.8 | 14.2 | 14.9 | 27.2 | 28.8 | 20.5 | 15.9 | 19.6 | 22.8 | 7.5 | 12.0 |
| 45–54 | 24.7 | 26.1 | 23.2 | 15.1 | 25.8 | 26.8 | 27.7 | 17.0 | 19.9 | 22.3 | 18.5 | 9.9 |
| 55–64 | 16.2 | 16.3 | 26.6 | 12.0 | 15.8 | 15.8 | 24.3 | 13.3 | 18.1 | 18.8 | 29.0 | 8.3 |
| 65 and over | 6.1 | 5.4 | 26.0 | 4.7 | 3.8 | 3.7 | 11.7 | 3.2 | 16.2 | 14.4 | 41.1 | 8.9 |
| TOTAL | 100.0 | 100.0 | 100.0 | 100.0 | 100.0 | 100.0 | 100.0 | 100.0 | 100.0 | 100.0 | 100.0 | 100.0 |

TABLE 14. Age Distribution of Comprehensive Plan Sample Including Dependents, by Occupation Class of Subscriber (Full-Year and Part-Year Members)

| | | OCCUPATION CLASS OF SUBSCRIBER | | | | | | |
|---|---|---|---|---|---|---|---|---|
| AGE | Total | Professional and Executive | Sales | Clerical and White-collar Unspecified | All White-collar | Blue Collar | Student | Retired |
| | % | % | % | % | % | % | % | % |
| 19 and Under | 38.1 | 35.0 | 40.2 | 39.2 | 38.5 | 38.2 | 1.4 | 6.8 |
| 20–24 | 5.5 | 5.2 | 5.0 | 6.3 | 6.0 | 5.0 | 98.6 | 1.2 |
| 25–34 | 12.2 | 12.7 | 9.4 | 13.8 | 13.4 | 11.6 | 0 | 0 |
| 35–44 | 16.1 | 19.2 | 18.1 | 16.6 | 17.1 | 15.7 | 0 | 1.5 |
| 45–54 | 15.5 | 16.7 | 15.0 | 14.2 | 14.7 | 16.3 | 0 | 4.6 |
| 55–64 | 9.9 | 8.7 | 9.9 | 8.2 | 8.4 | 10.8 | 0 | 18.1 |
| 65 and Over | 2.7 | 2.5 | 2.4 | 1.7 | 1.9 | 2.4 | 0 | 67.8 |
| TOTAL | 100.0 | 100.0 | 100.0 | 100.0 | 100.0 | 100.0 | 100.0 | 100.0 |
| 44 and Under | 71.9 | 72.1 | 72.7 | 75.9 | 75.0 | 70.5 | 100.0 | 9.5 |
| 45 and Over | 28.1 | 27.9 | 27.3 | 24.1 | 25.0 | 29.5 | 0 | 90.5 |

TABLE 15. Age Distribution of Comprehensive Plan Sample Including Dependents, by Year of Enrollment (Full-Year and Part-Year Members)

| AGE | YEAR OF ENROLLMENT | | | | | | | |
|---|---|---|---|---|---|---|---|---|
| | 1964 | 1963 | 1962 | 1961 | 1960 | 1959 | 1958 | 1957 *or* *Before* |
| | % | % | % | % | % | % | % | % |
| 19 and Under | 39.1 | 39.2 | 36.8 | 37.1 | 39.8 | 37.3 | 39.0 | 36.3 |
| 20–24 | 10.8 | 9.2 | 5.8 | 5.0 | 3.9 | 3.3 | 3.7 | 2.6 |
| 25–34 | 18.4 | 17.3 | 15.4 | 13.9 | 12.0 | 8.4 | 8.6 | 4.6 |
| 35–44 | 14.8 | 14.9 | 15.6 | 16.4 | 16.6 | 16.5 | 17.8 | 16.7 |
| 45–54 | 9.8 | 11.9 | 14.7 | 14.7 | 15.3 | 18.1 | 19.1 | 20.4 |
| 55–64 | 5.7 | 6.3 | 9.5 | 10.6 | 9.6 | 11.8 | 10.3 | 14.6 |
| 65 and Over | 1.4 | 1.2 | 2.2 | 2.3 | 2.8 | 4.6 | 1.5 | 4.8 |
| TOTAL | 100.0 | 100.0 | 100.0 | 100.0 | 100.0 | 100.0 | 100.0 | 100.0 |

# Chapter 4

# THE SUPPLY OF
# PRACTICING PHYSICIANS

The New York metropolitan area has more physicians than any other community in the world. This may be one reason for the difficulty encountered in sorting out precisely where, to what extent, and in what fields of practice, physicians are available for the treatment of patients. Yet such background information is a prerequisite for realistic evaluation of medical care distribution patterns presently in use or proposed.

In the absence of published tabulations from other sources, GHI has been conducting its own annual surveys based on its own records. While complete accuracy in this sphere, as of any one time, is almost impossible because of constant changes in the status of a minority of physicians, adequate perspective can be attained as to the number, geographic distribution, age, type and field of practice, and qualifications of physicians in private practice. The surveys are conducted on the assumption that sooner or later most physicians treating patients in its areas of operation would have occasion to file a claim with GHI, since it covers a million people, the majority of whom have ambulatory as well as hospital coverage of physicians' services under a free-choice-of-doctor arrangement.

Data reported in the following pages are based on GHI's 1966 survey of practicing physicians * in its principal areas of

---

* The survey applies only to physicians with the M.D. degree and osteopaths who treat private patients, excludes podiatrists and optometrists who under State Insurance Law are paid for covered services in their fields. The extent to which listed physicians devote full time to private practice, or may have salaried full- or part-time positions, is not known.

operation—the five counties of New York City (Manhattan, Bronx, Brooklyn, Queens, Richmond) and the surrounding New York counties of Nassau, Suffolk, Westchester. In this eight-county area the population totals over 11,000,000, the number of private physicians on current record at GHI 22,900. ("Current record" includes total number ever filing, minus those known to have moved out of the area or died.)

## Geographic Distribution

Manhattan, the hub of the area, has many more physicians in relation to population than its neighboring counties: 15.3 per cent of the population, 31.5 per cent of the doctors in practice. Suburban Westchester—the highest per capita income county of the group—accounts for practically identical proportions of population and physicians. Bronx, Brooklyn and Queens —the closest commuting areas with respect to Manhattan—contain 54 per cent of the population, 42 per cent of the physicians. Thus there are wide variations in physician-population ratios: from 240 residents per physician in Manhattan, to 800 in Suffolk, with an overall eight-county average of 490. Stated another way, this indicates over 200 physicians per 100,000 population (Table 16).

Although the population-ratio method of measurement has

TABLE 16. Distribution of Physicians and Population, by Area

| COUNTY | Population | Physicians in Private Practice | Population Per Physician | Physicians Per 100,000 Population |
|---|---|---|---|---|
| | % | % | | |
| Manhattan | 15.3 | 31.5 | 240 | 419 |
| Bronx | 13.0 | 9.3 | 690 | 145 |
| Brooklyn | 23.5 | 18.9 | 610 | 164 |
| Queens | 17.4 | 13.6 | 630 | 159 |
| Richmond | 2.3 | 1.5 | 740 | 134 |
| Nassau | 12.5 | 12.0 | 510 | 196 |
| Suffolk | 8.3 | 5.1 | 800 | 126 |
| Westchester | 7.7 | 8.1 | 460 | 215 |
| TOTAL | 100.0 | 100.0 | 490 | 204 |

been criticized as an inadequate substitute for precise evaluation of physician resources, ratios are used as one approach to
analysis of the present data on the ground that they at least
provide an attainable common denominator for rough area-to-
area comparisons within and beyond the areas of this study.
It is recognized that such comparisons, to be of practical value,
must be supplemented by further detail on physician characteristics, particularly qualifications and field of practice.

## Type of Practice, Qualifications and Age

In the eight-county area surveyed, the proportion of physicians classified as general practitioners—that is, without recorded indication of specialist qualifications—decreased from
49 per cent in 1964 and 48 per cent in 1965 to 45 per cent in
1966.

GHI's definition of a specialist recognizes any of the following qualifications: Diplomate of an American Specialty Board;
Fellow of a recognized American Specialty College; specialty
designation by the New York State Workmen's Compensation
Board; an outstanding hospital or teaching appointment de-
noting peer recognition; in psychiatry, full-time practice limited
to this field.

The elasticity of the GHI definition of specialist stops short
of self-designation—the method used in derivation of national
statistics [1] to produce the figure 61 specialists per hundred
private practitioners. On the other hand, the GHI definition is
too liberal for those who feel that only Diplomates of American
Specialty Boards and perhaps Fellows of recognized national
professional societies should be recognized. If the definition
were thus limited, the proportion classified as specialists in the
present survey would drop to 37 per cent, including Fellows,
or 32.8 per cent excluding all but Diplomates. These figures are
averages for the eight-county area. As shown in Table 17, there
is substantial variation from county to county.

---

[1] U.S. Department of Health, Education and Welfare, *Health Manpower Source
Book, Section 18, Manpower in the 1960's,* Washington, D.C., 1964, p. 28.

TABLE 17. Distribution of Physicians in Private Practice by Type of Practice and Qualifications, by County

| COUNTY | TOTAL | SPECIALISTS (COUNTED UNDER HIGHEST RATING) | | | | | NON-SPECIALISTS | | |
|---|---|---|---|---|---|---|---|---|---|
| | | All | Diplomates | Fellows | Workmen's Compensation Specialist Rating | Other | All | M.D. | D.O. |
| | % | % | % | % | % | % | % | % | % |
| 8-COUNTY AREA | 100.0 | 55.3 | 32.8 | 4.2 | 15.4 | 2.9 | 44.7 | 42.9 | 1.8 |
| Manhattan | 100.0 | 64.7 | 41.6 | 4.1 | 15.2 | 3.8 | 35.3 | 34.5 | .8 |
| Bronx | 100.0 | 44.3 | 23.2 | 4.4 | 14.1 | 2.6 | 55.7 | 53.9 | 1.8 |
| Brooklyn | 100.0 | 48.7 | 28.0 | 5.0 | 13.6 | 2.1 | 51.3 | 48.4 | 2.9 |
| Queens | 100.0 | 46.2 | 25.5 | 4.1 | 14.5 | 2.1 | 53.8 | 51.6 | 2.2 |
| Richmond | 100.0 | 53.9 | 24.9 | 4.9 | 21.8 | 2.3 | 46.1 | 45.3 | .8 |
| Nassau | 100.0 | 56.6 | 35.1 | 3.3 | 15.7 | 2.5 | 43.4 | 40.9 | 2.5 |
| Suffolk | 100.0 | 56.1 | 23.6 | 3.0 | 23.7 | 5.8 | 43.9 | 40.5 | 3.4 |
| Westchester | 100.0 | 59.3 | 36.6 | 4.5 | 15.9 | 2.3 | 40.7 | 39.6 | 1.1 |

## Comparison with Other Countries

For additional perspective in viewing the overall division of the practicing profession as between specialists and non-specialists, it is of interest to note the proportions reported for other countries with generally comparable experience on available health indices.

Published statistics reveal that in most of the countries listed (Table 18), the proportion of specialists is far below both the 61 per cent reported for the United States on the basis of self-designation and the 55 per cent found in the present survey. It ranges from 20 to 39 per cent in the British Isles, France, Scandinavia and West Germany.

TABLE 18.   Specialists as a Proportion of All Practicing Physicians in 11 Countries [1]

| Country | % Specialists |
|---|---|
| England and Wales | 20.5 |
| Scotland | 31.5 |
| Northern Ireland | 24.0 |
| France | 33.9 |
| West Germany | 39.2 |
| Netherlands | 29.6 |
| Denmark | 29.1 |
| Norway | 35.0 |
| Sweden | 35.9 |
| Canada | 45.7 |

[1] Charron, K. C., *Health Services, Health Insurance, and Their Inter-Relationship*, Department of National Health and Welfare, Ottawa, Canada, November 1963, p. 45 (citing World Health Organization figures).

If the U.S. definition of specialist were limited to Diplomates of Specialty Boards, however, the apparently unique position of the U.S. with respect to proportion of specialists would be considerably softened. The number of physicians self-classified as specialists appears to be about 70 per cent higher than the number of Board-certified specialists. Approximately a third of all active physicians are listed as Diplomates [1]—a figure closer to the proportion of specialists reported in other countries.

[1] Marquis—Who's Who, *Directory of Medical Specialists*, Volume 12 (1965–66), Chicago.

## Age Trends

The finding that 45 per cent of the physicians in the present study (including osteopaths) are listed as general practitioners seems to be at odds with statements proclaiming their disappearance. Such statements are premature; they are based not on today's levels but on the assumption that the rate of decrease over the past few years will continue, or on surveys of intentions to specialize, conducted among medical students.

Analysis of the GHI data on specialization among physicians of various ages provides further evidence of this trend. Among physicians aged 55 and over, the proportion listed as specialists in the present survey is 53 per cent; among those 35 to 54, the proportion rises to 63 per cent (Table 19).

TABLE 19. Type of Private Practice, by Age, Physicians in 8-County Area

| PHYSICIAN AGE | Number of Physicians | PROPORTION CLASSIFIED AS | | | | |
|---|---|---|---|---|---|---|
| | | | | NON-SPECIALISTS | | |
| | | TOTAL | SPECIALISTS | All | M.D. | D.O. |
| | | % | % | % | % | % |
| 29 and Under | 213 | 100 | 5.6 | 94.4 | 74.7 | 19.7 |
| 30–34 | 2,052 | 100 | 33.6 | 66.4 | 62.1 | 4.3 |
| 35–44 | 5,100 | 100 | 62.3 | 37.7 | 35.6 | 2.1 |
| 45–54 | 5,986 | 100 | 62.8 | 37.2 | 35.8 | 1.4 |
| 55–64 | 5,752 | 100 | 53.0 | 47.0 | 45.9 | 1.1 |
| 65 and Over | 3,829 | 100 | 52.0 | 48.0 | 47.2 | .8 |
| TOTAL | 22,932 | 100 | 55.3 | 44.7 | 42.9 | 1.8 |

When specialists are divided according to their levels of qualifications, marked variations are observed as to age-level concentration of the different groups. The concentration of Diplomates is highest at ages 45 to 54, where they comprise 46 per cent of the listed physicians, and next highest at ages 55 to 64; four out of five Diplomates are in the 45-plus bracket, compared to 68 per cent of all listed physicians.

Those who are not Diplomates but are Fellows account for only a small minority of the listed physicians and their proportion is constantly declining. Nearly 70 per cent are already past age 55.

In contrast to these two groups, specialists whose highest listed qualification is the "S" rating of the New York State Workmen's Compensation Board are generally younger—53.5 per cent under 45. At ages under 34 this segment accounts for the majority of all specialists; at ages 35 to 44, it still accounts for nearly half. A sudden dropping-off occurs at age 45, accompanying the spurt in the Diplomate class. In the 55-plus group of all specialists, the "S" rating is listed as the top qualification for about one fifth (Table 20).

TABLE 20.  Distribution of Physicians by Type of Practice and Qualifications, by Age Group

**A.**

| AGE | All Physicians | SPECIALISTS * | | | | NON-SPECIALISTS | | |
|---|---|---|---|---|---|---|---|---|
| | | All † | D ‡ | F § | S ‖ | All | M.D. | D.O. |
| | % | % | % | % | % | % | % | % |
| All Ages | 100.0 | 55.3 | 32.8 | 4.2 | 15.4 | 44.7 | 42.9 | 1.8 |
| 29 and Under | 100.0 | 5.6 | .5 | 0 | 3.7 | 94.4 | 74.7 | 19.7 |
| 30–34 | 100.0 | 33.6 | 1.8 | .3 | 28.1 | 66.4 | 62.1 | 4.3 |
| 35–44 | 100.0 | 62.3 | 29.3 | 1.4 | 25.5 | 37.7 | 35.6 | 2.1 |
| 45–54 | 100.0 | 62.8 | 46.0 | 3.9 | 9.7 | 37.2 | 35.8 | 1.4 |
| 55–64 | 100.0 | 53.0 | 35.0 | 6.5 | 10.3 | 47.0 | 45.9 | 1.1 |
| 65 and Over | 100.0 | 52.0 | 31.6 | 7.5 | 12.1 | 48.0 | 47.2 | .8 |

**B.**

| AGE | All Physicians | SPECIALISTS | | | | NON-SPECIALISTS | | |
|---|---|---|---|---|---|---|---|---|
| | | All | D | F | S | All | M.D. | D.O. |
| | % | % | % | % | % | % | % | % |
| 29 and Under | .9 | .1 | — | 0 | .2 | 2.0 | 1.6 | 10.0 |
| 30–34 | 9.0 | 5.4 | .5 | .6 | 16.4 | 13.3 | 13.0 | 21.0 |
| 35–44 | 22.2 | 25.1 | 19.9 | 7.2 | 36.9 | 18.7 | 18.4 | 26.1 |
| 45–54 | 26.1 | 29.6 | 36.7 | 23.9 | 16.5 | 21.7 | 21.8 | 20.6 |
| 55–64 | 25.1 | 24.1 | 26.8 | 38.7 | 16.8 | 26.4 | 26.8 | 15.1 |
| 65 and Over | 16.7 | 15.7 | 16.1 | 29.6 | 13.2 | 17.9 | 18.4 | 7.2 |
| TOTAL | 100.0 | 100.0 | 100.0 | 100.0 | 100.0 | 100.0 | 100.0 | 100.0 |

* Classified according to highest qualification.
† Includes specialists with unknown qualifications.
‡ Diplomates of American Specialty Boards.
§ Fellows of recognized American Colleges of medicine or surgery.
‖ Classified as specialists by New York State Workmen's Compensation Board.

Aside from the question of specialist qualifications at various age levels, Table 20B also brings out the age distribution of the entire group of physicians in practice. Comparison of the three ten-year intervals between ages 35 and 64 reveals similar proportions (26 and 25 per cent) of the total accounted for by the intervals 45–54 and 55–64, and a slight drop in the group aged 35–44, to 22 per cent. This reflects a difference of about 900 fewer physicians in the 35–44 group as compared with the 45–54 group. The significance (if any) of the lower figure shown for the younger group, in terms of possible long-term connotations, would be worth pursuing.

*Local Patterns.* Although the proportion of specialists varies from 44 per cent in the Bronx to 65 per cent in Manhattan, the age pattern by type of practice is fairly consistent within the geographic subdivisions of the eight-county area. The highest degree of specialization is found between the ages of 35 and 54, in all areas. When qualifications are taken into account along with age, the proportion of Diplomates is highest in all areas at ages 45 to 54, while the proportion with only State Workmen's Compensation Board recognition is highest at ages 30 to 44.

One of the noteworthy observations incidental to the detailed analysis in Table 21 concerns the markedly higher proportions of physicians with the "S" rating in the two counties having the lowest physician-to-population ratios, Richmond and Suffolk.

## Generalists

A fourth of all specialists in the GHI survey are internists or pediatricians; and there are over three times again as many general practitioners listed as there are internists and pediatricians combined. These three categories comprise the group to be referred to here as generalists. They are the practitioners who are presumably available for the general care of the population.

TABLE 21. Per Cent of Private Practicing Physicians Listed as Specialists in Each Area, by Age Group *

### A. ALL SPECIALISTS AS A PERCENTAGE OF ALL LISTED PHYSICIANS

| AGE GROUP | All Areas | Manhattan | Bronx | Brooklyn | Queens | Richmond | Nassau | Suffolk | Westchester |
|---|---|---|---|---|---|---|---|---|---|
| All Ages | 55 | 65 | 44 | 49 | 46 | 54 | 57 | 56 | 59 |
| 29 and Under | 6 | 17 | 5 | 2 | 2 | 11 | 3 | 0 | 11 |
| 30–34 | 34 | 35 | 36 | 27 | 34 | 33 | 33 | 43 | 32 |
| 35–44 | 62 | 67 | 55 | 54 | 58 | 64 | 63 | 66 | 66 |
| 45–54 | 63 | 76 | 48 | 55 | 49 | 65 | 67 | 61 | 66 |
| 55–64 | 53 | 67 | 40 | 47 | 45 | 43 | 47 | 49 | 61 |
| 65 and Over | 52 | 60 | 42 | 52 | 37 | 60 | 43 | 46 | 47 |

### B. DIPLOMATE-SPECIALISTS AS A PERCENTAGE OF ALL LISTED PHYSICIANS

| AGE GROUP | All Areas | Manhattan | Bronx | Brooklyn | Queens | Richmond | Nassau | Suffolk | Westchester |
|---|---|---|---|---|---|---|---|---|---|
| All Ages | 33 | 42 | 23 | 28 | 26 | 25 | 35 | 24 | 37 |
| 29 and Under | .5 | 0 | 0 | 0 | 0 | 11 | 0 | 0 | 0 |
| 30–34 | 2 | 2 | 3 | .6 | 2 | 5 | 3 | 3 | 1 |
| 35–44 | 29 | 34 | 28 | 22 | 23 | 24 | 34 | 24 | 32 |
| 45–54 | 46 | 58 | 32 | 37 | 36 | 42 | 50 | 41 | 52 |
| 55–64 | 35 | 49 | 22 | 30 | 27 | 24 | 32 | 21 | 42 |
| 65 and Over | 32 | 39 | 20 | 32 | 21 | 14 | 24 | 25 | 27 |

### C. "S" (WORKMEN'S COMPENSATION RATING)– SPECIALISTS AS A PERCENTAGE OF ALL LISTED PHYSICIANS

| AGE GROUP | All Areas | Manhattan | Bronx | Brooklyn | Queens | Richmond | Nassau | Suffolk | Westchester |
|---|---|---|---|---|---|---|---|---|---|
| All Ages | 15 | 15 | 14 | 14 | 15 | 22 | 16 | 24 | 16 |
| 29 and Under | 4 | 11 | 5 | 0 | 2 | 0 | 3 | 0 | 11 |
| 30–34 | 28 | 30 | 29 | 23 | 30 | 26 | 27 | 34 | 28 |
| 35–44 | 26 | 23 | 21 | 26 | 28 | 36 | 23 | 35 | 28 |
| 45–54 | 10 | 9 | 8 | 11 | 9 | 14 | 11 | 12 | 8 |
| 55–64 | 10 | 11 | 11 | 10 | 9 | 16 | 10 | 15 | 8 |
| 65 and Over | 12 | 13 | 12 | 11 | 10 | 24 | 9 | 12 | 12 |

* Specialists whose highest rating is Fellow or "other" are included in Part A but are not listed separately; they comprise only 7 percent of all listed physicians.

When the three types of generalists are analyzed as a separate unit, they total 13,400. In the eight-county area as a whole, 77 per cent of the practicing generalists are listed as general practitioners; the proportion varies little from county to county, amounting to 71 per cent in Manhattan and Westchester, as compared to 80 or 81 per cent in the four counties with the highest proportion (Table 22).

TABLE 22.  Distribution of Generalists in Each Area,
by Field of Practice

| AREA | All Generalists | Internists | Pediatricians | General Practitioners * |
|------|------|------|------|------|
| | % | % | % | % |
| Manhattan | 100.0 | 24.1 | 5.0 | 70.9 |
| Bronx | 100.0 | 13.2 | 5.6 | 81.2 |
| Brooklyn | 100.0 | 12.0 | 6.9 | 81.1 |
| Queens | 100.0 | 12.0 | 7.1 | 80.9 |
| Richmond | 100.0 | 14.5 | 7.7 | 77.8 |
| Nassau | 100.0 | 15.7 | 10.2 | 74.1 |
| Suffolk | 100.0 | 12.3 | 7.4 | 80.3 |
| Westchester | 100.0 | 19.5 | 9.1 | 71.4 |
| 8-COUNTY AREA | 100.0 | 16.5 | 6.9 | 76.6 |

* Includes M.D.'s and D.O.'s.

Thus the practical prospects for switching the entire burden of general medical care to internists and pediatricians, a proposal advanced in the interests of improved quality of care, must be viewed with certain population ratios in mind (Table 23).

For those who will recognize only Diplomates or Fellows as specialists in internal medicine or pediatrics, the first two columns of Table 23 require adjustment upward and the third downward, since, as previously indicated, GHI also classifies as specialists those with only the State Workmen's Compensation specialist rating or high-ranking hospital appointments. About 23 per cent of the internist-pediatrician list is in this non-Diplomate-or-Fellow category.

It is perhaps worth mentioning that the "S" (Workmen's Compensation) rating in internal medicine is more prevalent

TABLE 23. Population Per Practicing Generalist, by Area

| AREA | Internists | Internists and Pediatricians Combined | General Practitioners * | All Generalists Combined |
|---|---|---|---|---|
| Manhattan | 2,000 | 1,700 | 700 | 500 |
| Bronx | 7,600 | 5,300 | 1,200 | 1,000 |
| Brooklyn | 8,000 | 5,100 | 1,200 | 1,000 |
| Queens | 7,900 | 4,900 | 1,200 | 900 |
| Richmond | 8,700 | 5,700 | 1,600 | 1,300 |
| Nassau | 5,600 | 3,400 | 1,200 | 900 |
| Suffolk | 11,900 | 7,400 | 1,800 | 1,500 |
| Westchester | 4,200 | 2,800 | 1,100 | 800 |
| 8-COUNTY AREA | 5,100 | 3,600 | 1,100 | 800 |

* Includes M.D.'s and D.O.'s.

in the three outlying counties of Nassau, Suffolk and West-chester, than in New York City proper. These three counties account for 33 per cent of the "SJ" ratings (internal medicine) in the eight counties, but for only 20 per cent of the Internist-Diplomates or Fellows. This may well be attributable to differing practices or standards between New York City and suburban certifiers. Such variations within a relatively small area would presumably be multiplied many times over, if attempts at nation-wide standards short of the Diplomate rating were to be required.

It is apparent from the previous table that the notion of employing internists and pediatricians as family physicians, to the exclusion of general practitioners, is not feasible under present circumstances. The overall figure of 3,600 persons per internist-or-pediatrician is unthinkable; but the situation is actually worse than that, since people would not travel out of their counties for general office care—not to mention the problem of home visits, or hospitalization. While the ratios will gradually change if present trends continue, it is clearly unrealistic—apart from the debatable question of medical necessity—to suggest that medical insurance plans use their influence to insist now on specialist care for all services, just as it is an exercise in futility for "auditors" to use specialty status as an indiscriminate criterion for qualitative review of ambulatory services.

## Relative Importance of Different
## Specialty Fields

In the eight-county area surveyed, four specialties each account for ten or more per cent of all listed privately practicing specialists—internal medicine, general surgery, psychiatry, and obstetrics-gynecology. Over half the specialists are in these fields.

The next four specialties in relative numerical importance are pediatrics, ophthalmology, anesthesiology, and otolaryngology. When these are added to the leading four, the combination accounts for 75 per cent of all the specialists. After that come orthopedic surgery, radiology, dermatology and urology, comprising another 14 per cent, leaving only 11 per cent to be accounted for by all other specialties.

### Comparison with National Estimates

The twelve leading specialty fields among physicians in private practice in the New York metropolitan area are the same as the national leaders. Only minor shifts in position occur

TABLE 24. Rank of Leading Specialty Fields
of Physicians in Private Practice

| SPECIALTY FIELD | New York Metropolitan Area (1966) | United States [1] (1963) |
|---|---|---|
| | Rank | Rank |
| Internal Medicine | 1 | 1 |
| General Surgery | 2 | 2 |
| Psychiatry | 3 | 5 |
| Obstetrics-Gynecology | 4 | 3 |
| Pediatrics | 5 | 4 |
| Ophthalmology | 6 | 6 |
| Anesthesiology | 7 | 7 |
| Otolaryngology | 8 | 10 |
| Orthopedic Surgery | 9 | 9 |
| Radiology | 10 | 8 |
| Dermatology | 11 | 12 |
| Urology | 12 | 11 |

[1] U.S. Department of Health, Education, and Welfare, *Health Manpower Source Book,* op. cit.

when specialists are numerically ranked for the two sets of data (Table 24). The percentage of all privately practicing specialists accounted for by the twelve fields is also similar—89 per cent in the present study, 91 per cent nationally.

From the similarities in distribution of specialists in private practice, it may be inferred that patterns of relative use of the different types of specialists in the metropolitan New York area (discussed elsewhere) are in general indicative of national patterns.

### Local Variations

The twelve leading specialty fields in the eight-county area as a whole are also, with few exceptions, the leaders in each county. As expected, however, there are local differences in relative rank of the different specialties.

Psychiatry is in second place in Manhattan, just below internal medicine. It ranks third in Suffolk County, where there is a tremendous concentration of mental hospital beds, and also third in Westchester, where the proportion of psychiatrically oriented people who can afford such treatment is highest. In the remaining counties, as in the United States overall, psychiatry is in fifth or sixth place.

Pediatrics ranks relatively low in Manhattan, seventh among its specialty fields compared with fourth in most other areas, although on a population basis Manhattan still ranks higher than five other counties.

Internal medicine, the overall leader, ranks first in five counties, second in two, and fourth in Suffolk; general surgery is first in these latter three.

Obstetrics takes third or fourth place except for two counties—Suffolk, where it is second only to general surgery, and Westchester, where it is outranked by four specialty fields.

Ophthalmology and anesthesiology generally occupy ranks sixth or seventh within each county and orthopedic surgery is seventh or eighth except in Brooklyn and Queens, while otolaryngology, dermatology and urology are most frequently in ninth to twelfth place (Table 25).

TABLE 25.  Distribution of Specialists by Field of Practice, by Area

| SPECIALTY FIELD | Manhattan | Bronx | Brooklyn | Queens | Richmond | Nassau | Suffolk | Westchester |
|---|---|---|---|---|---|---|---|---|
| | % | % | % | % | % | % | % | % |
| Internal Medicine | 18.5 | 20.5 | 15.5 | 17.3 | 16.0 | 16.3 | 12.0 | 18.8 |
| General Surgery | 14.4 | 15.2 | 16.8 | 13.3 | 17.5 | 11.5 | 14.1 | 12.3 |
| Obstetrics and Gynecology | 8.4 | 8.7 | 12.0 | 12.1 | 13.8 | 11.0 | 13.2 | 8.2 |
| Psychiatry | 15.8 | 6.0 | 7.5 | 7.3 | 6.9 | 9.7 | 12.3 | 10.8 |
| Pediatrics | 3.8 | 8.6 | 9.0 | 10.2 | 8.5 | 10.6 | 7.3 | 8.8 |
| Ophthalmology | 5.6 | 3.9 | 5.9 | 5.7 | 4.3 | 6.4 | 6.0 | 5.9 |
| Anesthesiology | 3.3 | 4.7 | 4.9 | 7.4 | 5.8 | 5.3 | 7.3 | 6.5 |
| Orthopedic Surgery | 3.8 | 4.3 | 3.0 | 3.2 | 4.3 | 5.1 | 5.0 | 4.7 |
| Otolaryngology | 4.4 | 3.0 | 3.9 | 3.4 | 3.7 | 4.3 | 3.6 | 4.1 |
| Radiology | 2.7 | 4.0 | 3.2 | 5.1 | 2.1 | 4.2 | 4.4 | 4.6 |
| Dermatology | 3.8 | 3.2 | 2.8 | 3.6 | 2.7 | 3.9 | 2.1 | 2.9 |
| Urology | 3.3 | 2.5 | 2.7 | 2.4 | 3.7 | 2.2 | 3.2 | 2.4 |
| Other Specialties | 12.2 | 15.4 | 12.8 | 9.0 | 10.7 | 9.5 | 9.5 | 10.0 |
| TOTAL | 100.0 | 100.0 | 100.0 | 100.0 | 100.0 | 100.0 | 100.0 | 100.0 |

TABLE 26. Inter-County Rank, Ratio of Specialists to Population

| SPECIALTY FIELD | Manhattan | Westchester | Nassau | Brooklyn | Queens | Richmond | Suffolk | Bronx |
|---|---|---|---|---|---|---|---|---|
| | | | | | AREA | | | |
| Internal Medicine | 1 | 2 | 3 | 5-6 | 5-6 | 7 | 8 | 4 |
| General Surgery | 1 | 2 | 4-5 | 3 | 6-7-8 | 4-5 | 6-7-8 | 6-7-8 |
| Psychiatry | 1 | 2 | 3 | 5 | 6 | 7 | 4 | 8 |
| Obstetrics-Gynecology | 1 | 3 | 2 | 5 | 6-7 | 4 | 6-7 | 8 |
| Pediatrics | 3 | 2 | 1 | 5 | 4 | 6 | 8 | 7 |
| Ophthalmology | 1 | 2 | 3 | 4 | 6 | 7 | 8 | 8 |
| Anesthesiology | 1 | 2 | 3 | 7 | 4 | 6 | 5 | 8 |
| Otolaryngology | 1 | 2 | 3 | 4 | 7 | 5 | 6 | 8 |
| Orthopedic Surgery | 1 | 2 | 3 | 7 | 8 | 5 | 4 | 8 |
| Radiology | 1 | 2 | 3 | 7 | 4 | 8 | 5 | 6 |
| Dermatology | 1 | 3 | 2 | 5 | 4 | 7 | 8 | 6 |
| Urology | 1 | 2 | 4 | 6 | 7 | 3 | 5 | 8 |

On an inter-county basis, when specialists are related to population, Manhattan leads in all fields except pediatrics, where Westchester and Nassau have slightly higher ratios of physicians to population. This is not surprising since Manhattan has a lower proportion of children than the suburban areas. But in the other five counties which also have more children than Manhattan, the ratio of pediatricians is lower.

Of the other eleven leading fields of specialty practice, Westchester occupies second rank in nine fields and third rank in two (obstetrics and dermatology) with respect to specialist-population ratios, while Nassau is second in these two fields and third in seven others. Bronx County is at or next to the bottom in eight of the twelve fields. Suffolk shares this distinction in five fields (Table 26).

## Physician-Population Ratios

The range in actual numbers of population per specialist is of course broad both within each area, by type of specialist, and within each specialty from one area to the next. For internal medicine and general surgery, the population per specialist is around 10,000 or below, in most areas. In the more specialized fields, the ratio rises, for example, to an average of 31,500 persons per urologist, overall, and 63,500 in Bronx County (Table 27).

In Table 28, the ratios are reversed and stated in terms of number of physicians of each type per 100,000 population.

It is curious that despite the wide range in general practitioner ratios, from 148 in Manhattan to 55 in Suffolk, per 100,000 population, five of the eight counties seem to have found a "normal" level within a much smaller range, varying only between 81 and 87.5 general practitioners per 100,000 population in Bronx, Brooklyn, Queens, Nassau and Westchester. In these same five counties, on the other hand, the range in specialist ratios is much greater—from 64 specialists in Bronx to 128 in Westchester.

## TABLE 27. Population Per Practicing Specialist: 12 Leading Specialty Fields, by County

| | Internal Medicine | General Surgery | Psychiatry | Obstetrics-Gynecology | Pediatrics | Ophthalmology | Anesthesiology | Otolaryngology | Orthopedic Surgery | Radiology | Dermatology | Urology |
|---|---|---|---|---|---|---|---|---|---|---|---|---|
| 8-COUNTY AREA | 5,000 | 6,000 | 8,000 | 9,000 | 12,000 | 15,500 | 18,000 | 22,000 | 22,000 | 25,000 | 26,500 | 31,500 |
| Manhattan | 2,000 | 2,500 | 2,500 | 4,500 | 9,500 | 6,500 | 11,500 | 8,500 | 9,500 | 13,500 | 10,000 | 11,500 |
| Westchester | 4,000 | 6,500 | 7,000 | 9,500 | 9,000 | 13,000 | 12,000 | 19,000 | 16,500 | 17,000 | 27,000 | 33,000 |
| Nassau | 5,500 | 8,000 | 9,500 | 8,000 | 8,500 | 14,000 | 17,000 | 21,000 | 17,500 | 21,500 | 23,500 | 41,500 |
| Brooklyn | 8,000 | 7,500 | 16,500 | 10,500 | 14,000 | 21,500 | 25,500 | 32,000 | 41,500 | 39,500 | 44,500 | 45,500 |
| Queens | 8,000 | 10,000 | 18,500 | 11,000 | 13,500 | 24,000 | 18,500 | 40,000 | 42,500 | 27,000 | 37,500 | 56,000 |
| Richmond | 8,500 | 8,000 | 20,000 | 10,000 | 16,500 | 32,500 | 23,500 | 37,000 | 32,500 | 65,000 | 52,000 | 37,000 |
| Suffolk | 12,000 | 10,000 | 11,500 | 11,000 | 19,500 | 23,500 | 19,500 | 39,000 | 28,500 | 32,500 | 67,000 | 44,500 |
| Bronx | 7,500 | 10,000 | 26,000 | 18,000 | 18,000 | 39,500 | 33,000 | 52,000 | 36,500 | 38,500 | 48,500 | 63,500 |

## TABLE 28. Number of Physicians Per 100,000 Population, by Type and Specialty Field of Practice, by Area

| TYPE AND FIELD OF PRACTICE | Total All Areas | Manhattan | Bronx | Brooklyn | Queens | Richmond | Nassau | Suffolk | Westchester |
|---|---|---|---|---|---|---|---|---|---|
| POPULATION * | 11,248 | 1,725 | 1,460 | 2,640 | 1,955 | 260 | 1,410 | 938 | 860 |
| *Specialty Field* | | | | | | | | | |
| Internal Medicine | 19.6 | 50.1 | 13.2 | 12.4 | 12.7 | 11.5 | 18.0 | 8.4 | 24.0 |
| General Surgery | 16.0 | 39.0 | 9.8 | 13.5 | 9.8 | 12.7 | 12.8 | 9.9 | 15.7 |
| Obstetrics and Gynecology | 11.4 | 22.7 | 5.6 | 9.6 | 9.0 | 10.0 | 12.2 | 9.3 | 10.5 |
| Psychiatry | 12.7 | 43.0 | 3.9 | 6.0 | 5.4 | 5.0 | 10.8 | 8.7 | 13.8 |
| Pediatrics | 8.2 | 10.4 | 5.6 | 7.2 | 7.5 | 6.1 | 11.7 | 5.1 | 11.2 |
| Ophthalmology | 6.4 | 15.2 | 2.5 | 4.7 | 4.2 | 3.1 | 7.0 | 4.3 | 7.6 |
| Anesthesiology | 5.5 | 8.9 | 3.0 | 4.0 | 5.4 | 4.2 | 5.9 | 5.1 | 8.3 |
| Orthopedic Surgery | 4.5 | 10.3 | 2.8 | 2.4 | 2.4 | 3.1 | 5.7 | 3.5 | 6.1 |
| Otolaryngology | 4.5 | 12.0 | 1.9 | 3.1 | 2.5 | 2.7 | 4.7 | 2.6 | 5.2 |
| Radiology | 4.0 | 7.4 | 2.6 | 2.5 | 3.7 | 1.5 | 4.6 | 3.1 | 5.8 |
| Dermatology | 3.8 | 10.2 | 2.1 | 2.2 | 2.7 | 1.9 | 4.3 | 1.5 | 3.7 |
| Urology | 3.2 | 8.9 | 1.6 | 2.2 | 1.8 | 2.7 | 2.4 | 2.2 | 3.0 |
| Other Specialties | 12.9 | 33.0 | 9.8 | 10.3 | 6.6 | 7.8 | 10.5 | 6.7 | 12.7 |
| SUB-TOTAL ALL SPECIALTIES | 112.7 | 271.1 | 64.4 | 80.1 | 73.7 | 72.3 | 110.6 | 70.4 | 127.6 |
| GENERAL PRACTICE † | 91.2 | 147.6 | 81.0 | 84.2 | 85.7 | 61.9 | 84.9 | 55.1 | 87.5 |
| TOTAL | 203.9 | 418.7 | 145.4 | 164.3 | 159.4 | 134.2 | 195.5 | 125.5 | 215.1 |

* 1966 estimated population, in thousands.
† Includes M.D.'s and D.O.'s.

## Hospital Staff Appointments

It has frequently been stated that the interests of good quality care demand a hospital staff appointment for every practicing physician. It is also generally acknowledged that a significant proportion of New York's practicing physicians have no such appointments. The extent of the exclusion has not been pinpointed, however, and inasmuch as this was regarded as a matter of importance, GHI's planning of physicians' individual records provided for entries indicating the highest-ranking hospital, if any, at which each physician held an appointment.

Since then, the situation has been complicated by the changing organization of municipal hospitals in New York City. Many physicians formerly donating their services at these institutions resigned or were released when voluntary hospitals assumed control. The extent to which such displacements occurred and the proportion of these which represented the only hospital connection of the physicians involved, are not reflected in the figures shown here. The same applies to possible displacements from voluntary hospitals resulting from the drive toward full-time salaried staff physicians. In short, the proportion with appointments may be even lower than that shown.

In recording highest hospital-staff status of physicians, hospitals were ranked according to type of sponsorship (voluntary vs. municipal or county) and extent of medical training facilities (affiliated with medical school, approved for training residents or interns, other). Proprietary hospitals were excluded. Only one appointment, at his highest-ranking hospital, was entered for each physician, and his particular rank at that hospital was not considered at all.

Survey findings for the eight-county New York metropolitan area are summarized in Table 29.

Four of the eight counties, including three of the five counties of New York City, showed fewer than half their physicians as having voluntary hospital staff appointments.

Aside from Manhattan, physicians in outlying areas—Rich-

TABLE 29.  Hospital Appointment Status, Physicians in Eight-County Area *

| COUNTY | PER CENT WITH NO APPOINT-MENT † | PER CENT WITH NO VOLUNTARY HOSPITAL APPOINT-MENT | PER CENT WITH APPOINTMENT | | | | | At Government Hospital ‖ |
|---|---|---|---|---|---|---|---|---|
| | | | Total | AT VOLUNTARY HOSPITAL | | | | |
| | | | | Total | Affiliated ‡ | Approved § | Other | |
| All | 38.9 | 53.1 | 61.1 | 46.9 | 19.8 | 20.9 | 6.2 | 14.2 |
| Manhattan | 36.3 | 47.4 | 63.7 | 52.6 | 31.5 | 19.3 | 1.8 | 11.1 |
| Bronx | 40.4 | 63.5 | 59.6 | 36.5 | 12.8 | 22.3 | 1.4 | 23.1 |
| Brooklyn | 36.1 | 52.3 | 63.9 | 47.7 | 26.8 | 12.7 | 8.2 | 16.2 |
| Queens | 43.3 | 60.7 | 56.7 | 39.3 | 8.4 | 26.2 | 4.7 | 17.4 |
| Richmond | 37.8 | 42.2 | 62.2 | 57.8 | 9.1 | 36.1 | 12.6 | 4.4 |
| Nassau | 43.7 | 60.8 | 56.3 | 39.2 | 12.1 | 23.1 | 4.0 | 17.1 |
| Suffolk | 44.1 | 49.1 | 55.9 | 50.9 | 4.0 | 6.2 | 40.7 | 5.0 |
| Westchester | 36.0 | 45.6 | 64.0 | 54.4 | 9.1 | 38.8 | 6.5 | 9.6 |

* Each physician counted once, at highest status hospital.
† Excluding proprietary hospitals.
‡ Affiliated with medical school.
§ Approved for resident or intern training.
‖ Municipal or County.

86

mond, Suffolk, Westchester—were shown as the likeliest holders of voluntary staff appointments.

With municipal and county hospitals included, the inter-county range in total proportion of physicians with some appointments was relatively small, from 56 to 64 per cent. This indicates that where the practical possibilities of voluntary hospital appointments are lowest, the proportion joining municipal or county staffs had been high enough in every county to bring the total participation level to around the three-out-of-five eight-county average.

A corollary interpretation might infer a fairly constant ratio of two out of five in each area as representing those unconcerned with hospital status, or at least not concerned enough to work gratis in government institutions.

In the area as a whole, one out of five physicians was listed with an appointment at a medical-school-affiliated voluntary hospital. This overall figure, however, is heavily influenced by highly atypical Manhattan, nearly a third of whose physicians were listed with such appointments. In four counties—Suffolk, Westchester, Richmond, Queens—the proportion was lower than one out of ten.

The three counties shown as having the lowest proportions (i.e. under 40 per cent) of their physicians on any voluntary staff—Bronx, Queens, Nassau—also have extremely low voluntary bed-to-population ratios. The counties shown as having highest proportions of their physicians on voluntary staffs —Richmond, Westchester, Manhattan—have the highest bed ratios. Suffolk County is the exception to this pattern, showing 51 per cent of its physicians with voluntary hospital appointments despite a low voluntary bed ratio; the explanation here probably is connected with the relatively low ratio of physicians to population, which would of itself create openings for a higher proportion on hospital staffs, and with a relatively favorable attitude in the medical community toward hospital capabilities of family physicians.

On the general question of physician hospital appointments and their relationship to bed facilities, it may be pertinent that the voluntary bed-facility situation in much of the eight-county area discussed here is well below national averages. While the question of optimum bed ratios is always avoided in published reports, inadequacies in some areas can be inferred by inspection of comparative data. In the case of New York City, the inclusion of municipal beds in estimates of adequacy of resources confuses the issue for a number of reasons—the admitted obsolescence of many municipal facilities, the substantial proportion of beds accounted for by municipal facilities, and the fact that municipal beds cannot be used by physicians to hospitalize their private patients. On many occasions physicians, including those with appointments at voluntary hospitals, cannot find beds for patients in need of hospitalization. The situation in shortage areas has become more acute with the advent of Medicare and Medicaid.

In addition to the shortage of satisfactory facilities, the trend toward full-time salaried staffs further depresses the number of staff appointment opportunities for physicians practicing in the community.

Unless the lag in community efforts to offset these factors can be corrected by means of a bold new approach, it would appear that the objective of universal appointments is not likely of realization soon.

# UTILIZATION STUDIES: PHYSICIAN AND LABORATORY SERVICES

Chapter 5

# GENERAL PATTERNS OF
# MEDICAL SERVICE USE

## How Many Used Their Medical Insurance?

### Comprehensive vs. Limited Plan Membership

The great majority of subscribers with comprehensive coverage for the full year submitted at least one claim for themselves or their families, while over half of those with limited coverage received no benefits beyond the sense of security derived from possessing the insurance policy.

The general outline of this high-low pattern was of course anticipated, since the most frequent services to members with comprehensive coverage are outside the scope of the limited contract. There was no previous knowledge, however, of the exact form the pattern would assume.

The fact that the proportion of comprehensive contract holders filing claims reached 86 per cent reflects majority awareness of their coverage among all classes of members, leaving little room for conjecture as to possible sociological causes of non-use.

The proportion of an insured population which uses service during a given period of time can be expressed either in terms of family units, as above, to indicate subscriber awareness (and possibly to facilitate comparison with experience elsewhere); or in terms of persons, i.e. subscribers plus dependents, to permit detailed analysis of users-nonusers by age, sex, and other variables. The family (or contract holder) index of use will show proportionately fewer non-users, and more multiple users, than the person index: Any user in a family places that family in the user class, although there may be non-users covered by the same contract. Thus, 10 per cent of the individuals with comprehensive coverage, and 45 per cent of the family units, incurred at least seven claims; 80 per cent of the individuals and 86 per cent of the contract holders incurred one or more claims. Of those eligible only for limited coverage, 76 per cent of the individuals and 61 per cent of the family units incurred no claims (Table 30).

TABLE 30.   Proportion of Insured Population Incurring Indicated Number of Claims,* by Type of Coverage

| NUMBER OF CLAIMS INCURRED | COMPREHENSIVE COVERAGE | | LIMITED COVERAGE | |
|---|---|---|---|---|
| | *Persons* | *Contracts* | *Persons* | *Contracts* |
| | % | % | % | % |
| 0 | 19.8 | 13.6 | 76.4 | 60.5 |
| 1 | 26.6 | 10.0 | 15.5 | 19.5 |
| 2 | 15.6 | 7.6 | 4.7 | 10.2 |
| 3 | 10.9 | 7.2 | 1.9 | 4.9 |
| 4 | 7.6 | 6.2 | .6 | 2.1 |
| 5 | 5.3 | 5.5 | .3 | .8 |
| 6 | 3.8 | 4.9 | .1 | .4 |
| 7 or more | 10.4 | 45.0 | .5 | 1.6 |
| TOTAL | 100.0 | 100.0 | 100.0 | 100.0 |

* One claim may include any number of services.

The average number of claims per person eligible for comprehensive coverage was seven times the average under the limited contract—2.8 as against .4.

The comprehensive plan users of one or more services divide roughly into thirds—those with one claim, those with two or three claims, and those with four or more. Of the limited plan claimants, two thirds incurred only one claim (Table 31).

TABLE 31. Distribution of Individual Claimants,
by Number of Claims Incurred

| | INDIVIDUAL CLAIMANTS | |
|---|---|---|
| NUMBER OF CLAIMS | Comprehensive Coverage | Limited Coverage |
| | % | % |
| 1 | 33 | 66 |
| 2 or 3 | 33 | 28 |
| 4, 5, or 6 | 21 | 4 |
| 7 or more | 13 | 2 |
| 1 or more | 100 | 100 |

## Comprehensive Plan: Concentration of Claims and Claimants *

Despite the fact that 80 per cent of the individuals with comprehensive coverage used it, most of the claims were incurred by a minority of the membership.

Ten per cent of the eligible population accounted for nearly 40 per cent of the total number of claims incurred.

TABLE 32. Proportion of Membership Incurring
Specified Proportion of Claims

| CLAIMS PER MEMBER | Per Cent of Eligible Members | Accounting for | Per Cent of All Claims |
|---|---|---|---|
| 7 or more | 10.4 | | 38.5 |
| 6 or more | 14.2 | | 46.8 |
| 5 or more | 19.5 | | 56.4 |
| 4 or more | 27.1 | | 67.4 |
| 3 or more | 38.0 | | 79.2 |
| 2 or more | 53.6 | | 90.5 |
| 1 or more | 80.2 | | 100.0 |
| NONE | 19.8 | | 0.0 |

These are the people classified as having "7 or more" claims; actually they averaged 10.2 claims each for the year. Individuals filing four or more claims accounted for 27 per cent of the eligible population and 67 per cent of all claims incurred.

*From this point on, all data refer to comprehensive plan experience unless otherwise noted.

Table 32 provides a clear demonstration of the insurance principle in action.

As further experience accumulates and is retrieved for analysis, it is possible to determine the proportion of "high risk" individuals of different ages who remain in that category from year to year.

It cannot be inferred that the members with multiple claims are necessarily the same as those incurring the greatest expense, since it is theoretically possible to submit either a series of claims for relatively minor inexpensive services or one claim for a major service. Nevertheless, comparison of the two measurements indicates probable rough correlation between number of claims and claims dollars per member (Table 33).

TABLE 33.   Distribution of Membership (Persons), by Number and Amount of Claims Incurred

| CLAIMS EXPENDITURES PER MEMBER | | NUMBER OF CLAIMS PER MEMBER | |
|---|---|---|---|
| Range | Per Cent of Members Incurring | Range | Per Cent of Members Incurring |
| $ 0 | 19.8 | 0 | 19.8 |
| 1–24 | 42.3 | 1 or 2 | 42.2 |
| 25–99 | 27.2 | 3–6 | 27.6 |
| 100 and Over | 10.7 | 7 and Over | 10.4 |

# Who?

## (Users vs. Non-Users)

As previously stated, the high overall proportion of users in the eligible population indicates majority awareness of the coverage among all classes of subscribers. This was generally verified by further examination of the data for purposes of identifying non-users.

Non-users were of course found among all population segments. A composite of the person most likely to have been a non-user would call for a 45-year-old widowed professional man, living in New Jersey or Manhattan, with GHI membership since 1963!

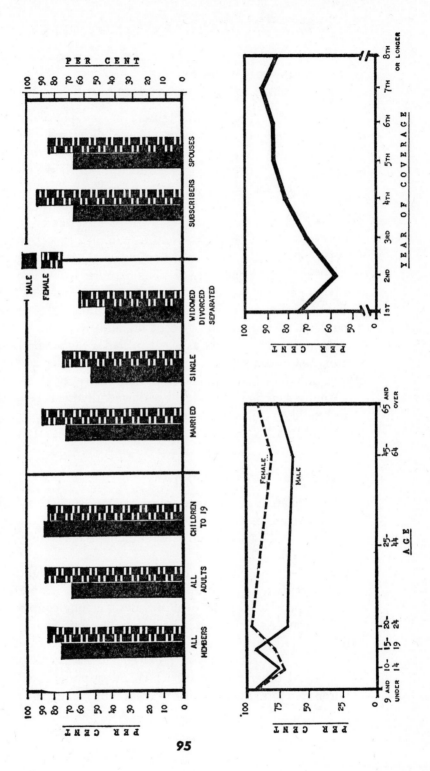

PROPORTION OF MEMBERS USING SERVICE
BY SEX, AGE, RELATIONSHIP,
MARITAL STATUS, AND YEAR OF ENROLLMENT

95

VARIATIONS IN USER RATES BY
AGE, SEX, MARITAL STATUS, RELATIONSHIP

The relative proportion of users in any population segment is not indicative of service volume, discussed elsewhere. Age groups past 45 had a lower proportion of users than those under 45 (except for those aged 10 to 14), but their volume of service was higher.

At all ages past 19, women were more likely to be users than men. This is true regardless of marital status or relationship to subscriber. During the entire span of their active working years, from 20 to 65, about two out of three men received at least one physician service. The pattern for women was nearly 50 per cent higher than for men at ages 20 to 24 (97 vs. 67 users per hundred eligibles), nearly a third higher from 25 through 44, and about 20 per cent higher after that.

Female policyholders as a group had a higher proportion of users than male subscribers and were also likelier users than other adult female segments except for those aged 20 to 24.

Unattached males (single, or widowed, divorced, separated) were less likely to use service than any other population segment (Table 34).

VARIATIONS BY SIZE OF FAMILY

The relatively low user rates among spouseless adults naturally recur in connection with analysis of variations by family size, to show a marked differential in usage by one-person families (Table 35).

Families with one, two or three children had highest user rates. After that, i.e. with four or more children, proportion of users dropped back to the level prevailing among couples without children. (As shown elsewhere, families with four or more children also used less service per capita, whereas families of two, once they became users, received more services per person than all other size families.) Whether parents with four children find less time to visit physicians, or feel expert enough

TABLE 34.  Proportion of Members Incurring One or More Claims, by Sex, Age, Relationship, and Marital Status

| MEMBER CATEGORY | USERS PER 100 ELIGIBLE MEMBERS | | |
| --- | --- | --- | --- |
| | *Total* | *Males* | *Females* |
| All Members | 80 | 75 | 85 |
| *Age* | | | |
| 9 and Under | 93 | 93 | 93 |
| 10–14 | 75 | 76 | 73 |
| 15–19 | 87 | 94 | 80 |
| 20–24 | 86 | 67 | 97 |
| 25–44 | 78 | 67 | 88 |
| 45–64 | 73 | 66 | 81 |
| 65 and Over | 80 | 75 | 90 |
| *Marital Status* | | | |
| All Adults | 77 | 68 | 86 |
| Married | 79 | 71 | 88 |
| Single | 60 | 52 | 73 |
| Widowed, Divorced, Separated | 56 | 46 | 63 |
| *Relationship* | | | |
| Subscribers | 72 | 68 | 93 |
| Spouses | 83 | 68 | 85 |
| Children to 19 | 85 | 87 | 84 |

to handle situations formerly requiring outside help, are two of many possible hypotheses for the explanation of family patterns.

AREA VARIATIONS

The proportion of users in most areas varied only within a small range, from 82 to 88 per cent. Chief exceptions were Manhattan and New Jersey, each showing only 67 per cent of their resident members using some service (Table 35). The explanation for Manhattan is related to its comparatively large spouseless population, which as shown above generally had fewer users. No explanation comes to mind for the low user rate in New Jersey.

When New Jersey is excluded from the total, the proportion of users rises slightly, from 80 to 82 per cent, for the eight-county metropolitan and other New York areas.

There is no indication within the metropolitan area of any relationship between availability of physicians and proportion of users in each county.

OCCUPATION CLASS VARIATIONS

Among the families of subscribers in blue-collar occupations, the proportion of users was close to average—79 per cent. This is slightly lower than the experience of the white-collar groups combined and slightly higher than that of the professional group.

Whatever social significance may be ascribed to the occupational pattern of users-nonusers thus derives from negative findings: the similarities of usage rates among most classes apparently demonstrate the neutralizing effect of medical insurance on class differences, with respect to seeking medical care from private physicians.

VARIATIONS BY DURATION OF MEDICAL INSURANCE COVERAGE

Except for the earliest and latest enrollees, duration of coverage appeared to be associated with use of service: the longer they had been insured, the higher the rate at which members became claimants in the course of the year (Table 35).

Among those for whom the study period represented their initial year of exposure, three of four enrollees incurred claims. For those in their second year, the proportion of users was 58 per cent. It jumped to 71 per cent in the third year, 82 per cent in the fourth, 88 per cent in the fifth and sixth, and reached 94 per cent in the seventh year before dropping back to 87 per cent among those enrolled over seven years.

The pattern of increasing proportions of users as coverage continued requires further investigation to determine how much of the increase occurred independently of the age distribution of each year's enrollees.

TABLE 35. Proportion of Members Incurring One or More
Claims, by Family Size, Subscriber Occupation Class,
Area of Residence, Duration of Enrollment

| MEMBER CATEGORY | Users Per 100 Eligible Members |
|---|---|
| *Family Size* | |
| 1 | 60 |
| 2 | 76 |
| 3 | 86 |
| 4 | 88 |
| 5 | 81 |
| 6 or more | 75 |
| | |
| *Subscriber Occupation Class* * | |
| Professional | 75 |
| Executive | 81 |
| Sales | 89 |
| Clerical and White-Collar Unspecified | 82 |
| Blue-Collar | 79 |
| | |
| *Area of Residence* | |
| Manhattan | 67 |
| Bronx | 79 |
| Brooklyn | 83 |
| Queens | 84 |
| Richmond | 87 |
| Nassau | 83 |
| Suffolk | 88 |
| Westchester | 86 |
| Other New York | 82 |
| New Jersey | 67 |
| | |
| *Year of Coverage* | |
| 1st | 75 |
| 2nd | 58 |
| 3rd | 71 |
| 4th | 82 |
| 5th | 88 |
| 6th | 88 |
| 7th | 94 |
| 8th or longer | 87 |

* Including dependents.

## Where?

The emphasis in medical care research and medical insurance, as well as in the training of physicians, is almost universally on hospitalized illness.

One of the purposes of the present report is to document the importance of the neglected sector of service, ambulatory care, to all segments of the population. In this section, the broad topic of service locale is introduced by showing the distribution of GHI-insured services as between office, home, and hospital.

The overall division of services received under the comprehensive plan was as follows:

| | |
|---|---|
| Office Services | 72.8 per cent |
| Home Visits | 11.9 per cent |
| Total Out-of-Hospital | 84.7 per cent |
| Hospital Visits | 15.3 per cent |
| Total | 100.0 per cent |

The proportion of out-of-hospital care would be even larger if hospital services were counted in terms of admissions (as they are generally billed) instead of visits.

### Variations Among Population Subgroups

Hospital service was more important to some population segments than others, but never accounted for more than 31 per cent of all services to any segment.

The greatest variations were associated with age, especially among males, for whom the proportion of hospital service rose steadily, from 9 per cent before age 19, to 12 per cent at ages 20 to 34, to 16 per cent at ages 35 to 54, to 22 per cent at ages 55 to 64, to 27 per cent at 65-plus. The age pattern for women contrasted markedly, with hospital services accounting for 18 to 21 per cent of total services at all ages past 19 (Table 36).

TABLE 36. Distribution of Insured Services
by Place Rendered, by Age and Sex

| MEMBER CATEGORY | TOTAL | HOSPITAL | OUT-OF-HOSPITAL | | |
| | | | TOTAL | *Office* | *Home* |
| --- | --- | --- | --- | --- | --- |
| | % | % | % | % | % |
| All Persons | 100 | 15.3 | 84.7 | 72.8 | 11.9 |
| Male | 100 | 14.6 | 85.4 | 73.3 | 12.1 |
| Female | 100 | 15.8 | 84.2 | 72.4 | 11.8 |
| 19 and Under | 100 | 8.1 | 91.9 | 70.6 | 21.3 |
| Male | 100 | 8.7 | 91.3 | 70.9 | 20.4 |
| Female | 100 | 7.5 | 92.5 | 70.3 | 22.2 |
| 20–34 | 100 | 18.0 | 82.0 | 74.6 | 7.4 |
| Male | 100 | 11.8 | 88.2 | 79.0 | 9.2 |
| Female | 100 | 20.2 | 79.8 | 73.0 | 6.8 |
| 35–54 | 100 | 17.0 | 83.0 | 74.9 | 8.1 |
| Male | 100 | 16.0 | 84.0 | 76.6 | 7.4 |
| Female | 100 | 17.7 | 82.3 | 73.7 | 8.6 |
| 55–64 | 100 | 20.6 | 79.4 | 70.9 | 8.5 |
| Male | 100 | 22.1 | 77.9 | 71.1 | 6.8 |
| Female | 100 | 18.7 | 81.3 | 70.8 | 10.5 |
| 65 and Over | 100 | 25.0 | 75.0 | 68.1 | 6.9 |
| Male | 100 | 27.4 | 72.6 | 65.8 | 6.8 |
| Female | 100 | 20.9 | 79.1 | 72.1 | 7.0 |
| All Adults | 100 | 18.3 | 81.7 | 73.7 | 8.0 |
| Male | 100 | 17.8 | 82.2 | 74.7 | 7.5 |
| Female | 100 | 18.6 | 81.4 | 73.1 | 8.3 |

As expected, the proportion of services accounted for by
home visits also varied markedly by age—8 per cent for adults,
21 per cent for children; within adult age categories, however,
differences were relatively minor.

Spouses of female subscribers, as well as males who were
widowed, divorced or separated, showed a much higher-than-
average proportion of hospital service, 28 to 31 per cent, as
compared with the overall male adult figure of 18 per cent
(Table 37).

TABLE 37.   Distribution of Insured Services by Place
Rendered, by Marital Status and Relationship
to Subscriber

| ADULT MEMBER CATEGORY | TOTAL | HOSPITAL | OUT-OF-HOSPITAL | | |
|---|---|---|---|---|---|
| | | | TOTAL | *Office* | *Home* |
| | % | % | % | % | % |
| Subscribers (Policyholders) | 100 | 16.6 | 83.4 | 76.0 | 7.4 |
| Male | 100 | 16.8 | 83.2 | 75.8 | 7.4 |
| Female | 100 | 15.8 | 84.2 | 76.8 | 7.4 |
| Spouses of Policyholders | 100 | 19.8 | 80.2 | 71.7 | 8.5 |
| Male | 100 | 30.8 | 69.2 | 60.6 | 8.6 |
| Female | 100 | 19.8 | 80.2 | 71.7 | 8.5 |
| Married Adults | 100 | 18.4 | 81.6 | 73.5 | 8.1 |
| Male | 100 | 17.7 | 82.3 | 74.6 | 7.7 |
| Female | 100 | 18.9 | 81.1 | 72.8 | 8.3 |
| Single Adults | 100 | 16.2 | 83.8 | 76.7 | 7.1 |
| Male | 100 | 16.3 | 83.7 | 77.9 | 5.8 |
| Female | 100 | 16.1 | 83.9 | 75.6 | 8.3 |
| Widowed, Divorced, Separated Adults | 100 | 19.8 | 80.2 | 72.4 | 7.8 |
| Male | 100 | 27.7 | 72.3 | 66.8 | 5.5 |
| Female | 100 | 15.4 | 84.6 | 75.6 | 9.0 |

Except for the retired, no relationship was shown between
occupation class and proportion of services rendered at the
hospital. There was some variation within white-collar categories, but none between white-collar and blue-collar (Table
38). Similarly, duration of enrollment was not a factor.

Variations of interest were observed in some geographic
areas. Within the eight-county New York metropolitan area,
two counties showed significantly higher proportions of services rendered in hospitals (Table 39). These two counties, Richmond and Westchester, also have far more private general beds
in relation to population than the other counties (excluding
Manhattan). The relationship between hospital utilization and
facilities is discussed in greater detail elsewhere. (See Chapter 18.)

TABLE 38.  Distribution of Insured Services by Place
Rendered, by Subscriber Occupation Class

| SUBSCRIBER OCCUPATION CLASS * | TOTAL | HOSPITAL | OUT-OF-HOSPITAL | | |
|---|---|---|---|---|---|
| | | | TOTAL | *Office* | *Home* |
| | % | % | % | % | % |
| Professional | 100 | 12.5 | 87.5 | 77.1 | 10.4 |
| Executive | 100 | 15.7 | 84.3 | 72.7 | 11.6 |
| Sales | 100 | 10.6 | 89.4 | 78.2 | 11.2 |
| Clerical and White-Collar Unspecified | 100 | 15.5 | 84.5 | 74.4 | 10.1 |
| All White-Collar | 100 | 15.0 | 85.0 | 74.7 | 10.3 |
| Blue-Collar | 100 | 15.0 | 85.0 | 72.0 | 13.0 |
| Student | 100 | 5.1 | 94.9 | 91.1 | 3.8 |
| Retired | 100 | 26.8 | 73.2 | 62.8 | 10.4 |

* Including dependents.

The area variation in per cent of services at the patient's home is also noteworthy. Despite the fact that children showed a much higher proportion of home calls than adults, areas with the highest proportion of children—Nassau and Suffolk—showed low proportions of home calls. This topic will be explored further in discussion of utilization rates for different services.

TABLE 39.  Distribution of Insured Services by Place
Rendered, by Subscriber Residence Area

| SUBSCRIBER RESIDENCE AREA | TOTAL | HOSPITAL | OUT-OF-HOSPITAL | | |
|---|---|---|---|---|---|
| | | | TOTAL | *Office* | *Home* |
| | % | % | % | % | % |
| Manhattan | 100 | 15.5 | 84.5 | 74.9 | 9.6 |
| Bronx | 100 | 14.7 | 85.3 | 71.8 | 13.5 |
| Brooklyn | 100 | 13.2 | 86.8 | 69.5 | 17.3 |
| Queens | 100 | 14.4 | 85.6 | 73.3 | 12.3 |
| Richmond | 100 | 22.6 | 77.4 | 60.4 | 17.0 |
| Nassau | 100 | 13.1 | 86.9 | 77.3 | 9.6 |
| Suffolk | 100 | 13.3 | 86.7 | 79.5 | 7.2 |
| Westchester | 100 | 20.7 | 79.3 | 69.1 | 10.2 |
| New Jersey | 100 | 19.0 | 81.0 | 71.9 | 9.1 |

## For What Types of Service?

The simplest form of utilization index refers to proportion of a given population using the different types of services, as contrasted with indices showing volume of services rendered.

With all indices, the analyst may employ either or both of two population bases as denominators in calculating use rates: total number of members eligible for service; and total number of users, or patients. Thus for the present type of index it is possible to study how many of a given population cohort had, say, ambulatory diagnostic x-rays in the course of a year; or alternatively, how many of those who saw a doctor were x-rayed. (The latter type of index has the further advantage of offering comparability with other data based only on patient populations, e.g. studies of physicians' practices, which cannot consider the population at risk.) The two ratios are given in Table 40 for various types of services.

TABLE 40.   Proportions of Eligible Population and Patient Population Using Various Types of Service

| TYPE OF SERVICE | Eligible Population | Patient Population |
|---|---|---|
| | % | % |
| Any Service | 80.2 | 100.0 |
| Office Service, General | 78.9 | 98.4 |
| Home Call | 27.8 | 34.7 |
| Hospital Care | 9.7 | 12.1 |
| Preventive Service | 14.1 | 17.6 |
| Out-of-Hospital Diagnostic Aids: | | |
|    Consultations | 6.8 | 8.5 |
|    X-rays | 13.3 | 16.6 |
|    Laboratory Tests | 16.5 | 20.6 |

When similar ratios are calculated for each segment of the population significant variations appear, particularly with respect to diagnostic services. Apart from the expected differences between adults and children, there were noteworthy differences among geographic subdivisions and among occupational groups (Table 41) which illustrate how quantitative

TABLE 41. Proportion of All Patients in Selected Categories Using Indicated Type of Service

| | NUMBER RECEIVING SPECIFIED TYPE OF SERVICE, PER 1000 PATIENTS | | | | | |
|---|---|---|---|---|---|---|
| | OUT-OF-HOSPITAL SERVICES | | | | | |
| PATIENT CATEGORY | Diagnostic X-ray | Laboratory Test | Consul- tation | Preventive Service | Home Call | Hospital Admission |
| ALL CATEGORIES | 166 | 206 | 85 | 176 | 347 | 121 |
| Age | | | | | | |
| 4 and Under | 50 | 80 | 57 | 472 | 512 | 83 |
| 5–14 | 86 | 116 | 65 | 300 | 447 | 68 |
| 15–24 | 148 | 163 | 75 | 169 | 278 | 110 |
| 25–44 | 199 | 252 | 88 | 73 | 283 | 163 |
| 45–64 | 263 | 278 | 115 | 45 | 263 | 140 |
| 65 and Over | 261 | 324 | 114 | 34 | 291 | 182 |
| Residents of: | | | | | | |
| Manhattan | 208 | 251 | 104 | 110 | 297 | 119 |
| Bronx | 178 | 202 | 99 | 127 | 404 | 120 |
| Brooklyn | 167 | 197 | 89 | 133 | 464 | 105 |
| Queens | 175 | 217 | 100 | 167 | 370 | 115 |
| Richmond | 133 | 147 | 80 | 147 | 398 | 140 |
| Nassau | 180 | 233 | 88 | 252 | 307 | 115 |
| Suffolk | 142 | 187 | 94 | 233 | 235 | 123 |
| Westchester | 163 | 236 | 53 | 243 | 317 | 152 |
| New Jersey | 158 | 190 | 40 | 180 | 286 | 140 |
| Subscriber Occupation Class * | | | | | | |
| Professional | 219 | 286 | 123 | 201 | 306 | 106 |
| Executive | 198 | 279 | 112 | 181 | 333 | 113 |
| Sales | 227 | 284 | 165 | 219 | 328 | 98 |
| Clerical and White-Collar Unspecified | 142 | 193 | 84 | 207 | 297 | 124 |
| Blue-Collar | 171 | 201 | 77 | 157 | 376 | 119 |

* Including dependents.

measurements can suggest paths to studies with qualitative connotations.

For example, the membership residing in Manhattan had fewer users, proportionately, than the membership of other areas; but of those who were users, the proportion having out-of-hospital consultations and diagnostic procedures was higher than in any other area. After further investigation, such usage might prove to be associated with some now-submerged artifact of the Manhattan situation; on the other hand, the elusive question of quality might explain some of the differences.

The variations in usage illustrated in Table 41 raise many questions for possible further investigation.

Why was the proportion of patients x-rayed in Manhattan 25 per cent higher than average, and over 50 per cent higher than in Richmond? Perhaps in Richmond, with its high hospitalization rate, more x-rays are done in the hospital. But Westchester, with an even higher proportion of hospitalized patients, was about average on out-of-hospital x-rayed patients. The same general type of question would apply to relative use of laboratory tests.

Why did Suffolk, with the highest proportion of children, have the lowest proportion of patients receiving home calls? Why was Brooklyn so high on this item, with double the proportion shown for Suffolk? Why did professional and sales categories show a 50 per cent higher ratio of x-ray users than patients from the clerical category? Why was the proportion of blue-collar patients having consultations and preventive services so much lower, and why were they highest on proportion receiving home visits?

To some of such questions, the answers may lie in further cross-tabulations of data already available, while others would involve obtaining additional information. This is the expected pattern for medical insurance data.

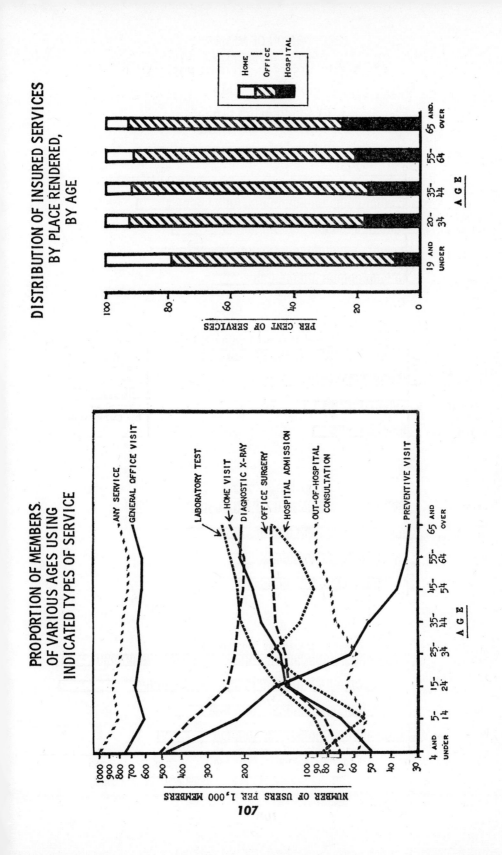

DISTRIBUTION OF INSURED SERVICES
BY PLACE RENDERED,
BY AGE

PROPORTION OF MEMBERS
OF VARIOUS AGES USING
INDICATED TYPES OF SERVICE

107

# PROPORTION OF MEMBERS
## AND PATIENTS USING
## PREVENTIVE VISITS AND OUT-OF-HOSPITAL
## DIAGNOSTIC TESTS

### BY OCCUPATION CLASS
·(Including Dependents)

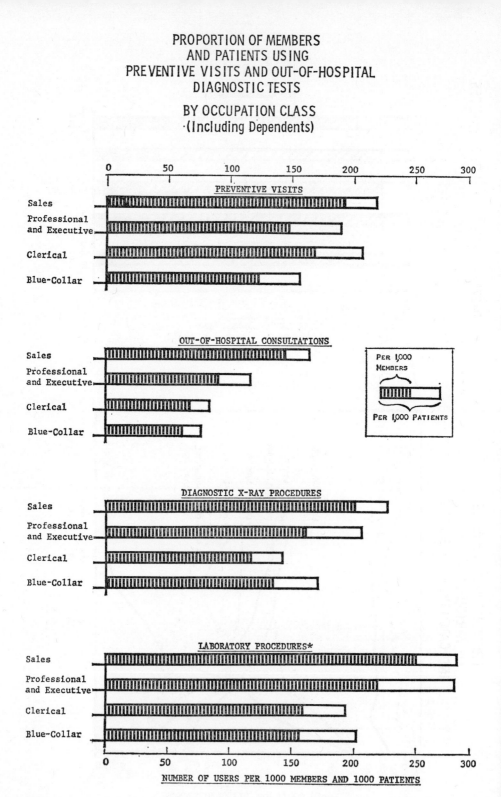

*EXCLUDES SIMPLE URINALYSIS AND HEMOGLOBIN TESTS.

# PROPORTIONS OF MEMBERS AND PATIENTS USING PREVENTIVE VISITS AND OUT-OF-HOSPITAL DIAGNOSTIC TESTS

## By Area of Residence

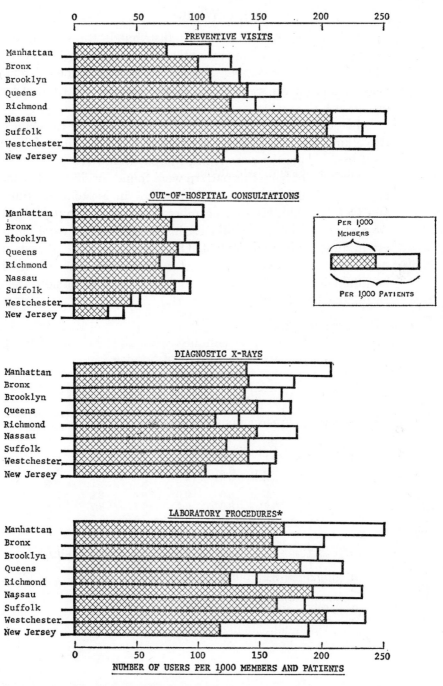

*EXCLUDING SIMPLE URINALYSIS AND HEMOGLOBIN TESTS.

## When?

Volume of service was well distributed throughout the year, except for the summer months of July and August and the Christmas lull in December. The first six months of the calendar year accounted for 53 per cent of the volume, distributed by first month of service (Table 42).

January was the top month; with 9.3 per cent of the claims, its volume was at a level 37 per cent higher than that of July. Next busiest months were April, March, October.

Departures from this pattern were found for different types of service. Preventive care was heaviest in September, June, and October, lightest in December. December through April were relatively heavy months for home calls, which were lightest in June, July and August. Office surgery was highest in April, May and November, lowest in December. The timing of hospital admissions varied according to type of admission. (See Hospitalization Studies, Chapter 18.)

TABLE 42. Distribution of Volume of Principal Services Classified by First Month of Service

| | All Services | Office Visits | Home Visits | Preventive Visits | Surgery | Diagnostic x-rays | Laboratory Tests | Consultations | Hospital Admissions |
|---|---|---|---|---|---|---|---|---|---|
| | | | | AMBULATORY CARE | | | | | |
| | % | % | % | % | % | % | % | % | % |
| January | 9.3 | 9.7 | 10.1 | 7.2 | 7.8 | 8.1 | 8.0 | 9.2 | 9.0 |
| February | 8.6 | 8.4 | 10.4 | 6.3 | 8.2 | 8.4 | 8.5 | 8.4 | 7.2 |
| March | 9.1 | 9.1 | 10.9 | 7.3 | 7.9 | 8.2 | 8.2 | 9.5 | 8.1 |
| April | 9.1 | 9.0 | 9.8 | 8.0 | 9.0 | 9.4 | 8.9 | 8.9 | 8.9 |
| May | 8.8 | 9.0 | 8.2 | 8.2 | 9.2 | 9.1 | 8.7 | 9.4 | 8.7 |
| June | 8.0 | 8.2 | 6.3 | 11.1 | 8.5 | 7.6 | 7.7 | 7.8 | 8.5 |
| July | 6.8 | 7.1 | 5.3 | 7.4 | 8.2 | 7.1 | 6.9 | 7.1 | 7.9 |
| August | 7.3 | 7.3 | 6.2 | 8.0 | 8.2 | 7.4 | 8.3 | 7.2 | 6.9 |
| September | 8.0 | 8.1 | 7.1 | 12.4 | 8.6 | 7.6 | 7.3 | 8.0 | 8.2 |
| October | 9.1 | 9.1 | 8.0 | 11.0 | 8.1 | 10.0 | 9.9 | 8.8 | 9.3 |
| November | 8.4 | 7.8 | 8.2 | 7.5 | 9.0 | 9.6 | 10.8 | 8.0 | 9.1 |
| December | 7.5 | 7.2 | 9.5 | 5.6 | 7.3 | 7.5 | 6.8 | 7.7 | 8.2 |
| TOTAL | 100.0 | 100.0 | 100.0 | 100.0 | 100.0 | 100.0 | 100.0 | 100.0 | 100.0 |

Chapter 6

# PATTERNS OF PHYSICIAN USE

## Operation of Free-Choice Principle

The sample population, narrowed to include only those protected for the full study year covered under the comprehensive "Family Doctor Plan," numbered some 42,600 persons. The working of the free-choice-of-physician principle is well illustrated by the number of physicians submitting claims for medical service rendered this relatively small population.

In the eight-county New York metropolitan area alone, the number of physicians serving one or more members of the sample at least once totaled 10,347. In addition, there were 2,856 physicians in this category with offices in other New York areas, in New Jersey, and in other states, bringing the grand total to 13,203 treating the study population—or nearly one treating physician to every three persons in the sample!

These physicians represented about two out of five physicians on GHI's register during the study year. The ratio of physicians used to physicians listed varied by area: In the eight-county New York metropolitan area, the range was from 30 per cent in Manhattan and 42 per cent in Westchester to 60.5 per cent in Suffolk, with the other five counties all past the 50 per cent level (Table 43).

TABLE 43. Per Cent of Listed Physicians Used
by Study Sample in One Year, by Area

| Area | Per Cent of Physicians Used |
|---|---|
| All Areas | 40.2 |
| 8-County New York Metropolitan Area | 47.3 |
| New York City | 45.5 |
|   Manhattan | 30.3 |
|   Bronx | 51.9 |
|   Brooklyn | 58.9 |
|   Queens | 56.3 |
|   Richmond | 55.2 |
| Nassau | 56.3 |
| Suffolk | 60.5 |
| Westchester | 41.9 |
| Other New York | 28.9 |
| New Jersey | 24.9 |
| Other | 8.2 |

The proportion of physicians used did not vary with type of practice: 40 per cent of general practitioners, 39 per cent of specialists were used by the sample population during the study year.

The average number of claims signed for members of the study sample by the 13,000 treating physicians was nine per

TABLE 44. Dispersion of Sample Patients, and Remuneration
for Their Services, Among Physicians

| Number of Patients from Sample Per Treating Physician | Per Cent of Treating Physicians | Dollars Received | Per Cent of Treating Physicians Receiving, for Services to Patients in Sample |
|---|---|---|---|
| 1 | 33.9 | Under 25 | 30.5 |
| 2 | 17.9 | 25–49 | 15.0 |
| 3–5 | 25.3 | 50–99 | 16.9 |
| 6–10 | 13.9 | 100–199 | 17.5 |
| 11–25 | 7.8 | 200–299 | 8.2 |
| 26 or more | 1.2 | 300–499 | 7.4 |
| | ——— | 500–999 | 4.0 |
| | 100.0 | 1000 or Over | .5 |
| | | | ——— |
| | | | 100.0 |

Average number of claims per physician for patients in sample: 9
Average dollars collected per physician for patients in sample: $131

physician, but for the majority the number was under five. Most physicians treated one, two, or three patients from the sample, and most collected under $100 for such services from GHI.

It should be clear that these figures cannot be used to estimate individual physicians' total patient load and income from GHI. They are principally indicative of the dispersion of patients and resources occurring under the free-choice system which permits a population of 40,000 to receive care without making much of a ripple in any segment of the medical community.

Another way of looking at the results of unlimited free choice offered at GHI is to examine the number of different physicians used per family or individual. It is perhaps as eloquent a commentary on today's medicine as has been revealed by any aspect of the present study, that half the families using any service used three or more different physicians during the study year. Only 27 per cent of the user families limited themselves to one physician, and one out of seven user families used six or more different physicians. These findings are apparently part of the modern pattern requiring different doctors for different family members; individuals were more likely to have had only one physician treating them. Even among individuals, however, a sizable minority, amounting to over 40 per cent of the individuals treated, went to more than one physician, and 18 per cent went to three or more (Table 45).

TABLE 45. Number of Different Physicians Used Per Family and Per Individual Using Any Physician

| Number of Physicians Used During Study Year | PER CENT OF USERS | |
|:---:|:---:|:---:|
| | Families | Individuals |
| 1 | 27.2 | 57.8 |
| 2 | 22.0 | 23.8 |
| 3 | 16.8 | 10.6 |
| 4 | 12.4 | 4.5 |
| 5 | 7.8 | 1.8 |
| 6 or more | 13.8 | 1.5 |
| | 100.0 | 100.0 |

Additional details on individual use of different physicians will be found in the second study on "Diagnosis and Treatment," Chapter 17.

## The Relative Roles of General Practitioner and Specialist

The overall pattern emerging from the study of one year's * experience showed out-of-hospital care rendered mainly by general practitioners—two of three office services, four of five home calls—while for three of five hospital services the attending physician was a specialist (Table 46).

TABLE 46.  Type of Attending Physician,
by Place Service Rendered

| PLACE OF PHYSICIAN SERVICE | TYPE OF ATTENDING PHYSICIAN | | | |
|---|---|---|---|---|
| | All | Specialist * | General Practitioner | Other † |
| | % | % | % | % |
| Hospital | 100 | 59.9 | 39.9 | .2 |
| Office | 100 | 35.1 | 63.8 | 1.1 |
| Home | 100 | 18.9 | 81.0 | .1 |
| TOTAL ‡ | 100 | 37.4 | 61.8 | .8 |

* A specialist is defined by GHI as a physician M.D. who is a Diplomate of an American Specialty Board, or a Fellow of an American College of Medicine or Surgery, or is recognized as a specialist by the New York State Workmen's Compensation Board, or in the absence of any of the foregoing has an outstanding hospital or teaching appointment attesting to his acceptance by his peers as a specialist; except for psychiatry, where any M.D. devoting full time to this specialty is recognized.
† Podiatrist or optometrist.
‡ Excluding hospital x-ray services, services administered by salaried hospital employees (e.g. anesthesia), and all laboratory tests.

Within the "hospital" and "office" service categories there were wide variations as to types of service for which specialists

* In interpreting data on proportions of services rendered by specialists, it is important to remember that changes are occurring steadily and probably have already altered the patterns shown for 1964 in the direction of higher proportions of specialist service.

were used. They provided the majority of surgical, anesthesiological, radiological, psychiatric, obstetrical services, and consultations, while general practitioners were in attendance for most of the non-surgical hospital admissions, as well as office and home calls (Table 47).

TABLE 47.   Attending Physician Type of Practice, by Type of Service Rendered

| TYPE OF SERVICE | PROPORTION OF SERVICE RENDERED BY | | | |
|---|---|---|---|---|
| | *All* | *Specialists* | *General Practitioners* | *Other* * |
| | % | % | % | % |
| *Hospital Attendance* | | | | |
| Surgical | 100 | 78 | 22 | † |
| Medical | 100 | 42 | 58 | † |
| Psychiatric | 100 | 100 | 0 | 0 |
| Obstetrical | 100 | 51 | 49 | 0 |
| Anesthesiological | 100 | 68 | 32 | 0 |
| *Office Services* | | | | |
| General Visit | 100 | 31 | 68 | 1 |
| Preventive Service | 100 | 38 | 62 | 0 |
| Surgery | 100 | 50 | 44 | 6 |
| Diagnostic X-ray | 100 | 65 | 31 | 4 |
| Other (Including Radiotherapy and Electroshock Treatment) | 100 | 81 | 19 | 0 |
| *Home Visit* | 100 | 19 | 81 | † |

\* Podiatrist, optometrist or laboratory.
† Less than .5 per cent.

## Who Used Specialists?

Aside from type of service, the measurable factors most strongly related to use of specialists were age, occupation class, and area of residence. Family size was a possible factor while sex, marital status, and number of years of GHI coverage showed little or no relationship.

In evaluating patterns of specialist use by various population segments, it should be remembered that differences of apparent significance are not necessarily indicative of consumer choice.

The fact that the use of surgical specialists increased sharply with age is less likely to be associated with the preferences of older people than with types of surgery predominating at various age levels.

Similarly, higher rates of specialist use in certain areas probably reflect local medical customs and facilities as much as individual residents' attitudes toward specialists.

The occupation category of the subscriber was associated with the most consistent variations in use of specialists. Differences here probably reflect the exercise of consumer choice.

### NEGATIVE FACTORS: SEX, MARITAL STATUS, DURATION OF MEDICAL COVERAGE

The percentage of services rendered by specialists was identical, or nearly so, for males and females, with respect to all types of service.

Widowed, divorced, or separated women used specialists at a greater rate than married women, for surgery in or out of the hospital. Otherwise there were no notable differences related to marital status.

The length of time in GHI was entirely irrelevant to the degree of specialist use; newcomers and those with 8 years of coverage showed the same experience.

### VARIATIONS BY FAMILY SIZE

The highest proportion of surgery by specialists occurred among the smallest families, the lowest proportion among the largest families. Although the differences are not explained wholly on the basis of age, the pattern failed to hold for non-surgical services. The data would require further refinement, taking type of surgery as well as age into account, to determine the significance, if any, of the surgical findings (Table 48).

TABLE 48.  Proportion of Surgery Performed
by Specialists, by Family Size

| | PROPORTION PERFORMED BY SPECIALISTS | |
|---|---|---|
| ENROLLED FAMILY SIZE | *In-Hospital Surgery* | *Out-of-Hospital Surgery* |
| | % | % |
| 1 or 2 | 85 | 64 |
| 3 or 4 | 78 | 53 |
| 5 or more | 69 | 41 |

DIFFERENCES ASSOCIATED WITH AGE

The age pattern of specialist use varied by type of service. For surgery in or out of the hospital, specialist use increased steadily with increasing age.

For medical care at home or hospital, higher specialist use occurred at the youngest and oldest levels; for office calls this pattern was weakly repeated, while for diagnostic x-rays, age was not a factor (Table 49).

TABLE 49.  Proportion of Specified Types of Service Rendered
by Specialists, by Patient Age

| | PROPORTION RENDERED BY SPECIALISTS | | | | | |
|---|---|---|---|---|---|---|
| | SURGERY | | MEDICAL VISITS | | | DIAGNOSTIC X-RAYS |
| AGE | *Hospital* | *Office* | *Hospital* | *Office* | *Home* | |
| | % | % | % | % | % | % |
| Under 10 | 68 | 35 | 48 | 30 | 26 | 67 |
| 10–44 | 76 | 50 | 42 | 25 | 14 | 65 |
| 45–64 | 85 | 63 | 38 | 28 | 13 | 70 |
| 65 and Over | 93 | 66 | 50 | 33 | 28 | 70 |

Since surgery and diagnostic x-rays constitute a relatively minor part of all physician services, the general practitioner's role was clearly important at all ages. Specialists provided about every third service up to age 45, after which their responsibility increased, to 42 per cent of services received at age 65 or over. The increase is largely related to the more serious nature of the surgery undertaken at older ages.

LOCAL DIFFERENCES

Inter-county differences found in degree of specialist use may be related to local facilities and medical customs as well as to population characteristics. For example, the fact that Suffolk County showed the highest percentage of surgery by general practitioners, both in and out of the hospital, may have resulted from its young population and from the relative freedom enjoyed by non-specialists with respect to hospital privileges, at least up to the time of the present study. Even here, however, 71 per cent of the hospital surgery was done by specialists.

In general, patterns of specialist use were similar within each county: the overall finding of high specialist use for surgery and x-rays, low for medical care in office, home, or hospital, holds throughout the areas surveyed, varying only in degree.

The greatest variation occurred with respect to medical service in the hospital: specialists attended 56 per cent of Manhattanites, 29 per cent of Queens-ites.

Office surgery also varied broadly by area, with specialists performing 62 per cent of such services in Manhattan as against 41 per cent in Suffolk.

The lowest degree of geographic variation occurred with repect to home visits and diagnostic x-rays. In all areas, close to 80 per cent of the home visits were by general practitioners, ranging from 75 per cent in upstate New York to 84 per cent in Queens; while the range for x-rays performed by non-specialists was from 29 per cent in Richmond and Queens to 38 per cent in the Bronx (Table 50).

It is of interest that Queens showed the lowest proportion of specialist responsibility for all three medical indices—office, home, and hospital visits—while Suffolk had this distinction with respect to both surgical indices. Data on type-of-physician availability only partially explain these rankings.

TABLE 50. Proportion of Specified Types of Service Rendered by Specialists, in Different Areas

| | PROPORTION RENDERED BY SPECIALISTS | | | | | |
|---|---|---|---|---|---|---|
| | SURGERY | | MEDICAL VISITS | | | DIAGNOSTIC X-RAYS |
| AREA | *Hospital* | *Office* | *Hospital* | *Office* | *Home* | |
| | % | % | % | % | % | % |
| Manhattan | 83 | 62 | 56 | 28 | 20 | 63 |
| Bronx | 81 | 54 | 50 | 26 | 19 | 62 |
| Westchester | 82 | 59 | 40 | 37 | 23 | 68 |
| Other New York | 83 | 55 | 52 | 34 | 25 | 69 |
| Brooklyn | 78 | 56 | 40 | 27 | 18 | 69 |
| Queens | 78 | 54 | 29 | 23 | 16 | 71 |
| Richmond | 76 | 55 | 29 | 30 | 24 | 71 |
| Nassau | 75 | 47 | 37 | 25 | 18 | 65 |
| New Jersey | 72 | 46 | 46 | 32 | 22 | 68 |
| Suffolk | 69 | 41 | 34 | 24 | 23 | 70 |

DIFFERENCES ASSOCIATED WITH SUBSCRIBER OCCUPATION CLASS

To the extent that the decision to consult specialists is initiated by the medical consumer, it is logical to hypothesize that socioeconomic status plays an important role in such decisions.

As previously explained, subscriber occupation is the only "class" index available to GHI, as to most medical insurance organizations. Occupation categories, however, have been found satisfactory, even preferable in some cases, as a rough "status" gauge. (See p. 40.)

The expected patterns emerged from the present data, although not to the expected extent. That is, there was a definite class difference in the use of specialists, but the differences were neither as large nor as consistent as might have been anticipated.

For example, a reasonable hypothesis would assume that the most likely users of specialists would be families of those in professional occupations, and this in fact proved to be the case. But the pattern of choice was spotty—even though their use of specialists for office care was nearly twice that of blue-collar families, the professional class among GHI members received over half of such care from general practitioners. When it came to medical care in the hospital, however, this class received seven out of ten services from specialists, a much higher proportion than all other classes.

The data demonstrate the inaccurate impression that can result from grouping all white-collar occupations and comparing them, as though they were a homogeneous class, with the blue-collar groups. The experience of the clerical group was closer to that of blue-collar groups than to higher-ranking white-collar occupations (Table 51).

TABLE 51. Proportion of Specified Types of Service Rendered by Specialists, by Subscriber Occupation Class

| | PROPORTION RENDERED BY SPECIALISTS | | | | | | |
|---|---|---|---|---|---|---|---|
| OCCUPATION CLASS * | SURGERY | | MEDICAL VISITS | | | DIAGNOSTIC X-RAYS | OBSTETRICAL CARE |
| | *Hospital* | *Office* | *Hospital* | *Office* | *Home* | | |
| | % | % | % | % | % | % | % |
| Professional | 91 | 69 | 72 | 44 | 25 | 72 | 88 |
| Executive | 86 | 65 | 37 | 36 | 28 | 73 | 65 |
| Sales | 78 | 63 | 47 | 37 | 30 | 71 | 85 |
| Clerical and White-Collar Unspecified | 79 | 49 | 44 | 29 | 20 | 66 | 46 |
| Blue-Collar | 76 | 53 | 39 | 24 | 17 | 67 | 52 |

* Including dependents.

## Patterns of Specialist Use

Four specialty fields—internal medicine, pediatrics, general surgery, and obstetrics—accounted for five of every eight specialist services rendered to the GHI study population.

Surgical subspecialties provided another 19 per cent, the other non-surgical specialties 18 per cent.

Surgical and non-surgical fields were almost equally represented in volume of service provided—49 per cent and 51 per cent, respectively. These proportions, however, exclude such non-surgical services as laboratory procedures (usually claimed by internists) and hospital services rendered by radiologists, pathologists, salaried anesthesiologists, and salaried physiatrists. Furthermore, not all services rendered by surgeons were connected with surgical cases; surgeons were responsible for 39 per cent of the medical admissions treated by specialists.

The relative use of specialists in various fields of practice naturally depends at least in part on the service sought. Patterns experienced by GHI members are discussed below for each type of service.

### Consultations

A marked difference emerged between the distribution of hospital and office consultations among the various specialty fields.

In the hospital, four fields accounted for three-fourths of the consultations, with internal medicine far in the lead, followed by general surgery, pediatrics, and psychiatry.

| Consultant Field | Proportion of Hospital Consultations |
|---|---|
|  | % |
| Internal Medicine | 44.5 |
| General Surgery | 16.0 |
| Pediatrics | 8.4 |
| Psychiatry | 5.6 |
|  | 74.5 |

Except for internal medicine, the predominating specialty fields for office consultations were all different from the hospital leaders, and five fields were listed to account for three-fourths of the consultations. Ophthalmology ranked first—ahead of internal medicine by a significant margin; these were followed by otolaryngology, orthopedic surgery, and dermatology.

| Consultant Field | Proportion of Office Consultations |
|---|---|
|  | % |
| Ophthalmology | 25.4 |
| Internal Medicine | 18.3 |
| Otolaryngology | 12.8 |
| Orthopedic Surgery | 9.0 |
| Dermatology | 8.4 |
|  | 73.9 |

*Office Visits*

The term "office visits" as used here refers to physician office services not otherwise classified under preventive care, office surgery, consultations, or diagnostic x-rays. (Included are follow-up visits for surgical cases and pre- and postnatal maternity visits, distributed by field of practice of physician attending patient in hospital.)

Over half of all physician services fell into this category (laboratory tests are excluded); and of these, 68.9 per cent represented non-specialist visits (62.7 per cent to MD-general practitioners, 5.4 per cent to osteopaths, .7 per cent to podiatrists, .1 per cent to optometrists).

The 31.1 per cent of office visits involving specialists were chiefly in the fields of internal medicine, general surgery, obstetrics-gynecology, and pediatrics. Together these accounted for nearly two thirds of specialist office visits (Table 52).

TABLE 52.  Distribution of Specialist Office Visits, by Specialist Field of Practice

| SPECIALTY FIELD | Proportion of Specialist Office Visits |
|---|---|
| | % |
| Internal Medicine | 19.9 |
| General Surgery | 16.7 |
| Obstetrics-Gynecology | 15.0 |
| Pediatrics | 13.2 |
| Otolaryngology | 5.6 |
| Dermatology | 4.6 |
| Ophthalmology | 4.3 |
| Allergy | 3.7 |
| Cardiology | 2.6 |
| Orthopedic Surgery | 2.6 |
| Urology | 2.3 |
| Other Surgery | 1.9 |
| Psychiatry | 1.6 |
| Gastroenterology | .9 |
| Other Non-Surgical Fields | 5.1 |
| TOTAL | 100.0 |

### Preventive Services

Immunizations and well-baby care are the main components of this category.

Physical checkups are included if so designated by the physician, but this is believed to be a weak spot in the classification system. Probably many such services are included with general office visits.

General practitioners were responsible for 62 per cent of preventive visits, pediatricians for another 31 per cent. Most of the remaining 7 per cent was rendered by internists, obstetricians, and general surgeons.

### Diagnostic X-rays (Office)

For 65 per cent of their out-of-hospital x-rays, subscribers went to specialists' offices. Another 31 per cent of the x-rays were taken by general practitioners (including 3 per cent by osteopaths), 2 per cent were by podiatrists, and the remainder by laboratories.

Of procedures by specialists, radiologists accounted for slightly less than half, with internists occupying a strong second place (Table 53).

TABLE 53. Distribution of Diagnostic X-rays Performed in Specialists' Offices, by Specialist Field of Practice

| SPECIALTY FIELD | Proportion of X-rays |
|---|---|
| | % |
| Radiology | 46.5 |
| Internal Medicine | 31.2 |
| Orthopedic Surgery | 6.1 |
| Pediatrics | 3.0 |
| General Surgery | 2.8 |
| Gastroenterology | 2.5 |
| Urology | 2.3 |
| Cardiology | 1.5 |
| All Other | 4.1 |
| TOTAL | 100.0 |

## Office Surgery

Half the surgical procedures performed on an ambulatory basis were by specialists. The other half were divided among MD-general practitioners (40 per cent), osteopaths (4 per cent) and podiatrists (6 per cent).

The fact that podiatrists were responsible for 6 per cent of all office surgery by 1964 is somewhat startling since they were not accepted as "physicians" by GHI until 1959, when a revision in the New York State Insurance Law made this policy change mandatory.

A large proportion of the procedures performed by specialists involved non-surgeons—chiefly internists and dermatologists (Table 54). Presumably these were of a diagnostic nature (endoscopy) in the case of internists.

TABLE 54. Distribution of Ambulatory Surgery Performed by Specialists, by Specialist Field of Practice

| SPECIALTY FIELD | Proportion of Ambulatory Surgical Procedures |
|---|---|
| | % |
| Internal Medicine | 24.1 |
| Dermatology | 17.5 |
| General Surgery | 14.6 |
| Obstetrics-Gynecology | 8.3 |
| Otolaryngology | 7.5 |
| Urology | 6.6 |
| Ophthalmology | 5.5 |
| Orthopedic Surgery | 4.0 |
| Proctology | 3.8 |
| Pediatrics | 3.5 |
| Gastroenterology | 1.1 |
| All Other | 3.5 |
| TOTAL | 100.0 |

## Hospital Surgery

Specialists were credited with 77.5 per cent of hospital surgery. General practitioners (MD's) were responsible for most of the rest, 21 per cent, osteopaths for 1.3 per cent and podiatrists for .2 per cent.

General surgeons performed less than half the procedures done by specialists—44 per cent; the five leading surgical sub-specialties accounted for another 46 per cent; while the remainder, 10 per cent, was divided between other surgeons (6 per cent) and medical specialists performing mainly diagnostic or dermatological surgical procedures (Table 55).

TABLE 55.   Distribution of Hospital Surgery Performed by Specialists, by Specialist Field of Practice

| SPECIALTY FIELD | Proportion of Surgery |
|---|---|
| | % |
| General Surgery | 44.0 |
| Otolaryngology | 14.4 |
| Gynecology | 12.1 * |
| Urology | 8.7 |
| Orthopedic Surgery | 6.5 |
| Ophthalmology | 5.5 |
| Proctology | 1.8 |
| Plastic Surgery | 1.7 |
| Neurosurgery | 1.3 |
| Thoracic Surgery | 1.1 |
| Other Surgery | .1 |
| Medical Specialties | 4.1 |
| TOTAL | 100.0 |

* Obstetrical services are not included.

The distribution of surgery by type of specialist of course reflects the distribution of surgical procedures (discussed elsewhere), which in turn relates to the age-sex distribution of the population. If children were excluded, otolaryngologists, who are apparently still inclined toward tonsillectomies, would take a minor place on the list. Similarly, if the proportion of persons past 65 were higher, the urologists, proctologists, ophthalmologists and orthopedic surgeons would rank higher.

*Relation of Type of Practice to Type of Hospital Used for Surgery.*   The fact that surgeons other than general surgeons performed over half of all procedures done by specialists is noteworthy of itself, but particularly with respect to the type of hospital in which they predominate.

In a separate tabulation of hospital surgery by type of hospital, the operating physicians were divided into three categories: general practitioners, general surgeons, and other specialists. The analysis revealed a marked rise in proportion of surgery performed by specialists other than general surgeons, corresponding to steps in the hospital hierarchy—from 27 per cent at the lowest to 53 per cent at the highest hospital level—and a concomitant decrease in the role of general practitioners, from 41 per cent to 9 per cent; while the proportion performed by general surgeons remained comparatively constant at 32 to 38 per cent irrespective of hospital type (Table 56).

TABLE 56.   Type of Physicians Performing Surgery, by Type of Hospital

| | PROPORTION OF SURGERY PERFORMED | | | |
| TYPE OF HOSPITAL | All Physicians | General Practitioners | General Surgeons | Other Specialists |
|---|---|---|---|---|
| | % | % | % | % |
| *Voluntary* | | | | |
| Affiliated * | 100 | 9 | 38 | 53 |
| Approved † | 100 | 19 | 36 | 45 |
| Other | 100 | 24 | 38 | 38 |
| | | | | |
| *Proprietary* | | | | |
| Accredited | 100 | 26 | 35 | 39 |
| Unaccredited | 100 | 41 | 32 | 27 |

* Affiliated with medical school.
† Approved for resident or intern training.

### Hospital Medical Care

The majority of the medical patients hospitalized were served by general practitioners—58.4 per cent, including 3.6 per cent by osteopaths.

Of the cases under specialist care, 53 per cent were admitted by internists, pediatricians, allergists, cardiologists, gastroenterologists; 39 per cent by surgeons of various types; 3 per cent by psychiatrists (Table 57).

TABLE 57.   Distribution of Hospital Medical Cases Under the Care of Specialists, by Specialist Field of Practice

| SPECIALTY FIELD | Proportion of Specialist Admissions |
|---|---|
| | % |
| Internal Medicine | 32.0 |
| General Surgery | 24.1 |
| Pediatrics | 14.9 |
| Urology | 3.9 |
| Cardiology | 3.7 |
| Orthopedic Surgery | 3.6 |
| Psychiatry | 3.0 |
| Otolaryngology | 2.1 |
| Gynecology | 1.8 |
| Gastroenterology | 1.6 |
| Ophthalmology | 1.5 |
| Other Surgical Fields | 2.4 |
| Other Non-Surgical Fields | 5.4 |
| TOTAL | 100.0 |

*Relation of Type of Practice to Type of Hospital Used for Medical Cases.*   To determine the influence of the hospital on categories of physicians admitting medical patients, a tabulation similar to that given above for hospital surgery was made, substituting internists for general surgeons.

Despite the large overall proportion of medical admissions by general practitioners, the differences by type of hospital emerge even more strongly than for surgical admissions. The line of demarcation between voluntary and proprietary hospitals was more definite, as was that between medical school affiliates and other voluntary hospitals.

While the proprietary hospital was clearly the domain of the general practitioner, however, it is also apparent that non-specialists still occupied an important place in hospitals of all types (Table 58).

## Obstetrical Care

Forty-nine per cent of obstetrical care was rendered by obstetricians, 2 per cent by surgeons, 47 per cent by MD-general practitioners, and 2 per cent by osteopaths.

TABLE 58.   Type of Physicians Admitting Medical Patients,
by Type of Hospital

| | PROPORTION OF MEDICAL ADMISSIONS | | | |
| TYPE OF HOSPITAL | All Physicians | General Practitioners | Internists | Other Specialists |
|---|---|---|---|---|
| | % | % | % | % |
| *Voluntary* | | | | |
| Affiliated * | 100 | 32 | 30 | 38 |
| Approved † | 100 | 50 | 17 | 33 |
| Other | 100 | 56 | 16 | 28 |
| *Proprietary* | | | | |
| Accredited | 100 | 74 | 6 | 20 |
| Unaccredited | 100 | 82 | 5 | 13 |

* Affiliated with medical school.
† Approved for resident or intern training.

## Anesthesia

Anesthesiologists administered anesthesia in 66 per cent of the cases for which GHI was billed. Non-specialists assumed responsibility for 32 per cent, and specialists in fields other than anesthesia accounted for 2 per cent.

## Home Calls

General practitioners made 81 per cent of all home visits, including 5 per cent by osteopaths. Another 10 per cent involved pediatricians, 3 per cent internists, 2 per cent general surgeons. No other specialty field accounted for as much as one per cent of all home calls.

## Field of Physician Practice vs. Locale of Services

In the course of examining relative responsibilities for the various types of service, another pattern emerged demonstrating broad differences among specialties as to locale in which services were concentrated.

As shown in Table 59, surgeons characteristically rendered much higher proportions of service in the hospital than non-surgeons.

TABLE 59.  Distribution of Physician Services by Locale, by Selected Fields of Practice

| FIELD OF PRACTICE | TOTAL | HOSPITAL | OUT-OF-HOSPITAL | | |
|---|---|---|---|---|---|
| | | | Total | Office † | Home |
| | % | % | % | % | % |
| *Surgical Specialties* | | | | | |
| General Surgery | 100 | 48 | 52 | 48 | 4 |
| Obstetrics-Gynecology | 100 | 34 | 66 | 65 | 1 |
| Ophthalmology | 100 | 20 | 80 | 79 | 1 |
| Otolaryngology | 100 | 41 | 59 | 59 | — |
| Urology | 100 | 52 | 48 | 48 | — |
| Orthopedic Surgery | 100 | 39 | 61 | 61 | — |
| Proctology | 100 | 41 | 59 | 59 | — |
| Neurosurgery | 100 | 70 | 30 | 30 | 0 |
| Plastic Surgery | 100 | 56 | 44 | 43 | 1 |
| Thoracic Surgery | 100 | 71 | 29 | 29 | 0 |
| *Non-Surgical Specialties* | | | | | |
| General Internal Medicine | 100 | 18 | 82 | 76 | 6 |
| Pediatrics | 100 | 9 | 91 | 67 | 24 |
| Allergy | 100 | 3 | 97 | 92 | 5 |
| Cardiology | 100 | 17 | 83 | 68 | 15 |
| Dermatology | 100 | 2 | 98 | 98 | — |
| Endocrinology | 100 | 0 | 100 | 80 | 20 |
| Gastroenterology | 100 | 19 | 81 | 69 | 12 |
| Neurology | 100 | 65 | 35 | 35 | 0 |
| Psychiatry | 100 | 41 | 59 | 53 | 6 |
| *General Practice-M.D.'s* | 100 | 12 | 88 | 71 | 17 |
| *Non-M.D.'s* | | | | | |
| Osteopathy | 100 | 9 | 91 | 76 | 15 |
| Podiatry | 100 | 4 | 96 | 94 | 2 |

\* Including only services rendered under GHI contracts, thus excluding routine refractions, most ambulatory psychotherapy, and all services remunerated from other sources or ren-- dered without charge. In calculating percentage of services rendered at each locale, no consideration of time per service could be undertaken.
† Including follow-up care of surgical patients, and pre- and postnatal maternity visits.
— = Less than .5 per cent.

Some medical specialists—pediatricians, allergists, derma- tologists, endocrinologists—performed practically all their serv- ices out of the hospital, exceeding general practitioners in this respect.

Pediatricians also exceeded non-specialists in proportion of home calls to total number of services: every fourth service they rendered was in this category. (As previously noted, telephone calls are not included in the service count.) The only other specialists showing home calls as more than 10 per cent of all their services were cardiologists, endocrinologists, and gastroenterologists; in actual volume, however, none of these subspecialists was responsible for a significant proportion of house calls.

## Chapter 7

# HOW MANY SERVICES?

The number of physician and laboratory services rendered under their comprehensive coverage averaged 6.7 per eligible member for the year, of which one service represented in-hospital physician care. Among those who used any service, the average was 8.4 services per user.

In order to give a reasonably fair picture of the number of physician services rendered hospitalized cases, thus creating a common denominator for ambulatory and hospital contacts, claims data were adjusted to allow one physician service per contact, rather than per claim, plus office care for obstetrical and surgical cases. (See Chapter 2 for details.) Allowance was also made for the fact that GHI counts both day of admission and day of discharge, in remunerating physicians, whereas hospital insurance is paid on the basis of number of nights in hospital, thus in effect producing a stay one day shorter than that recorded by GHI. In interpreting the data, physicians' hospital services were counted according to the GHI method. Hospitalization studies, however, calculated length of stay in accordance with number of nights, to conform with payment practice.

The utilization rate of physician and laboratory services, before adjustment, was 5.4 services per capita, as against the 6.7 adjusted rate.

Demographic variations in unadjusted use rates followed patterns similar to the adjusted rates given in this report with the exceptions caused by high or low hospital-use tendencies of some population segments.

Adjusted utilization rates are presented in succeeding sections for all services combined, for all ambulatory services combined, and separately for the principal ambulatory components. Since the later chapter on hospitalization studies analyzes demographic and type-of-admission patterns in some detail, utilization rates of physicians' hospital services are not discussed separately; these may be calculated, using the tables presented in the next section, by subtracting total ambulatory from total services.

## Utilization Rates—All Services Combined

Utilization rates, stated as the number of services per eligible member or per thousand "exposure years", * varied broadly among the different segments of the population.

Age was the single most important factor associated with different volumes of service use. Occupation class (excluding students and retired) was the least important, at the overall level of comparison.

Since medical needs are known to increase with age and are not known to vary by broad occupation categories, such findings may indicate the positive social role played by comprehensive medical insurance in leveling off class differences formerly associated with the seeking of private medical care. This question is considered in further detail under analyses of component services.

---

* An "exposure year" (or "person year" or "member year") represents the insurance coverage of one person for one year.

## Variations in Total Service Volume
## Among Population Subgroups

VARIATIONS BY AGE AND SEX

The greatest range in service utilization rates was observed among the various age levels of females, who showed both the lowest and the highest extremes of use: 3,550 services per thousand girls aged 10 to 14, vs. a rate more than three times that level, 11,247 services per thousand women past 64.

Among males, the extremes occurred at the same age levels as for females, but within a smaller range: boys used more services than girls, while men past 64 used service at about the level of women aged 55 to 64, i.e. one fewer service per capita than women 65 and over (Table 60).

TABLE 60. Number of Services Per 1000 Exposure Years, by Age and Sex

| | SERVICE UTILIZATION RATE | | | |
|---|---|---|---|---|
| | | | Females | |
| AGE | Males and Females | Males | TOTAL | Excluding Obstetrics |
| Under 5 | 6,661.8 | 6,795.5 | 6,519.8 | |
| 5–9 | 4,764.8 | 4,955.7 | 4,572.2 | |
| 10–14 | 3,871.9 | 4,179.4 | 3,549.8 | |
| 15–19 | 4,939.7 | 5,267.8 | 4,636.7 | 4,557.7 |
| 20–24 | 8,407.8 | 4,149.8 | 11,070.6 | 7,069.2 |
| 25–34 | 7,387.1 | 4,438.0 | 10,032.2 | 7,253.8 |
| 35–44 | 7,214.5 | 5,432.8 | 9,021.5 | 8,325.2 |
| 45–54 | 7,696.4 | 6,422.1 | 8,991.1 | 8,970.4 |
| 55–64 | 9,157.5 | 8,442.2 | 10,194.0 | |
| 65 and Over | 10,558.8 | 10,208.6 | 11,247.1 | |
| All Under 65 | 6,638.3 | 5,749.8 | 7,547.3 | |
| All Adults | 7,915.1 | 6,337.5 | 9,574.7 | |
| All Children | 4,966.3 | 5,208.1 | 4,720.0 | |

VARIATIONS ASSOCIATED WITH MARITAL STATUS
AND RELATIONSHIP TO SUBSCRIBER

The wide disparities in use rates between men and women past 20 were only partially accounted for by maternity care.

Women generally used more service at all ages, whether single or married, and regardless of subscriber-dependent status. Single women used nearly 60 per cent more services than single men. The category widowed-divorced-or-separated females, using less service than either single or married women, still used more than any of the male marital categories; while female subscribers and spouses used one third to one half more services than males in corresponding categories (Table 61).

TABLE 61. Number of Services Per 1000 Adult Exposure Years, by Marital Status and Relationship to Subscriber, by Sex

| | SERVICE UTILIZATION RATE | | | |
|---|---|---|---|---|
| | *Males and Females* | *Males* | *Females* | |
| | | | TOTAL | Excluding Obstetrics |
| *Marital Status* | | | | |
| Married | 8,158.2 | 6,537.9 | 9,814.2 | 8,680.0 |
| Single | 6,095.0 | 4,968.0 | 7,784.9 | |
| Widowed, Divorced, Separated | 6,170.1 | 5,258.2 | 6,840.4 | |
| *Relationship to Subscriber* | | | | |
| Self | 6,725.9 | 6,346.9 | 8,709.4 | 8,371.7 |
| Spouse | 9,486.2 | 6,208.3 | 9,774.3 | 8,603.8 |

VARIATIONS BY FAMILY SIZE

Analysis of use rates by families of different sizes shows an inverse relationship: the larger the family, the fewer the services per person.

Since service utilization rates among children are so much lower than among adults, additional children in a family would be expected to decrease the average use per person. But the age factor is not sufficient to explain the use levels shown in Table 62. Among families of six or more, services per person were even lower than the average for all children. If the use rates for a family of two parents and four children were consistent with the general use rates of adults and children, they would average 6.0 services per person instead of the 4.9 services actually experienced. Interestingly enough, a decrease in maternity care was *not* one of the reasons for decreased service utilization, among families which already had four children; the volume of such service was actually higher, for such families.

The finding of decreasing per capita use of service with family increments does not mean lower aggregate family use, but merely signals a smaller increment in services with each successive increment in family size (Table 62).

TABLE 62.  Number of Services Per Person and Per Family of Two or More, by Family Size

| FAMILY SIZE | Services Per Family Member | Services Per Family |
|---|---|---|
| 2 | 8.7 | 17.4 |
| 3 | 7.6 | 22.8 |
| 4 | 6.8 | 27.1 |
| 5 | 5.6 | 28.2 |
| 6 or more | 4.9 | 30.4 |

GEOGRAPHIC VARIATIONS

Services per person ranged from 5.0 for New Jersey residents to 7.4 for Brooklynites—a difference of nearly 50 per cent.

In most areas, however, utilization hovered within 9 per cent of the overall average. The three counties of New York City with the largest membership—Bronx, Brooklyn, Queens—showed almost identical volume of services per person (7.2 to 7.4), while suburban Westchester was in the same category with a rate of 7.2. In the remaining New York counties, the range was from 6.2 in Suffolk to 6.7 in Nassau, with Manhattan,

# FREQUENCY OF
## PHYSICIAN AND LABORATORY SERVICES
## BY SUBSCRIBER OCCUPATION CLASS

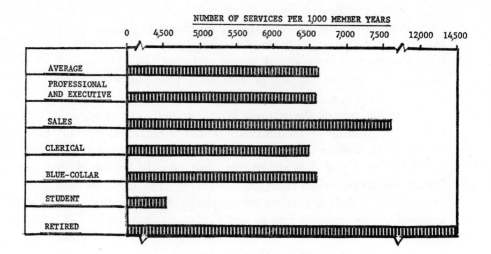

NUMBER OF SERVICES PER 1,000 MEMBER YEARS

## NUMBER OF SERVICES PER PERSON AND
## PER FAMILY OF TWO OR MORE,
### By Family Size

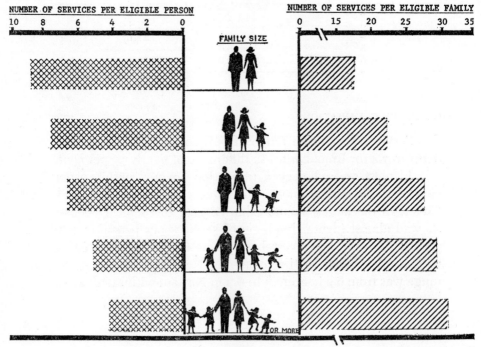

NUMBER OF SERVICES PER ELIGIBLE PERSON

NUMBER OF SERVICES PER ELIGIBLE FAMILY

FAMILY SIZE

Richmond and upstate areas in intermediate positions (Table 63).

TABLE 63.  Number of Services Per 1000 Members
Residing in Each Area

| AREA | Service Utilization Rate |
|---|---|
| New York City | 7,166.1 |
| Manhattan | 6,391.9 |
| Bronx | 7,260.9 |
| Brooklyn | 7,405.1 |
| Queens | 7,210.0 |
| Richmond | 6,633.9 |
| Nassau | 6,744.4 |
| Suffolk | 6,154.5 |
| Westchester | 7,169.8 |
| Other New York | 6,303.0 |
| New Jersey | 5,002.8 |

When these service utilization rates are compared with other indices of use, the positions of the different areas relative to each other change. Manhattan members, for example, showed below-average service utilization rates only because fewer eligibles used any service; once they became patients, they received a greater number of services (9.5) than patients in any other area (Table 64). Suffolk residents showed the highest proportion using service, but the lowest number of services per eligible member in the entire New York area, because of a

TABLE 64.  Number of Services Per Patient, by Area

| AREA | Services Per Patient |
|---|---|
| New York City | 8.9 |
| Manhattan | 9.5 |
| Bronx | 9.1 |
| Brooklyn | 8.9 |
| Queens | 8.5 |
| Richmond | 7.7 |
| Nassau | 8.2 |
| Suffolk | 7.0 |
| Westchester | 8.3 |
| Other New York | 7.7 |
| New Jersey | 7.4 |

relatively low (7.0) number of services per patient. New Jersey was low both as to proportion of users (67 per cent) and services per user (7.4), hence its comparatively low service utilization rate shown in the previous table.

OCCUPATION CLASS VARIATIONS

Blue-collar workers and their families used services at precisely the combined rate of the professional-executive classes— 6.7 services per member. Moreover, there was very little difference between these groups and the families of clerical workers, with their rate of 6.5 services per eligible member.

Separate analysis of the professional and executive categories showed a somewhat higher utilization rate for the executive class, while the professional class was closest to the clerical group.

Of all employed categories, the sales category stood out, with a service utilization rate 16 per cent higher than the average for the membership as a whole. This group was also highest on proportion of users (88.5 per cent) and services per user (8.8).

The non-working categories, students and retired, showed the extremes in service use rates expected because of the age factor. Although 88 per cent of the students took advantage of their coverage, the users from this group averaged only 5.2

TABLE 65. Number of Services Per 1000 Exposure Years,* by Subscriber Occupation Class

| OCCUPATION CLASS | Service Utilization Rate |
|---|---|
| Professional and Executive | 6,693.3 |
| Professional | (6,384.9) |
| Executive | (6,926.5) |
| Sales | 7,815.3 |
| Clerical and White-Collar Unspecified | 6,483.3 |
| Blue-Collar | 6,744.3 |
| Student | 4,588.2 |
| Retired | 14,176.0 |

* Including dependents.

services as against the average of 8.4 for all patients, with the result that their utilization rate for all eligibles was only 68 per cent of that experienced by the membership as a whole. The retired group used over two services for every service used by the rest of the membership (Table 65).

VARIATIONS WITH DURATION OF ENROLLMENT

The longer the period of coverage, the higher the service utilization rate. This applied from the second through the seventh year of enrollment, after which a slight falling-off was observed (Table 66).

TABLE 66.  Number of Services Per 1000 Exposure Years, by Duration of Enrollment

| YEAR OF COVERAGE | Service Utilization Rate |
|---|---|
| 1st | 4,629.4 |
| 2nd | 4,436.3 |
| 3rd | 5,796.2 |
| 4th | 6,843.1 |
| 5th | 7,414.7 |
| 6th | 7,703.5 |
| 7th | 7,872.7 |
| 8th or Longer | 7,641.3 |

Part of the apparent trend toward greater use, as members became accustomed to their coverage, was attributable to variations in age distribution. The newer members and their dependents were more heavily concentrated in the younger, lower-utilizing brackets.

But judging purely by the age factor, one would expect those in their third, fourth and fifth year of coverage to have shown similar rates of service use, which they failed to do; fifth-year members were closer to sixth-year members in utilization levels, although closer to fourth-year members as to age distribution. Similarly, those in their sixth, seventh or eighth year of coverage produced use rates much closer to each other than would have been predicted on the basis of their respective age distributions.

The evidence leaves unresolved the question of a causal relationship between duration of insurance coverage and increased use of service.

# Chapter 8

# GENERAL OFFICE VISITS

## Ambulatory Services

As previously noted, the great majority of services, 5.7 of 6.7 per member, were rendered to non-hospitalized patients. The volume of out-of-hospital care was in turn concentrated in the category of general office visits, which accounted for three fifths of non-hospital services (Table 67). The ratio of all office services to reported home calls was about six to one. The combined frequency of out-of-hospital consultations, diagnostic x-rays, and laboratory tests (excluding routine urinalysis and

TABLE 67. Out-of-Hospital Physician and Laboratory
Services: Frequency Per 1000 Exposure Years,
by Type of Service

| TYPE OF SERVICE | Utilization Rate |
|---|---|
| *Physician Services* | |
| General Office Visits | 3,522.5 |
| Consultations | 77.8 |
| Preventive Visits | 230.3 |
| Surgery | 157.3 |
| Diagnostic X-rays | 202.6 |
| Radiotherapy and All Other | 15.3 |
| Home Visits | 804.4 |
| *Laboratory Tests* * | 693.4 |
| TOTAL AMBULATORY SERVICES | 5,703.6 |

* Excluding simple urinalysis and hemoglobin tests.

# PER CENT DISTRIBUTION OF OUT-OF-HOSPITAL PHYSICIAN AND LABORATORY SERVICES BY TYPE OF SERVICE

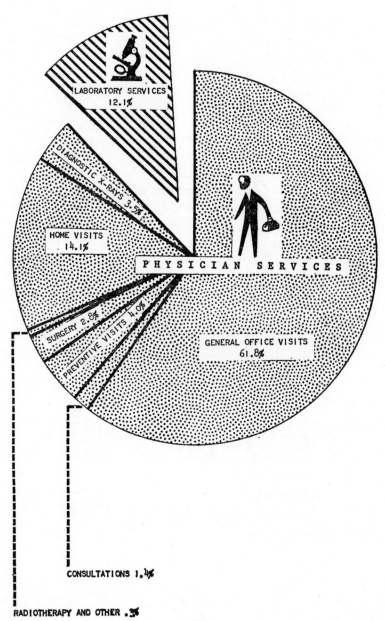

LABORATORY SERVICES 12.1%

DIAGNOSTIC X-RAYS 3.5%

HOME VISITS .14.1%

PHYSICIAN SERVICES

SURGERY 2.8%

PREVENTIVE VISITS 4.0%

GENERAL OFFICE VISITS 61.8%

CONSULTATIONS 1.4%

RADIOTHERAPY AND OTHER .3%

142

hemoglobin tests) amounted to nearly one service per member (974 per thousand), or 17 per cent of all covered ambulatory services.

These rates of utilization of each insured out-of-hospital service represent averages for the GHI study population enrolled for the full year under the comprehensive plan. Variations in use of the principal component services by population subgroups are introduced in this and following chapters.

Additional data, on variations in use of different types of service by diagnosis, are included under "Studies of Patient Care."

### Comparison of Three Indices of Service Volume, by Age, Marital Status, Relationship, Occupation Class, Area of Residence, Duration of Coverage

Of 5.7 non-hospital services per person eligible for service, 3.5 represented office visits not classified elsewhere. Since this category accounted for most out-of-hospital care, which in turn comprised 85 per cent of all services, demographic variations in all three of these indices of use are similar to those shown in the preceding section on combined utilization rates, varying mainly in degree. (See Table 68.)

The tendency toward greater use of service with increasing age applies to most types of service, but was much less pronounced with respect to ambulatory care. Members past 64 used about two and one-half times as much hospital care, 40 per cent more ambulatory care than the rest of the population.

The failure of overall blue-collar utilization rates to differ significantly from those of other groups, previously noted, continues in evidence in Table 68. Their total per capita out-of-hospital usage was the same as that of the combined professional-executive group, slightly higher than that of all white-collar groups. When the comparison is limited to general office visits, the positions are reversed, with blue-collar utilization somewhat lower than the combined white-collar rate. The differences are accounted for by other types of out-of-hospital service.

TABLE 68.   Comparison of Three Indices of Use Among
Population Subgroups: Total Services, Total Out-of-Hospital
Services, and General Office Visits

PART 1—MARITAL STATUS, SUBSCRIBER RELATIONSHIP
AND AGE

| | SERVICES PER ELIGIBLE MEMBER | | |
|---|---|---|---|
| | 1 | 2 * Total Out-of- | 3 * General Office |
| MEMBER CATEGORY | Total | Hospital | Visits |
| All | 6.73 | 5.70 | 3.52 |
| All Under 65 | 6.64 | 5.65 | 3.48 |
| All Adults | 7.92 | 6.47 | 4.23 |
| Married | 8.16 | 6.66 | 4.33 |
| Single | 6.10 | 5.11 | 3.51 |
| Widowed, Divorced, Separated | 6.17 | 4.95 | 3.30 |
| Subscriber | 6.73 | 5.61 | 3.59 |
| Spouse | 9.49 | 7.61 | 5.08 |
| All Children (to 19) | 4.97 | 4.56 | 2.46 |
| Age: | | | |
| Under 5 | 6.66 | 6.03 | 2.79 |
| 5–9 | 4.76 | 4.44 | 2.38 |
| 10–14 | 3.87 | 3.59 | 2.11 |
| 15–19 | 4.94 | 4.51 | 2.82 |
| 20–24 | 8.41 | 6.76 | 5.18 |
| 25–34 | 7.39 | 6.09 | 4.28 |
| 35–44 | 7.21 | 6.05 | 3.98 |
| 45–54 | 7.70 | 6.32 | 3.99 |
| 55–64 | 9.16 | 7.27 | 4.43 |
| 65 and Over | 10.56 | 7.91 | 5.20 |

* See footnote at end of table.

With two exceptions, Richmond County and New Jersey,
the inter-area range in number of general office visits per
eligible member rendered was remarkably small—from 3.42 in
Manhattan to 3.84 in the Bronx; in most areas, the experience
was within two tenths of a visit of the overall average. As will
be seen, geographic patterns of use showed wider variations
with respect to other types of out-of-hospital services.

### Male vs. Female Rates of General Office Visits

After the age of 19, female rates of general office visits
were substantially higher than those of all male categories.
The lowest female use rate for any class, 3.84 per person among

TABLE 68. *(Cont'd)*

## PART 2—OCCUPATION CLASS, DURATION OF ENROLLMENT, AREA OF RESIDENCE

| MEMBER CATEGORY | SERVICES PER ELIGIBLE MEMBER | | |
|---|---|---|---|
| | 1 | 2 * | 3 * |
| | | *Total Out-of-Hospital* | *General Office Visits* |
| | *Total* | | |
| *Subscriber Occupation Class* † | | | |
| Professional-Executive | 6.69 | 5.73 | 3.35 |
| Sales | 7.82 | 6.98 | 3.98 |
| Clerical and White-Collar Unspecified | 6.48 | 5.48 | 3.63 |
| All White-Collar | 6.59 | 5.60 | 3.60 |
| Blue-Collar | 6.74 | 5.73 | 3.44 |
| Student | 4.59 | 4.35 | 3.38 |
| Retired | 14.18 | 10.37 | 7.06 |
| *Year of Coverage* | | | |
| 1st | 4.63 | 3.86 | 2.31 |
| 2nd | 4.44 | 3.79 | 2.45 |
| 3rd | 5.80 | 4.93 | 3.12 |
| 4th | 6.84 | 5.85 | 3.58 |
| 5th | 7.41 | 6.38 | 3.99 |
| 6th | 7.70 | 6.49 | 3.91 |
| 7th | 7.87 | 6.69 | 4.07 |
| 8th or Longer | 7.64 | 6.30 | 3.83 |
| *Residence* | | | |
| Manhattan | 6.39 | 5.40 | 3.42 |
| Bronx | 7.26 | 6.19 | 3.84 |
| Brooklyn | 7.41 | 6.42 | 3.65 |
| Queens | 7.21 | 6.17 | 3.70 |
| Richmond | 6.63 | 5.13 | 2.93 |
| Nassau | 6.74 | 5.86 | 3.60 |
| Suffolk | 6.15 | 5.34 | 3.61 |
| Westchester | 7.17 | 5.68 | 3.44 |
| Other New York | 6.30 | 5.01 | 3.64 |
| New Jersey | 5.00 | 4.05 | 2.68 |

* Column 2 is a component of column 1 and column 3 is a component of column 2. Other components of column 2 are detailed in following sections.
† Including dependents.

the widowed, divorced or separated, was higher by half a visit than the highest use rate among male marital categories (married males, 3.32 general office visits per person).

Both female subscribers and wives of subscribers showed markedly higher rates than either male subscribers or spouses. Maternity care was only partially responsible for this disparity. At ages 20 to 44, the female rate, excluding obstetrics, was at

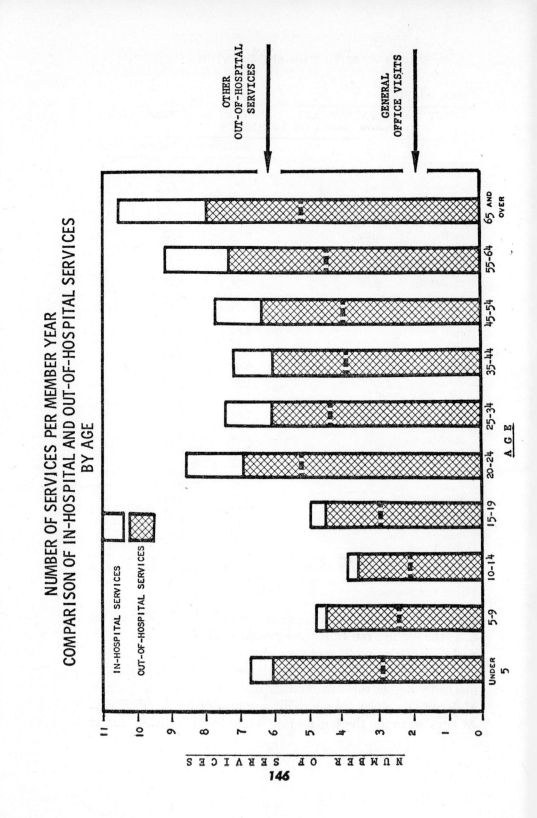

NUMBER OF SERVICES PER MEMBER YEAR
COMPARISON OF IN-HOSPITAL AND OUT-OF-HOSPITAL SERVICES
BY AGE

# NUMBER OF SERVICES PER MEMBER YEAR
## COMPARISON OF IN-HOSPITAL AND OUT-OF-HOSPITAL SERVICES
### By Marital Status, Subscriber Relationship, and Age Group

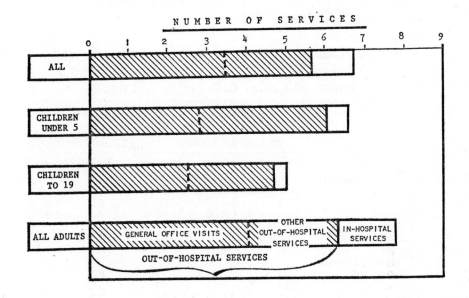

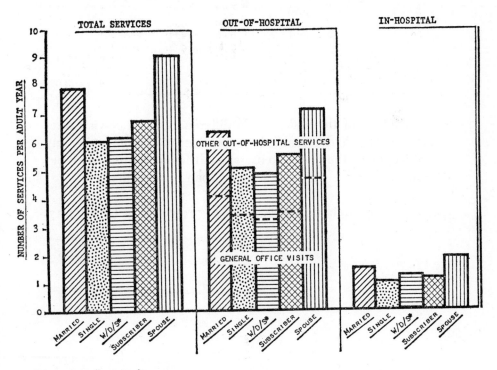

*W/D/S = WIDOWED/DIVORCED/SEPARATED

least 50 per cent higher than that of males. The ratio decreased at later age levels, but even at 65 the women's rate was 25 per cent higher (Table 69).

TABLE 69.   General Office Visits: Utilization Rates of Males and Females, Per Eligible and Per Patient, by Marital Status, Subscriber Relationship and Age

| | NUMBER OF GENERAL OFFICE VISITS PER YEAR | | | | |
|---|---|---|---|---|---|
| | PER ELIGIBLE MEMBER | | | PER PATIENT | |
| | *Males* | *Females* | | *Males* | *Females* |
| MEMBER CATEGORY | | TOTAL | *Excl. Obst.* | | |
| All | 2.99 | 4.07 | 3.68 | 4.9 | 5.9 |
| All Under 65 | 2.94 | 4.04 | 3.64 | 4.9 | 5.9 |
| All Adults | 3.25 | 5.26 | 4.60 | 5.7 | 7.3 |
| Married | 3.32 | 5.37 | 4.63 | 5.6 | 7.4 |
| Single | 2.85 | 4.49 | | 6.5 | 6.9 |
| Widowed, Divorced, Separated | 2.55 | 3.84 | | 6.3 | 6.8 |
| Subscriber | 3.29 | 5.11 | 4.89 | 5.7 | 6.5 |
| Spouse | 2.68 | 5.30 | 4.53 | 4.9 | 7.5 |
| Age: | | | | | |
| 20–24 | 2.63 | 6.77 | 4.15 | 4.7 | 9.2 |
| 25–34 | 2.49 | 5.90 | 4.09 | 4.5 | 8.2 |
| 35–44 | 2.91 | 5.06 | 4.60 | 5.1 | 6.9 |
| 45–54 | 3.30 | 4.69 | 4.68 | 6.0 | 6.7 |
| 55–64 | 3.97 | 5.08 | | 6.9 | 7.4 |
| 65 and Over | 4.79 | 6.00 | | 7.4 | 7.8 |
| Children to 19 | 2.60 | 2.30 | | 3.9 | 3.6 |

Not all of the male-female differences in office-visit rates are traceable to differences in proportions of eligibles using any service. Once they became users, adult females also had 28 per cent more office visits per patient, than male patients.

Further data on office visits are presented in Chapter 17.

# Chapter 9

# PREVENTIVE VISITS

The category "preventive visits" might be termed a residuary classification for services not associated with the diagnosis and treatment of specified illness.

It includes physical examinations, well-baby care, immunizations—unless the physician enters a diagnosis of illness on the claim form, in which case the service is classified as an office visit. Furthermore, any number of preventive services may be rendered during one visit. For these reasons the actual number of preventive *services* is never known, while the number of preventive *visits* is probably understated in the available material.

Nevertheless, comparative data for different population groups do serve the purpose of showing variations in volume of office visits reported as preventive: If it can be assumed that underreporting is likely to occur at the same level for all membership subgroups—and there is no reason to believe otherwise —then significant variations in reported use rates of preventive care can validly be characterized as indications of differing medical consumption habits.

Variables showing a positive association with the use of preventive service were age, sex, marital status, family size, and subscriber occupation class.

VARIATIONS ASSOCIATED WITH AGE AND SEX

As expected, the greatest use of preventive service was recorded for young children (under 5). They averaged 1,158 visits per thousand eligibles, which was five times the rate for the population as a whole (Table 70). A significant share of this differential is attributable to the number of preventive visits per user, which in the group under 5 averaged 2.5, as against 1.2 or fewer among users in other age groups.

After the age of 4, there was a tremendous falling-off in claims for preventive service, to 373 visits per thousand exposure years at ages 5 to 9, and thereafter a steady decline with each age increment.

This is the only service category in which the oldest group showed the least usage.

The usual pattern with other services—higher use rates for women—was also found for preventive services in each age, marital and subscriber relationship category. Aside from the group past 65, where male and female rates were about the same, the differences were of significance in all categories, with use rates of women averaging nearly 60 per cent higher than those of men.

Differences between rates for boys and girls were minor, never exceeding 7 per cent for any age subgroup.

VARIATIONS ASSOCIATED WITH MARITAL STATUS

Marital status may be of some importance in the decision to seek preventive service. Large differences in use rates between the spouseless and the married suggest marital concern with the partner's health as a possibly deciding factor. The rate for married members was 60 per cent higher than for single adults and 80 per cent higher than for the widowed-divorced-or-separated. Even the women in the latter category had a lower rate than that of married men. For single women, the rate was 10 per cent higher than that of married men, but far below that of married women (Table 70).

TABLE 70. Preventive Visits: Proportion of Users and
Utilization Rates, by Age, Sex, Marital Status,
Relationship and Family Size *

| MEMBER CATEGORY | Users Per 1000 Exposure Years | VISITS PER 1000 EXPOSURE YEARS | | |
|---|---|---|---|---|
| | | All | Male | Female |
| *All* | 141 | 230.3 | 220.9 | 240.0 |
| *All Under 65* | 144 | 235.3 | 227.1 | 243.6 |
| *Children* | 282 | 494.4 | 493.0 | 495.8 |
| Under 5 | 470 | 1158.2 | 1133.5 | 1184.3 |
| 5–9 | 279 | 373.1 | 366.9 | 379.4 |
| 10–14 | 199 | 247.2 | 251.2 | 243.0 |
| 15–19 | 173 | 198.6 | 206.2 | 191.6 |
| *Adults* | 46 | 53.4 | 41.5 | 65.9 |
| 20–24 | 65 | 74.5 | 43.8 | 93.6 |
| 25–34 | 63 | 74.3 | 52.2 | 94.2 |
| 35–44 | 52 | 62.5 | 50.5 | 74.7 |
| 45–54 | 36 | 39.5 | 34.2 | 44.8 |
| 55–64 | 28 | 31.8 | 25.9 | 40.4 |
| 65 and Over | 27 | 28.4 | 28.1 | 29.1 |
| Married | 48 | 56.0 | 43.8 | 68.4 |
| Single | 30 | 35.1 | 26.5 | 47.9 |
| Widowed, Divorced, Separated | 28 | 31.3 | 24.6 | 36.2 |
| Subscriber | 39 | 45.3 | 41.5 | 65.2 |
| Spouse | 55 | 64.1 | 41.7 | 66.1 |
| *Family Size* | | | | |
| 2 | 57 | 109.5 | | |
| 3 | 149 | 290.7 | | |
| 4 | 182 | 282.1 | | |
| 5 | 176 | 261.9 | | |
| 6 and Over | 178 | 277.2 | | |

* See also Chapter 5, Table 41

VARIATIONS ASSOCIATED WITH FAMILY SIZE

The use of preventive services by families of different size
was inconsistent with expectations based on experience shown
for adults and children. The average use rate of children was
nine times the average for adults. It might therefore be hypothesized that additional children in a family would raise the
per capita use of preventive services for that family. Such was
not the case. Although the differences were insignificant, they
occurred in the wrong direction, with families of five or more
showing lower per capita visits than families of three or four.

OCCUPATION CLASS VARIATIONS

Evidence of class differences in use of preventive service emerges in varying degrees depending on the type of analysis employed.

Altogether, four indices of use are available: the proportion of *patients* using preventive care (see Table 41); the number of such visits per user; the proportion of eligible *members* using; and the utilization rate—the number of preventive visits per thousand eligible members.

On all but one of these indices, the blue-collar segment of the membership placed lowest in claims for preventive service.

The greatest class differences were found in proportion of membership using any preventive service. In this respect the experience of all other occupation groups appears to have been significantly higher than that of the blue-collar category: the sales category showed 56 per cent more preventive service users, the clerical category 37 per cent, and the professional-executive class 19 per cent more than the blue-collar category. The combined white-collar proportion of preventive care users was 35 per cent higher than the blue-collar (Table 71).

TABLE 71. Proportion of Members Having One or More Preventive Service Visits, by Occupation Class of Subscriber

| OCCUPATION CLASS | *Users Per* 1000 *Exposure Years* * |
|---|---|
| Professional-Executive | 148 |
| Sales | 194 |
| Clerical and White-Collar Unspecified | 170 |
| Combined White-Collar | 168 |
| Blue-Collar | 124 |

* Including dependents.

The class differences in proportion of preventive service users assume greater significance when contrasted with the minor differences previously shown in proportions of the different classes using service of any kind (Table 35).

While the direction of the variations shown in the above table persists in the index of service utilization rates (Table 72),

TABLE 72. Preventive Visits Per 1000 Exposure Years,[*]
by Occupation Class of Subscriber

| OCCUPATION CLASS | Utilization Rate |
|---|---|
| Professional-Executive | 225.7 |
| Sales | 265.7 |
| Clerical and White-Collar Unspecified | 276.6 |
| Combined White-Collar | 267.0 |
| Blue-Collar | 206.8 |

[*] Including dependents.

the degree of variation is modified because blue-collar members, once they became users of preventive service, had somewhat more such visits per user—1.7 as against 1.4 for the sales category, 1.5 for the professional-executive category, and 1.6 for the clerical category. These variations counterbalance some of those in the previous index, reducing the class differences: Preventive visit utilization rates of sales and clerical groups were 28 per cent higher than blue-collar rates, and the professional-executive differential falls to 9 per cent.

GEOGRAPHIC VARIATIONS

Preventive service utilization ranged from 121 visits per thousand Manhattan residents to 335 for Suffolk members. The wide variation in this instance was consistent with expectations based on the age and marital distribution of the resident population in the two counties; the GHI Manhattan membership had a larger than average percentage of subgroups characterized by low preventive service use (adults in general and especially spouseless adults), while Suffolk had the highest percentage of children of any area.

Variations in other areas, however, are not so readily explained by demography. Nassau and Westchester showed almost identical utilization rates for differing populations. Westchester and New Jersey, with similar age distribution of members, showed a broad range of utilization, 324 visits in Westchester vs. 188 in New Jersey, per thousand members.

Two other indices of preventive care use—users per thousand eligibles and per thousand patients—generally followed geographic patterns similar to those shown for visit utilization rates. The fourth index, number of visits per user, was remarkably consistent from one area to the next, with Brooklyn the only area to depart from the average by as much as 13 per cent.

TABLE 73. Preventive Visit Indices of Use, by Area of Subscriber Residence *

| AREA | Users Per 1000 Exposure Years | Visits Per 1000 Exposure Years | Visits Per User |
|---|---|---|---|
| Manhattan | 74 | 121.4 | 1.6 |
| Bronx | 101 | 167.4 | 1.7 |
| New Jersey | 121 | 188.1 | 1.6 |
| Brooklyn | 111 | 197.1 | 1.8 |
| Richmond | 127 | 203.0 | 1.6 |
| Queens | 141 | 232.2 | 1.6 |
| Other New York | 169 | 274.9 | 1.6 |
| Westchester | 210 | 324.3 | 1.5 |
| Nassau | 208 | 327.3 | 1.6 |
| Suffolk | 204 | 335.1 | 1.6 |

* See also Chapter 5, Table 41

VARIATIONS WITH DURATION OF ENROLLMENT

No relationship between duration of enrollment and use of preventive service is evident in any of the indices of use.

Those in their first, third, fourth, sixth and seventh year of coverage used almost the same amounts of service, fifth-year members used 15 to 20 per cent more, second- and eighth-year members showed the lowest use (Table 74). Such findings would not be expected on the basis of the age distribution of the population enrolled in different years. The general consistency of utilization rates among enrollees of most years appears to indicate the likelihood of incurring such levels irrespective of years covered, but even if true, the significance of this finding is obscure.

TABLE 74. Preventive Visits Per 1000 Exposure Years, by Duration of Enrollment

| YEAR OF COVERAGE | Utilization Rate |
|---|---|
| 1st | 235.3 |
| 2nd | 180.8 |
| 3rd | 238.3 |
| 4th | 243.6 |
| 5th | 277.9 |
| 6th | 239.7 |
| 7th | 239.4 |
| 8th or Longer | 194.9 |
| AVERAGE | 230.3 |

# Chapter 10

# SPECIALIST CONSULTATIONS

Comprehensive plan subscribers are allowed consultations in all fields of medical and surgical practice, both in and out of the hospital. The fields in which these occurred have been discussed elsewhere (Chapter 6).

The present section presents data on frequency rates and variations—including in this case hospital services.

Nearly all consultations—86 per cent—occurred out of the hospital. The combined rate was 90.4 consultations per thousand members, of which 77.8 were office services.

Consultations represented only 1.4 per cent of office and hospital services. For this reason, variations in utilization by different segments of the population would not be expected to exert any significant influence on variations in utilization rates for all services combined. By the same token, it might be hypothesized that patterns of consultation use would not necessarily conform with the overall pattern applying to the more frequent services.

With respect to some variables, particularly occupation class and area of residence, this hypothesis was confirmed by the data; for other variables—age, sex, marital status, family size —tendencies previously noted in the overall utilization pattern appear to have been repeated and perhaps accentuated in the pattern of consultation use.

A second hypothesis posits a relationship between utiliza-

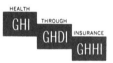

# Group Health Insurance, Inc.

221 Park Avenue South / New York, N. Y. 10003 / SPring 7-6000

GEORGE W. MELCHER, JR., M.D.
President

It is our pleasure to send you this report.
It is being distributed to individuals
professionally concerned with various phases
of health or medical care problems, in order
to implement one of the primary purposes of
the research project reported - i.e., to call
attention to an important data resource which
remains largely neglected despite continuing
scarcity of the information on disease rates
and medical care needed for rational appraisal
of a situation said to be in crisis.

We welcome comments. Please address them to
me or to Mrs. Helen H. Avnet at the above
address.

Thank you.

*George W. Melcher, Jr. M.D.*

A few findings ➜

# EXAMPLES OF FINDINGS:

ON ILLNESSES OF ADULT MALES:

Significantly more men than women were treated for the more serious conditions, e.g. most types of heart disease, malignant neoplasms of digestive, respiratory, urinary systems, and lung and liver disorders.

This finding, in conjunction with the finding that at all ages markedly lower proportions of men than women used any service, raised questions as to neglect or postponement as possible factors in the shorter life expectancy of men.

ON OUT-OF-HOSPITAL CARE:

The emphasis in discussions of medical care problems is generally directed toward hospitalized illness, but as this book reminds us, it is office-home service which represents the average person's contact with the medical profession. In the GHI experience, only 10 per cent of the membership was hospitalized, while 80 per cent incurred claims for out-of-hospital services in a single year.

ON HOSPITALIZATION:

Contrary to a hypothesis advanced by some, the inclusion of office care as an integral part of medical insurance coverage showed no apparent effect on hospital admission rates. Once admitted, however, GHI patients without office coverage tended to stay somewhat longer.

Frequency of GHI member admissions to PROPRIETARY hospitals was directly linked to relative scarcity of private VOLUNTARY beds in each area. This finding clearly indicated the limited options available to private patients and physicians and may explain why union "education" programs to change choice-of-hospital patterns have been ineffective.

ON PRIVATELY PRACTICING PHYSICIANS IN THE 8-COUNTY NEW YORK METROPOLITAN AREA:

Over half of these physicians were classified as specialists, but only 33 per cent had the Diplomate rating of an American Specialty Board.

Fewer than half the physicians were on the staff of a voluntary hospital.

ON DIAGNOSTIC X-RAYS:

NON-RADIOLOGIST SPECIALISTS PERFORMED MORE OFFICE X-RAYS THAN DID RADIOLOGISTS.

ON SURGERY:

IN-HOSPITAL SURGERY INVOLVED 370 DIFFERENT PROCEDURES FOR THE STUDY POPULATION, BUT THE 25 LEADING NON-MATERNITY PROCEDURES ACCOUNTED FOR MORE THAN HALF OF THE TOTAL VOLUME.

FOR EACH IN-HOSPITAL SURGICAL PROCEDURE, THERE WERE $2\frac{1}{2}$ OUT-OF-HOSPITAL PROCEDURES, OF WHICH 21 PER CENT WERE OF A DIAGNOSTIC NATURE.

ON AREA DIFFERENCES:

THE AVERAGE RATE OF HOME CALLS IN THE 5-COUNTY NEW YORK CITY AREA WAS 40 PER CENT HIGHER THAN THE HIGHEST RATE OUTSIDE NEW YORK CITY.

LOCAL VARIATIONS IN DIAGNOSTIC SERVICE RATES WERE AMONG THE MOST CHALLENGING FINDINGS, FROM A QUALITY STANDPOINT. THE FREQUENCY OF SPECIALIST OFFICE CONSULTATIONS IN THE AREA WITH THE HIGHEST RATE MORE THAN TRIPLED THE FREQUENCY FOUND IN THE AREA WITH THE LOWEST RATE.

FREQUENCIES OF AMBULATORY LABORATORY AND X-RAY TESTS WERE GENERALLY LOWEST IN OUTLYING AREAS.

SURGICAL PROCEDURE FREQUENCIES WERE GENERALLY HIGHEST IN OUTLYING AREAS.

HOSPITAL ADMISSION RATES OF GHI MEMBERS WERE ABOUT 50 PER CENT HIGHER IN THE TWO SUBURBAN AREAS HAVING THE HIGHEST RATIOS OF GENERAL PRIVATE BEDS TO POPULATION.

ON SOCIAL CLASS DIFFERENCES:

JUDGING BY THE PROPORTION OF MEMBERS USING INSURED SERVICES, BLUE-COLLAR FAMILIES DID NOT DIFFER SUBSTANTIALLY FROM OTHERS IN AWARENESS OF INSURANCE BENEFITS AND IN READINESS TO CALL ON THE SERVICES OF PRIVATE PHYSICIANS.

CLASS DIFFERENCES WERE APPARENT IN THE RATES OF USE OF PREVENTIVE, DIAGNOSTIC AND SPECIALIST SERVICES. SPECIALIST CONSULTATIONS WERE USED MUCH LESS FREQUENTLY BY CLERICAL AND BLUE-COLLAR FAMILIES THAN BY OTHERS.

THE RATE OF SURGICAL TREATMENT FOR LOCAL TUMORS AND CYSTS, INCLUDING BENIGN NEOPLASMS, WAS DOUBLE AMONG MALES AND MORE THAN DOUBLE AMONG FEMALES FROM PROFESSIONAL-OR-EXECUTIVE FAMILIES, AS COMPARED WITH CORRESPONDING CATEGORIES OF BLUE-COLLAR GROUPS.

THE RATE OF TREATMENT OF MALIGNANCIES AND GLAUCOMA AMONG MALES OF THE COMBINED PROFESSIONAL-EXECUTIVE-SALES CLASS WAS DOUBLE THE RATE FOUND AMONG MALES OF THE BLUE-COLLAR CLASS.

tion rates of office and hospital consultations, proposing either that a higher-than-average office consultation rate would occur in conjunction with a lower-than-average hospital consultation rate, for a given population segment; or alternatively that high rates in one index would be accompanied by high rates in the other.

Each of these propositions found some support. The high-high and low-low pattern applied in general to age, sex, family size, subscriber relationship, and in some degree to marital status. There was some evidence of a high-low pattern for certain areas and occupation classes; this was related generally to overall hospital use.

VARIATIONS BY AGE, SEX, MARITAL STATUS, SUBSCRIBER
RELATIONSHIP, FAMILY SIZE

With one exception (occupation class), the variables showing the greatest range in use of consultations were age and family size (Table 75).

While these two are related (the children's rate was two thirds of the adult rate), the number of children in the larger families was insufficient to account for the far-below-average use of consultations by such families. The rate of 53 consultations per thousand persons in families with four or more children was not only half the adult rate (105) but was lower than the rate for all children (69) and in fact lower than the lowest rate for any group of children (58, for those aged 10 to 14).

As with the overall pattern of service utilization, boys had more consultations (17 per cent more) than girls, while the women's rate was 37 per cent higher than that of the men. The only exception to the latter tendency was among the group aged 65 and over, where the men exceeded the women by 15 per cent. In the 20-to-24-year group, the number of consultations for women was two-and-one-half times the rate of the men—120 vs. 48.

Male and female patterns in general were dissimilar except for increases with age. The men's rate stabilized at a low level

TABLE 75. Specialist Consultations Per 1000 Exposure Years, by Age, Sex, Marital Status, Subscriber Relationship, and Family Size

| | CONSULTATION RATE | | | | |
| | TOTAL | | | MALE | FEMALE |
| MEMBER CATEGORY | *Office* | *Hospital* | TOTAL | TOTAL | TOTAL |
|---|---|---|---|---|---|
| All | 77.8 | 12.6 | 90.4 | 83.0 | 98.2 |
| All Under 65 | 77.1 | 12.2 | 89.3 | 81.2 | 97.9 |
| Children (to 19) | 62.1 | 6.7 | 68.8 | 74.1 | 63.4 |
| Adults | 88.4 | 16.6 | 105.0 | 88.9 | 122.0 |
| Married | 90.9 | 17.5 | 108.4 | 93.4 | 123.8 |
| Single | 69.7 | 9.0 | 78.7 | 62.5 | 103.0 |
| Widowed, Divorced, | | | | | |
| Separated | 69.4 | 15.6 | 85.0 | 41.0 | 117.5 |
| Subscriber | 80.9 | 13.5 | 94.4 | 88.7 | 124.5 |
| Spouse | 98.3 | 20.7 | 119.0 | 92.3 | 121.4 |
| Age | | | | | |
| 20–24 | 80.7 | 11.5 | 92.2 | 48.4 | 119.6 |
| 25–34 | 65.2 | 10.6 | 75.8 | 54.0 | 95.3 |
| 35–44 | 87.6 | 12.2 | , 99.8 | 83.4 | 116.5 |
| 45–54 | 91.9 | 18.5 | 110.4 | 87.9 | 133.3 |
| 55–64 | 107.7 | 26.6 | 134.3 | 124.3 | 149.0 |
| 65 and Over | 105.9 | 28.4 | 134.3 | 140.6 | 122.1 |
| Family Size | | | | | |
| 2 | 99.0 | 24.6 | 123.6 | | |
| 3 | 86.7 | 13.7 | 100.4 | | |
| 4 | 84.5 | 10.3 | 94.8 | | |
| 5 | 69.9 | 7.9 | 77.8 | | |
| 6 and Over | 45.8 | 6.9 | 52.7 | | |

from age 20 to 34, at an intermediate level from 35 to 54, then jumped 50 per cent. The women's rate started high, dipped at ages 25–34, started upward again at 35 and gradually reached a peak at 55–64, before returning nearly to the level of the youngest adult years.

Spouseless categories all had fewer consultations than the married, especially the men. This conforms with previous tendencies found applicable to overall service use rates.

Male subscribers and spouses of female subscribers showed exactly the same rates of office consultations and nearly the

# SPECIALIST CONSULTATIONS
## UTILIZATION RATES,
## BY AGE AND SEX

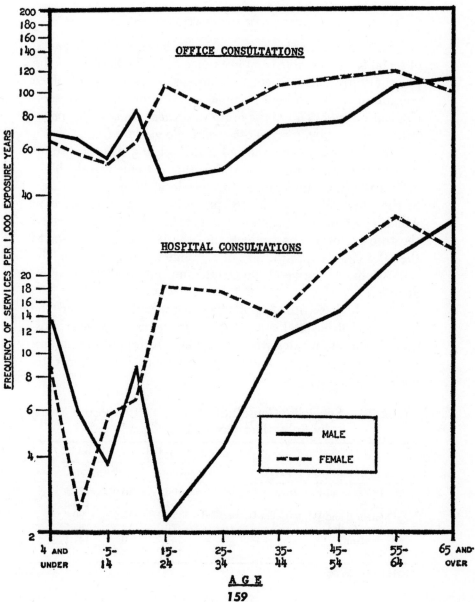

same rates of hospital consultations. Female subscribers showed a somewhat higher rate of office consultations than female spouses, while their hospital consultation rate was lower.

VARIATIONS ASSOCIATED WITH OCCUPATION CLASS

Since the subscriber's occupation is the only possible gauge of social level available from insurance data, the findings of the present study with respect to wide variations in use of office consultations by different occupational groups may be of sociological interest. *The range in use rates was broader for occupation classes than for any other variable analyzed.*

The sales category showed a rate of 185 office consultations per thousand members. At the other extreme was the blue-collar category, with a rate of 70. The clerical groups were close to the blue-collar level at 78 (providing another instance in which combining all white-collar groups would have masked the true picture). The students and the retired were closer to the sales category, with rates of 147 and 140 respectively. The professional-executive class occupied an intermediate position, at 106.

The highest utilizers of office consultations showed the lowest use of hospital consultations. In general, however, hospital consultation rates were more likely to follow the pattern of hospital use indices found for the various occupation categories.

TABLE 76. Specialist Consultations Per 1000 Exposure Years, by Subscriber Occupation Class *

| OCCUPATION CLASS | CONSULTATION RATE | | |
|---|---|---|---|
| | *Office* | *Hospital* | TOTAL |
| Professional-Executive | 106.1 | 15.0 | 121.1 |
| Sales | 184.7 | 9.1 | 193.8 |
| Clerical and White-Collar Unspecified | 78.4 | 12.2 | 90.6 |
| Blue-Collar | 70.2 | 12.3 | 82.5 |
| Student | 147.1 | 0 | 147.1 |
| Retired | 140.0 | 48.0 | 188.0 |

* Including dependents.

GEOGRAPHIC VARIATIONS

Members in the areas with the highest overall hospital use indices, Richmond and Westchester, had the highest hospital consultation rates and among the lowest office consultation rates—possibly indicating that the family physician in such areas hospitalizes first, then calls a consultant, while those with tighter bed situations may reverse the process.

This is only a theory, however; the data available suggest, but by no means confirm it. Three of the ten areas listed (Table 77) showed higher-than-average use rates for both indices. The

TABLE 77. Specialist Consultations Per 1000 Resident Members, by Area *

| | CONSULTATION RATE | | |
|---|---|---|---|
| AREA | Office | Hospital | TOTAL |
| Queens | 95.6 | 12.9 | 108.5 |
| Suffolk | 90.8 | 14.0 | 104.8 |
| Bronx | 90.4 | 15.0 | 105.4 |
| Brooklyn | 86.3 | 10.2 | 96.5 |
| Nassau | 82.9 | 11.4 | 94.3 |
| Manhattan | 82.6 | 10.1 | 92.7 |
| AVERAGE | 77.8 | 12.6 | 90.4 |
| Richmond | 71.0 | 21.2 | 92.2 |
| Westchester | 55.7 | 19.0 | 74.7 |
| Other New York | 54.8 | 13.2 | 68.0 |
| New Jersey | 30.9 | 15.0 | 45.9 |

* See also Chapter 5, Table 41.

other seven demonstrated different degrees of the high-low pattern—that is, higher-than-average on one index, lower-than-average on the other. But the range of experience was too great for ready acceptance of any theory. The highest area with respect to frequency of office consultations had a rate over three times as high as the lowest, for no known reason.

Another hypothesis which might logically be offered to explain area variations in the use of specialist consultations would introduce the question of general practitioner and specialist supply. Does the presence of more specialists encourage more consultations? Or is the opposite true—where the ratio of general practitioners is greater, are they more likely to seek the advice of consultants? There appears to be some justification for the latter theory: the areas with the highest office consultation rates—Queens, Suffolk, Bronx—have the highest ratios of general practitioners; while Westchester, with one of the lowest office consultation rates, has a high ratio of specialists. The other areas, however, failed to accommodate to this hypothesis.

VARIATIONS WITH DURATION OF ENROLLMENT

The pattern previously found in the overall service index—increasing use with longer coverage—applied, with reservations, to office consultations. The average rate of office consultations among those covered five years or more was 25 per cent higher than among those in their first four years of coverage. But members in their first, fifth, sixth and eighth years showed above-average use; fourth-year members showed about the same experience as seventh, and sixth as eighth (Table 78). The result was a see-saw pattern in use of office consultations which was not consistently related either to year of enrollment or to age characteristics of each year's enrollees.

TABLE 78. Specialist Consultations Per 1000 Exposure Years, by Duration of Enrollment

| YEAR OF COVERAGE | CONSULTATION RATE | | |
| | Office | Hospital | TOTAL |
| --- | --- | --- | --- |
| 1st | 82.3 | 8.8 | 91.1 |
| 2nd | 51.0 | 7.2 | 58.2 |
| 3rd | 70.2 | 10.8 | 81.0 |
| 4th | 75.4 | 15.2 | 90.6 |
| 5th | 96.7 | 11.6 | 108.3 |
| 6th | 87.8 | 12.8 | 100.6 |
| 7th | 76.0 | 15.1 | 91.1 |
| 8th or Longer | 87.8 | 17.1 | 104.9 |

# Chapter 11

# HOME VISITS

The 28 per cent of the study population for whom home call claims were paid accounted for 804 such calls per thousand members.

As with other types of service, these figures are weighted by the composition of the insured membership. Use of home calls was strongly related to age, sex, marital status and area of residence.

Home calls represented the second most frequent service to children—after office visits but ahead of laboratory tests, which ranked second among adults. Half the children under age 5 had home calls, averaging 3.3 calls each and producing a utilization rate of 1.7 visits per capita for this membership category.

The proportion of members receiving home calls declined steadily throughout the childhood years, reached 21 per cent at the 20-to-24-year level and varied only within 2 per cent of that level thereafter. The number of visits per user rose with age, however, peaking at ages 55 to 64 and producing the highest adult home visit utilization rate, 776 per thousand, for that age group.

Separate analysis of experience of males and females aged

20 or over revealed lower proportions of male users at every adult age level, resulting in a markedly different pattern of use for each sex. The proportion of female users varied only between 24 and 28 per cent, after the age of nine, whereas the proportion of male users showed a 100 per cent variation within the same age categories, from 14 to 29 per cent.

Throughout adulthood, women users also received more home calls per patient than men users (3.2 vs. 2.0); consequently, tremendous differences in home visit frequencies were found, the women's rate averaging 67 per cent higher than that of men (Table 79).

TABLE 79. Home Visits: Proportion of Users, Utilization Rates, and Visits Per User, by Age and Sex *

| AGE | PROPORTION OF MEMBERSHIP USING | | | UTILIZATION RATE: VISITS PER 1000 EXPOSURE YEARS | | | VISITS PER USER | |
|---|---|---|---|---|---|---|---|---|
| | All | Male | Female | All | Male | Female | Male | Female |
| | % | % | % | | | | | |
| Under 5 | 51.0 | 50.3 | 51.8 | 1699 | 1651 | 1750 | 3.3 | 3.4 |
| 5–9 | 44.0 | 43.0 | 45.0 | 1224 | 1237 | 1211 | 2.9 | 2.7 |
| 10–14 | 28.1 | 28.5 | 27.7 | 686 | 703 | 668 | 2.5 | 2.4 |
| 15–19 | 25.1 | 26.5 | 23.9 | 603 | 632 | 577 | 2.4 | 2.4 |
| 20–24 | 20.7 | 14.3 | 24.8 | 478 | 304 | 586 | 2.1 | 2.4 |
| 25–34 | 22.2 | 17.6 | 26.3 | 578 | 421 | 720 | 2.4 | 2.7 |
| 35–44 | 21.8 | 18.2 | 25.4 | 607 | 433 | 783 | 2.4 | 3.1 |
| 45–54 | 20.2 | 16.6 | 23.8 | 603 | 449 | 760 | 2.7 | 3.2 |
| 55-64 | 20.1 | 17.1 | 24.4 | 776 | 570 | 1073 | 3.3 | 4.4 |
| 65 and Over | 23.2 | 21.3 | 27.0 | 722 | 691 | 782 | 3.2 | 2.9 |
| All Adults | 21.4 | 17.8 | 25.3 | 632 | 476 | 796 | 2.0 | 3.2 |
| All Children | 37.2 | 37.2 | 37.2 | 1062 | 1069 | 1056 | 2.8 | 2.8 |

* See also Chapter 5, Table 41.

VARIATIONS BY MARITAL STATUS AND RELATIONSHIP

Spouseless males had the lowest use of home visits of any member category, irrespective of the variable analyzed—290 visits per thousand members.

Spouseless women incurred substantially lower use rates than married women—but considerably higher than those for

# OFFICE AND HOME VISITS: UTILIZATION RATES, BY AGE AND SEX

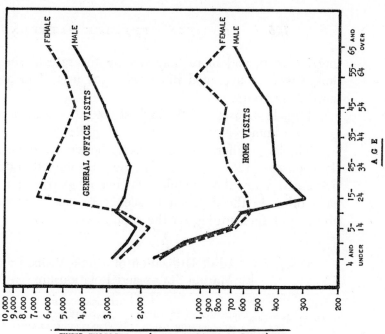

# PROPORTION OF MEMBERS AND PATIENTS: USING HOME VISITS BY AREA OF RESIDENCE AND OCCUPATION CLASS

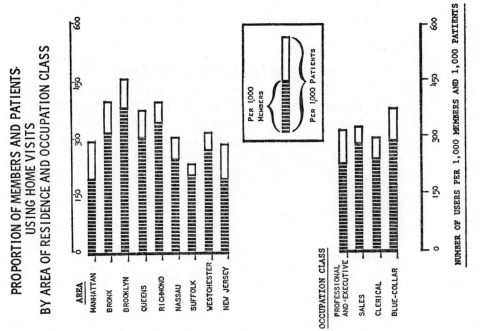

married men, and more than double the rate of single men. Single women averaged more calls per user than any other marital subgroup.

Female spouses had the highest use rates of any adult category, 831 home visits per thousand eligibles.

The large differences in use rates between the married and the spouseless raise again the question introduced in discussing preventive care—the possible influence of married partners on each other in the decision to seek care, and conversely the absence of such urging on the spouseless.

TABLE 80.   Adult Utilization of Home Visits, by Sex, by Marital Status and Relationship

| ADULT MEMBER CATEGORY | PROPORTION OF ADULT MEMBERSHIP USING | | | UTILIZATION RATE: VISITS PER 1000 EXPOSURE YEARS | | | VISITS PER USER | |
|---|---|---|---|---|---|---|---|---|
| | All | Male | Female | All | Male | Female | Male | Female |
| | % | % | % | | | | | |
| Married | 22.5 | 19.0 | 26.3 | 657 | 503 | 815 | 2.7 | 3.1 |
| Single | 12.7 | 10.1 | 16.5 | 433 | 290 | 646 | 2.9 | 3.9 |
| Widowed, Divorced, Separated | 14.9 | 9.8 | 18.7 | 479 | 291 | 618 | 2.7 | 3.3 |
| Subscriber | 18.5 | 17.9 | 21.4 | 499 | 471 | 647 | 2.6 | 3.0 |
| Spouse | 25.3 | 15.8 | 26.2 | 807 | 536 | 831 | 3.4 | 3.2 |

VARIATIONS BY FAMILY SIZE

The greatest use of home calls occurred among families of four, who averaged nearly one visit per person. Families of three or five had similar experience, with 877 and 894 calls per thousand members. But families of six or more, with four or more children, had a significantly lower rate of use, 692, contrary to what would have been expected on the basis of the higher rates found among children—but consistent with the emerging picture of low use rates among large families for other types of service such as office visits, preventive care and consultations.

TABLE 81.  Utilization of Home Visits, by Family Size

| FAMILY SIZE | Proportion of Family Members Using | Utilization Rate: Visits Per 1000 Exposure Years | Visits Per User |
|---|---|---|---|
| | % | | |
| 2 | 21.3 | 715 | 3.4 |
| 3 | 30.8 | 877 | 2.8 |
| 4 | 33.2 | 941 | 2.8 |
| 5 | 31.7 | 894 | 2.8 |
| 6 or More | 26.1 | 692 | 2.6 |

LOCAL VARIATIONS

The proportion of Brooklyn members who received home calls from their physicians during the study year was double that among the New Jersey members—38.6 per cent vs. 19.2 per cent. Another area with experience about as low as New Jersey was Suffolk County, where a high proportion of home-call users would have been expected because of its larger proportion of children.

The areas with lowest proportions of home call recipients also had the lowest number of calls per recipient and hence show only fractional utilization rates as compared with the highest areas. The rate in Suffolk was hardly more than a third of the Brooklyn rate and half or less than half the rates of Bronx, Queens, and Richmond.

In New York City proper (i.e. the five-county area as a whole), the average utilization rate of 1.03 home calls per capita was significantly higher than that in any of the outlying areas. With Manhattan excluded, the rate for the other four counties of the City rises to 1.09, as compared with a combined out-of-City rate of .52 home calls per eligible member.

The pattern suggests a definite cleavage between the attitudes of physicians in and outside the City with respect to home calls (Table 82).

TABLE 82. Utilization of Home Visits,
by Area of Subscriber Residence *

| AREA | Proportion of Resident Membership Using | Utilization Rate: Visits Per 1000 Exposure Years | Visits Per User |
|------|------|------|------|
| | % | | |
| New York City | 32.9 | 1028 | 3.1 |
| Manhattan | 20.0 | 610 | 3.1 |
| Bronx | 32.1 | 982 | 3.1 |
| Brooklyn | 38.6 | 1277 | 3.3 |
| Queens | 31.2 | 887 | 2.8 |
| Richmond | 34.5 | 1126 | 3.3 |
| Nassau | 25.4 | 651 | 2.6 |
| Suffolk | 20.6 | 446 | 2.2 |
| Westchester | 27.4 | 733 | 2.7 |
| Other New York | 16.8 | 390 | 2.3 |
| New Jersey | 19.2 | 457 | 2.4 |

* See also Chapter 5, Table 41.

VARIATIONS BY OCCUPATION CLASS

Blue-collar subscribers and their families had the highest proportion of home-call recipients—about on a par with the sales category, 20 per cent higher than the clerical group.

One explanation for the higher rate among blue-collar families could be that more of them reside in areas where the physicians are willing to make house calls (60 per cent of the

TABLE 83. Utilization of Home Visits,
by Occupation Class of Subscriber

| OCCUPATION CLASS | Proportion of Membership Using | Utilization Rate: Visits Per 1000 Exposure Years * | Visits Per User |
|------|------|------|------|
| | % | | |
| Professional | 22.9 | 663 | 2.9 |
| Executive | 26.8 | 805 | 3.0 |
| Sales | 29.0 | 878 | 3.0 |
| Clerical and White-Collar Unspecified | 24.4 | 652 | 2.7 |
| Blue-Collar | 29.6 | 878 | 3.0 |
| Student | 11.8 | 177 | 1.5 |
| Retired | 32.4 | 1480 | 4.6 |

* Including dependents.

blue-collar groups were listed as residents of Bronx, Brooklyn, Queens and Richmond, as against 34 per cent of white-collar groups).

VARIATIONS BY DURATION OF ENROLLMENT

Members in their fourth year of coverage received home calls at precisely double the rate of newcomers. Those covered less than four years showed markedly lower use—466 to 673 visits per thousand—than the more seasoned members covered for four or more years, whose rates varied between 836 and 985 visits per thousand.

Otherwise there appears to have been no pattern—the peak rates occurred among those in their fourth and seventh years of coverage.

In order to ascertain whether duration of coverage was in fact related to use of home calls, it would be necessary to rule out for each year's enrollees the effect of two strong variables previously demonstrated—age and area of residence.

TABLE 84.   Utilization of Home Visits,
by Duration of Enrollment

| YEAR OF COVERAGE | Proportion of Membership Using | Utilization Rate: Visits Per 1000 Exposure Years | Visits Per User |
|---|---|---|---|
| | % | | |
| 1st | 21.8 | 466 | 2.1 |
| 2nd | 17.9 | 523 | 2.9 |
| 3rd | 24.4 | 673 | 2.8 |
| 4th | 30.0 | 933 | 3.1 |
| 5th | 32.5 | 904 | 2.8 |
| 6th | 29.8 | 883 | 3.0 |
| 7th | 33.5 | 985 | 3.0 |
| 8th or Longer | 29.0 | 836 | 2.9 |

Further analysis of home-call use, by diagnosis, is included in the sections on "Studies of Patient Care," Chapter 17.

# Chapter 12

# DIAGNOSTIC X-RAYS

One hundred and thirty-three persons per thousand in the study population reported ambulatory diagnostic x-rays during the study year. They averaged about 1.5 procedures each, produced a utilization rate of 203 procedures per thousand. (This does not include x-rays of hospitalized patients, which are billed to the hospital insurer and therefore are not recordable by GHI.)

Most office x-rays were of the chest or extremities. Ranking next in frequency were x-rays of the gastrointestinal-abdominal tract, and the spinal-pelvic area. The four categories accounted for nine of ten procedures.

These averages reflect the composition of the GHI population. Demographic deviations in overall utilization rates, as well as in distribution by type of procedure, are discussed below.

## Variations in Overall Utilization

### VARIATIONS BY AGE AND SEX

Age was the most important factor in x-ray use (Table 85). With minor exceptions, the utilization curve climbed steadily from early childhood and then from early adulthood, through age 64. The rate at ages 55 to 64 was two-and-one-half times that of the early twenties.

TABLE 85. Out-of-Hospital Diagnostic X-rays: Proportion of
Users, Utilization Rates, and Number of Procedures
Per Patient, by Age, Sex, Marital Status,
Relationship and Family Size *

| MEMBER CATEGORY | PROPORTION OF MEMBERSHIP USING | | | PROCEDURES PER 1000 EXPOSURE YEARS | | | PROCEDURES PER PATIENT | |
|---|---|---|---|---|---|---|---|---|
| | *All* | *Male* | *Female* | *All* | *Male* | *Female* | *Male* | *Female* |
| | % | % | % | | | | | |
| *All* | 13.3 | 13.4 | 13.3 | 203 | 201 | 205 | 1.5 | 1.5 |
| Adults | 17.1 | 16.3 | 17.9 | 269 | 253 | 285 | 1.5 | 1.6 |
| Children | 7.7 | 8.9 | 6.6 | 104 | 122 | 86 | 1.4 | 1.3 |
| *Age* | | | | | | | | |
| Under 5 | 5.0 | 5.1 | 4.9 | 68 | 65 | 70 | 1.3 | 1.4 |
| 5–9 | 5.3 | 5.9 | 4.7 | 67 | 78 | 55 | 1.3 | 1.2 |
| 10–14 | 8.7 | 9.9 | 7.4 | 118 | 139 | 96 | 1.4 | 1.3 |
| 15–19 | 13.7 | 17.3 | 10.3 | 189 | 248 | 135 | 1.4 | 1.3 |
| 20–24 | 10.1 | 9.9 | 10.2 | 144 | 138 | 147 | 1.4 | 1.4 |
| 25–34 | 13.4 | 12.6 | 14.1 | 191 | 180 | 201 | 1.4 | 1.4 |
| 35–44 | 16.9 | 16.0 | 17.9 | 253 | 233 | 273 | 1.5 | 1.5 |
| 45–54 | 18.2 | 16.8 | 19.7 | 302 | 261 | 344 | 1.6 | 1.7 |
| 55–64 | 20.4 | 18.8 | 22.6 | 347 | 327 | 376 | 1.7 | 1.7 |
| 65 and Over | 20.8 | 21.6 | 19.2 | 321 | 336 | 291 | 1.6 | 1.5 |
| *Marital Status* | | | | | | | | |
| Married | 17.5 | 17.0 | 18.0 | 276 | 264 | 288 | 1.6 | 1.6 |
| Single | 14.0 | 12.0 | 17.1 | 206 | 175 | 253 | 1.5 | 1.5 |
| Widowed, Divorced, | | | | | | | | |
| Separated | 13.2 | 10.7 | 15.1 | 243 | 201 | 274 | 1.9 | 1.8 |
| *Relationship* | | | | | | | | |
| Subscriber | 17.0 | 16.6 | 19.1 | 261 | 256 | 285 | 1.5 | 1.5 |
| Spouse | 17.2 | 13.3 | 17.6 | 279 | 211 | 285 | 1.6 | 1.6 |
| *Family Size* | | | | | | | | |
| 2 | 18.8 | | | 302 | | | 1.6 | |
| 3 | 14.8 | | | 230 | | | 1.6 | |
| 4 | 13.3 | | | 197 | | | 1.5 | |
| 5 | 10.1 | | | 147 | | | 1.5 | |
| 6 or More | 8.5 | | | 119 | | | 1.4 | |

* See also Chapter 5, Table 41.

Overall rates for males and females were almost identical;
but this was more coincidence that consistency, resulting from
differences at one age balancing those of another.

Males aged 5 to 19 had substantially higher rates than
females, particularly during the late teens (248 procedures per
thousand boys vs. 135 for girls aged 15 to 19). Starting at age

20, the women's rate exceeded the men's at each level to age 65, at which point the male rate continued its steady increase while the female rate receded. From age 45 through 64, utilization among women topped the highest rate of men at any age. Male-female rates were closest before age 5, and proportionately close at ages 20 to 34.

The number of procedures per x-rayed patient was generally similar for males and females. It varied primarily by age, from 1.3 for children under 10 to 1.7 for adults aged 45 to 64.

### VARIATIONS ASSOCIATED WITH MARITAL STATUS

Spouseless males experienced markedly lower utilization than the married (Table 85). For single males, the rate was consistent with expectations based on age distribution. The low rate among the widowed-divorced-separated group, however, is not so readily explained. It reflects an extraordinarily low proportion of x-ray users—107 per thousand, vs. 170 among married males and 120 for single males. The utilization rate of 201 procedures per thousand, compared with 264 for married and 175 for single males, reached even this low level only because the number of x-rays per patient among widowed-divorced-separated males, 1.9, was exceptionally high.

Widowed-divorced-separated females showed markedly higher use indices than their male counterparts. Procedures per patient were somewhat lower, at 1.8, but their proportion of x-ray users ran 40 per cent higher, resulting in a procedure utilization rate of 274 vs. the male 201. There were about 20 per cent more users among the married women, but the effect of this was almost cancelled by a lower number of procedures per patient, so that the two female groups, unlike the corresponding groups of men, showed similar utilization rates.

### VARIATIONS BY FAMILY SIZE

Among families of two, three, and four persons, per capita use of x-rays decreased with increasing size, as expected based on age distribution of family members. The experience of families of five was only slightly below expected levels, while families of six, true to their usual pattern, used markedly fewer services than would have been anticipated on the basis of family composition.

GEOGRAPHIC VARIATIONS

Member residents of one of the areas highest in ratio of non-government hospital beds to population, Richmond, registered significantly lower ambulatory x-ray use rates than members in the other four boroughs of New York City and the adjacent counties of Westchester and Nassau. Since Richmond members experienced the highest use of hospitalization and the lowest use of office care in metropolitan New York, the explanation for their low office x-ray rate may lie in the same direction.

On the other hand, residents of New Jersey experienced even lower x-ray rates than Richmond, but their hospitalization rates were also low.

The comparatively low x-ray rate in Suffolk County would be expected on the basis of its high proportion of children.

The six more central geographic areas clustered at the upper level of use rates (i.e. above the overall average) within a relatively narrow range, from 207 to 229 procedures per thousand exposure years, as compared with the wide lower range, 135 to 183, demonstrated in the four outlying areas (Table 86).

A similar distribution was found when the different areas were ranged according to proportion of members having any office x-rays: 139 to 149 per thousand in the six more central counties; 93 to 124 in the other four areas listed.

As will be shown in the next chapter, utilization of laboratory tests tended to follow a geographic pattern similar to that shown for diagnostic x-rays.

TABLE 86. Out-of-Hospital Diagnostic X-ray Utilization, by Area of Subscriber Residence *

| AREA | Proportion of Membership Using | Procedures Per 1000 Exposure Years | Procedures Per Patient |
|---|---|---|---|
| | % | | |
| Queens | 14.8 | 229.0 | 1.5 |
| Nassau | 14.9 | 225.0 | 1.5 |
| Westchester | 14.1 | 219.6 | 1.6 |
| Brooklyn | 13.9 | 219.2 | 1.6 |
| Manhattan | 14.0 | 213.8 | 1.5 |
| Bronx | 14.1 | 207.2 | 1.5 |
| AVERAGE | 13.3 | 202.6 | 1.6 |
| Suffolk | 12.4 | 183.2 | 1.5 |
| Richmond | 11.5 | 170.6 | 1.5 |
| New Jersey | 10.6 | 150.7 | 1.4 |
| Other New York | 9.3 | 134.8 | 1.5 |

* See also Chapter 5, Table 41.

OCCUPATION CLASS VARIATIONS

The use of diagnostic x-rays among the professional-executive classes was 25 per cent higher than in the blue-collar groups. The latter in turn experienced a rate 22 per cent higher than the clerical groups.

As with other types of ambulatory services, the sales class had a higher x-ray rate than any other occupation category.

TABLE 87. Out-of-Hospital Diagnostic X-ray Utilization, by Occupation Class *

| OCCUPATION CLASS | Proportion of Membership Using | Procedures Per 1000 Exposure Years † | Procedures Per Patient |
|---|---|---|---|
| | % | | |
| Professional-Executive | 16.1 | 257.1 | 1.6 |
| Sales | 20.1 | 368.3 | 1.8 |
| Clerical and White-Collar Unspecified | 11.7 | 169.6 | 1.4 |
| Blue-Collar | 13.5 | 206.2 | 1.5 |
| Student | 17.7 | 205.9 | 1.2 |
| Retired | 21.6 | 312.0 | 1.4 |

* See also Chapter 5, Table 41.
† Including dependents.

Their utilization of 368 procedures per thousand was more than double the clerical rate and 30 per cent higher than the professional-executive rate. The extraordinary utilization by the sales class was associated with the compounding of two other high indices: 201 x-rayed persons per thousand members, compared with the average of 133; and 1.8 procedures per x-rayed patient, compared with the average of 1.5.

## Component X-Ray Procedures

The distribution of office x-rays among the various procedure categories is summarized in Table 88. Two out of three procedures involved the chest or extremities.

TABLE 88. Frequency and Distribution of Out-of-Hospital Diagnostic X-rays, by Procedure Category

| PROCEDURE CATEGORY | Procedures Per 1000 Exposure Years | Distribution |
|---|---|---|
| | | % |
| TOTAL | 202.6 | 100.0 |
| Chest | 74.9 | 38.6 |
| Extremities | 53.1 | 27.3 |
| Abdominal Tract | 29.2 | 15.0 |
| Spine and Pelvis | 19.8 | 10.2 |
| Head and Neck | 9.0 | 4.7 |
| Kidney | 6.2 | 3.2 |
| Other | 1.9 | 1.0 |
| Unclassified | 8.5 | — |

### Distribution by Age, Males and Females

When the distribution of procedures was analyzed in further detail at different age levels (Table 89), principal variations were noted for the younger generation.

Over half the x-rays of males under 25 involved the extremities, as against a range of 15 to 26 per cent after age 25. A similar pattern at a lower level was found for females. The chest x-ray ranked second for the young groups, did not assume first place until age 25.

TABLE 89. Distribution of Out-of-Hospital Diagnostic X-rays, by Procedure Category, Males and Females, by Age

| | Total * | Chest | Extrem-ities | Abdomen | Spine-Pelvis | Head-Neck | Kidney | Other † |
|---|---|---|---|---|---|---|---|---|
| | % | % | % | % | % | % | % | % |
| **MALES** | | | | | | | | |
| Under 5 | 100 | 22.1 | 50.7 | 1.4 | 7.4 | 18.4 | 0 | 0 |
| 5–14 | 100 | 26.6 | 56.4 | 3.5 | 4.1 | 7.2 | 1.8 | .4 |
| 15–24 | 100 | 31.7 | 49.5 | 3.5 | 6.6 | 7.2 | 1.3 | .2 |
| 25–34 | 100 | 40.5 | 25.9 | 14.2 | 12.7 | 4.7 | 2.0 | 0 |
| 35–44 | 100 | 44.1 | 18.4 | 19.6 | 8.9 | 4.8 | 4.1 | .1 |
| 45–54 | 100 | 44.4 | 20.8 | 14.8 | 11.1 | 3.7 | 5.1 | .1 |
| 55–64 | 100 | 47.4 | 14.9 | 19.7 | 9.5 | 2.0 | 6.4 | .1 |
| 65 and Over | 100 | 49.3 | 18.0 | 14.3 | 9.2 | 4.1 | 5.1 | 0 |
| **ALL MALES** | 100 | 40.5 | 28.0 | 13.5 | 9.0 | 5.0 | 3.9 | .1 |
| **FEMALES** | | | | | | | | |
| Under 5 | 100 | 23.7 | 45.3 | 3.6 | 6.5 | 18.8 | 1.4 | .7 |
| 5–14 | 100 | 38.5 | 47.6 | 2.7 | 3.8 | 6.2 | .3 | .9 |
| 15–24 | 100 | 31.2 | 37.6 | 9.7 | 11.8 | 4.2 | 3.7 | 1.8 |
| 25–34 | 100 | 35.0 | 20.8 | 17.7 | 12.2 | 4.7 | 4.3 | 5.3 |
| 35–44 | 100 | 36.6 | 20.8 | 20.6 | 12.7 | 3.9 | 3.0 | 2.4 |
| 45–54 | 100 | 37.4 | 25.6 | 17.3 | 13.8 | 3.2 | 1.6 | 1.1 |
| 55–64 | 100 | 39.4 | 22.0 | 22.4 | 9.9 | 2.4 | 3.1 | .8 |
| 65 and Over | 100 | 47.4 | 17.9 | 20.0 | 10.5 | 3.1 | 0 | 1.1 |
| **ALL FEMALES** | 100 | 36.6 | 26.7 | 16.6 | 11.4 | 4.3 | 2.5 | 1.9 |

* Excluding unclassified procedures.
† Principally gynecological procedures and mammography.

X-rays of the abdominal tract also became relatively more important after age 25, occasionally displacing x-rays of the extremities in second place.

Among children under 5, head x-rays (mainly skull studies) accounted for nearly every fifth procedure—in marked contrast to the population as a whole, with only one of twenty procedures in this category.

Procedures involving the extremities, spine or pelvic region, and abdomen generally accounted for a larger percentage of female than male x-rays after the age of 35, while chest x-rays were relatively somewhat more important to males than females after age 25.

## Utilization Rates

The over-all tendency toward increasing x-ray utilization with advancing years applies most dramatically to the largest category, *chest x-rays*, where the rate at 65 plus, 145 per thousand members, was nine to ten times that of the youngest group. Male use of chest x-rays generally exceeded that of females, although the differences were minor except at ages 15 to 24 and past 64.

Rates of *abdominal procedures* reached their highest level at ages 55 to 64, then returned to the level reached in the forties. For both males and females a decided jump in this category occurred at age 25, again at 35, and finally at 55. At all ages past 15, female rates exceeded male rates by at least 20 per cent.

From ages 35 to 64, women also experienced substantially higher rates of *spinal-pelvic* x-rays than men. The age pattern differed here—the men's rate neared its peak at 45 to 54 and remained around the same level thereafter; the women's rate peaked during the same years—at a level 60 per cent higher than the men's—but then decreased, meeting the male rate by age 65. Most of this category was accounted for by spinal x-rays (lumbo-sacral or cervical).

*Urological* procedures (mainly pyelography) for males were performed at increasing rates with each age increment to 65. The picture for females was less consistent, although the highest rate of use was also reached before age 65. Females aged 15 to 34 experienced higher rates than males of corresponding ages, but male rates after 45 were much higher than female, readily accounting for an overall male rate more than 50 per cent higher.

There was no discernible age pattern related to frequencies of *head or neck x-rays*. The rate for males averaged 25 per cent higher than that for females.

*X-rays of the extremities* headed the list for age groups through 24. The rates were substantially the same for males and females under 5, but diverged after that. Boys incurred

# UTILIZATION RATES OF
## COMPONENT DIAGNOSTIC X-RAY CATEGORIES
### BY AGE AND SEX

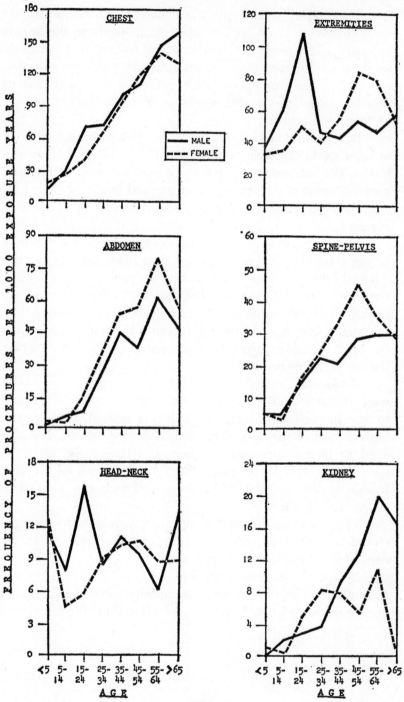

# DIAGNOSTIC X-RAY PROCEDURES: OUT-OF-HOSPITAL RATES, BY AGE AND SEX

# COMPARISON OF DIAGNOSTIC X-RAY UTILIZATION BY BLUE-COLLAR AND PROFESSIONAL-EXECUTIVE CLASSES, BY TYPE OF PROCEDURE AND BY SEX

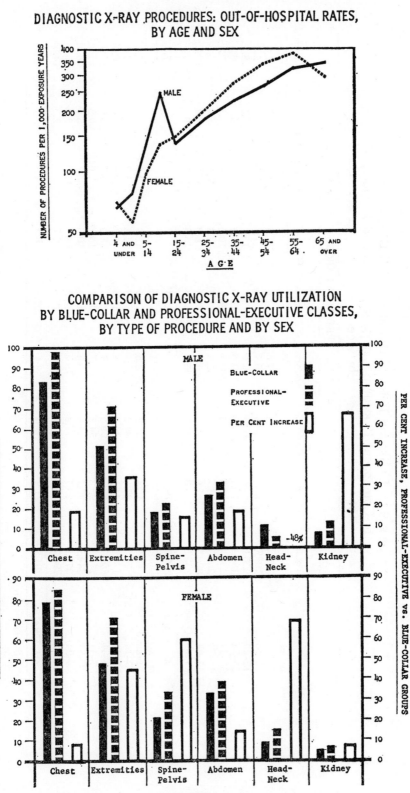

TABLE 90. Utilization Rates of Out-of-Hospital Diagnostic X-rays in Component Procedure Categories, Males and Females, by Age

| | Total | Chest* | Extremities | Abdomen | Spine-Pelvis | Head-Neck | Kidney | Other | Unclassified |
|---|---|---|---|---|---|---|---|---|---|
| | PROCEDURES PER 1000 EXPOSURE YEARS | | | | | | | | |
| **MALES** | | | | | | | | | |
| Under 5 | 65.4 | 14.0 | 32.2 | 1.0 | 4.6 | 11.7 | 0 | 0 | 1.9 |
| 5–14 | 107.9 | 28.1 | 59.5 | 3.7 | 4.3 | 7.7 | 1.9 | .4 | 2.3 |
| 15–24 | 225.0 | 68.8 | 107.3 | 7.6 | 14.2 | 15.7 | 2.8 | .5 | 8.1 |
| 25–34 | 180.1 | 70.4 | 44.9 | 24.6 | 22.0 | 8.2 | 3.5 | 0 | 6.5 |
| 35–44 | 233.4 | 99.5 | 41.5 | 44.1 | 20.1 | 10.9 | 9.2 | .3 | 7.8 |
| 45–54 | 260.7 | 111.7 | 52.3 | 37.3 | 28.0 | 9.3 | 12.7 | .3 | 9.1 |
| 55–64 | 326.7 | 147.0 | 46.2 | 61.0 | 29.5 | 6.0 | 19.9 | .4 | 16.7 |
| 65 and Over | 335.8 | 158.3 | 57.7 | 45.8 | 29.6 | 13.3 | 16.3 | 0 | 14.8 |
| ALL MALES | 200.8 | 78.4 | 54.2 | 26.1 | 17.4 | 9.7 | 7.4 | .3 | 7.3 |
| **FEMALES** | | | | | | | | | |
| Under 5 | 69.9 | 16.4 | 31.2 | 2.5 | 4.5 | 12.9 | 1.0 | .5 | 1.0 |
| 5–14 | 75.2 | 27.6 | 34.2 | 1.9 | 2.8 | 4.5 | .2 | .6 | 3.4 |
| 15–24 | 138.5 | 41.1 | 49.5 | 12.8 | 15.5 | 5.6 | 4.8 | 2.4 | 6.8 |
| 25–34 | 200.7 | 66.7 | 39.5 | 33.7 | 23.3 | 8.9 | 8.1 | 10.0 | 10.5 |
| 35–44 | 272.9 | 95.3 | 54.3 | 53.7 | 33.1 | 10.2 | 7.9 | 6.2 | 12.2 |
| 45–54 | 344.2 | 122.7 | 83.9 | 56.6 | 45.1 | 10.6 | 5.2 | 3.7 | 16.4 |
| 55–64 | 375.9 | 139.7 | 77.9 | 79.7 | 35.2 | 8.7 | 11.0 | 2.9 | 20.8 |
| 65 and Over | 290.7 | 130.8 | 49.4 | 55.3 | 29.1 | 8.7 | 0 | 2.9 | 14.5 |
| ALL FEMALES | 204.5 | 71.2 | 52.0 | 32.4 | 22.3 | 8.4 | 4.8 | 3.7 | 9.7 |

* Including rib x-rays.

over 70 per cent more such x-rays at ages 5 to 14. During the age interval 15 to 24, males more than doubled the female rate, with 107 x-rays per thousand. The latter figure far exceeds that incurred by any other age group for x-rays of extremities.

At age 35, the female rate for this type of procedure started to exceed the male rate. From 45 to 54 it was 60 per cent higher, from 55 to 64 it was 70 per cent higher, before returning to its young-adult rate, at age 65, and falling below the corresponding male rate.

Thus the women reached their highest use of this category at ages 45 to 54, with a frequency rate of 84 per thousand, while the males reached theirs 30 years earlier.

Differences between the sexes as to relative incidence of upper vs. lower extremity x-rays are noteworthy (Table 91). At

TABLE 91.  Frequency of Out-of-Hospital Diagnostic X-rays of Upper and Lower Extremities, by Age and Sex

| | PROCEDURES PER 1000 EXPOSURE YEARS | | | |
| | UPPER EXTREMITIES | | LOWER EXTREMITIES | |
| AGE | *Males* | *Females* | *Males* | *Females* |
|---|---|---|---|---|
| Under 5 | 14.9 | 18.3 | 17.3 | 12.9 |
| 5–14 | 34.7 | 17.2 | 24.8 | 17.0 |
| 15–24 | 54.1 | 15.2 | 53.2 | 34.3 |
| 25–34 | 25.5 | 18.2 | 19.4 | 21.3 |
| 35–44 | 24.0 | 26.3 | 17.5 | 28.0 |
| 45–54 | 25.7 | 39.9 | 26.6 | 44.0 |
| 55–64 | 26.3 | 28.3 | 19.9 | 49.6 |
| 65 and Over | 23.7 | 20.3 | 34.0 | 29.1 |

all ages past 15, women had more x-rays of lower than upper extremities—strikingly so at ages 15 to 24 and 55 to 64. Males, in contrast, generally had more x-rays of the upper extremities except at the youngest and oldest age levels.

During the age period 55 to 64, when the rates for upper extremity x-rays were almost the same for both sexes, the female rate for lower extremities climbed to two-and-one-half times the male rate.

Wide variations were also observed in rates of component abdominal procedures at various ages and between the sexes. Most notable was the marked excess in female over male rates of gall bladder x-rays, at all ages (Table 92).

TABLE 92. Frequency of Out-of-Hospital Component Abdominal X-ray Procedures Among Males and Females, by Age

| | PROCEDURES PER 1000 EXPOSURE YEARS | | | | | | | |
|---|---|---|---|---|---|---|---|---|
| | UPPER GI TRACT | | GALL BLADDER | | COLON BY BARIUM ENEMA | | FLAT PLATE | |
| AGE | Male | Female | Male | Female | Male | Female | Male | Female |
| Under 5 | 0 | 1.0 | 0 | 0 | 0 | 0 | .5 | 1.5 |
| 5–14 | 1.7 | .9 | 0 | 0 | .3 | .6 | 1.7 | .2 |
| 15–24 | 4.3 | 6.0 | .9 | 2.8 | .9 | 2.0 | .6 | 1.2 |
| 25–34 | 10.4 | 11.6 | 2.1 | 11.6 | 6.9 | 4.3 | 3.9 | 4.6 |
| 35–44 | 22.0 | 19.0 | 8.4 | 17.5 | 8.9 | 9.3 | 4.2 | 6.5 |
| 45–54 | 20.6 | 21.0 | 5.4 | 18.4 | 6.2 | 11.5 | 4.2 | 4.3 |
| 55–64 | 30.7 | 31.8 | 14.3 | 25.4 | 10.8 | 15.0 | 3.6 | 6.3 |
| 65 and Over | 28.1 | 23.3 | 4.4 | 5.8 | 11.8 | 14.6 | 1.5 | 8.7 |

Further details as to utilization rates of individual procedures are presented in Table 93, with some reclassification to separate skeletal from other x-rays.

### Occupation Class Variations in Type of X-ray Use

In a search for possible clarification of occupation-class differences in x-ray utilization rates, frequencies experienced for the different types of procedures have been compared.

Results are illustrated below in a comparison of blue-collar with professional-executive rates. As previously shown (Table 87) the latter groups experienced an overall x-ray use rate 25 per cent higher than the former.

One of the first findings is that the females of the two groups were further apart than the males. Females in professional-executive families experienced an overall rate 30 per cent higher than those in blue-collar families, as against a 20 per cent figure for the corresponding male groups.

Secondly, the analysis by x-ray site demonstrates substan-

TABLE 93. Individual X-ray Procedures: Out-of-Hospital Frequencies, by Sex

| TYPE OF PROCEDURE | NUMBER PER 1000 EXPOSURE YEARS | | |
|---|---|---|---|
| | *All* | *Male* | *Female* |
| Skeletal | | | |
| Skull | 5.1 | 5.6 | 4.6 |
| Nasal Bones | .8 | 1.1 | .5 |
| Other Head-Neck | 1.3 | 1.3 | 1.4 |
| Ribs | 1.6 | 1.4 | 1.7 |
| Spine | 18.1 | 16.3 | 20.1 |
| Lumbosacral | 7.0 | 6.2 | 7.7 |
| Cervical | 6.2 | 5.9 | 6.6 |
| Lumbar | 2.6 | 2.0 | 3.1 |
| Thoracic | 1.7 | 1.7 | 1.8 |
| Complete | .6 | .5 | .9 |
| Pelvis | 1.7 | 1.1 | 2.2 |
| Hip | 1.4 | 1.4 | 1.4 |
| Femur | .4 | .6 | .2 |
| Knee | 6.4 | 7.5 | 5.1 |
| Leg | 2.4 | 2.3 | 2.5 |
| Ankle | 5.2 | 4.1 | 6.3 |
| Foot | 9.9 | 8.3 | 11.6 |
| Toe | 1.0 | .7 | 1.4 |
| Shoulder, Clavicle, Scapula | 7.9 | 8.0 | 7.9 |
| Humerus | .7 | .8 | .6 |
| Elbow | 2.9 | 3.5 | 2.2 |
| Forearm | 2.0 | 1.8 | 2.2 |
| Wrist | 3.9 | 4.6 | 3.2 |
| Hand | 5.3 | 6.2 | 4.4 |
| Finger | 3.7 | 4.4 | 3.0 |
| Chest | 73.3 | 77.0 | 69.5 |
| Abdominal Tract | 29.2 | 26.1 | 32.4 |
| Flat Plate | 3.1 | 2.7 | 3.4 |
| Upper GI Series | 12.7 | 13.3 | 12.1 |
| Colon-Barium Enema | 5.4 | 5.0 | 5.9 |
| Gall Bladder | 7.1 | 4.4 | 10.0 |
| Other | .9 | .7 | 1.0 |
| Urological Tract | 6.2 | 7.4 | 4.8 |
| Kidney | 1.6 | 2.0 | 1.2 |
| Pyelography | 4.5 | 5.3 | 3.6 |
| Other | .1 | .1 | 0 |
| Gynecological-Mammary | 1.7 | — | 3.5 |
| Nasal-Sinus | 1.8 | 1.7 | 1.9 |
| All Other Known | .2 | .3 | .2 |
| Unclassified | 8.5 | 7.3 | 9.7 |
| TOTAL | 202.6 | 200.8 | 204.5 |

tially different patterns of class differences for males and females. Professional-executive class females had 60 to 69 per cent more x-rays of the spine, head-neck, and lower extremities than blue-collar group females. The corresponding differences among the males of the two classes were much lower—and in fact in the other direction with respect to head-neck x-rays.

The professional-executive class males experienced a chest x-ray rate 19 per cent higher than the blue-collar class males, but minimal differences were found between the two groups of females.

The data in Table 94, together with that presented in the analysis of component ambulatory surgical procedures by occupation class, represent a first step toward evaluation of possibly significant class differences in use of these services.

TABLE 94. Differences in X-ray Utilization of Blue-Collar and Professional-Executive Classes, by Type of Procedure, by Sex

| | MALES | | | FEMALES | | |
|---|---|---|---|---|---|---|
| | Number of Procedures Per 1000 Exposure Years | | | Number of Procedures Per 1000 Exposure Years | | |
| TYPE OF PROCEDURE | (Col. 1) | (Col. 2) | % Increase Col. 2/1 | (Col. 4) | (Col. 5) | % Increase Col. 5/4 |
| | Blue Collar Families | Professional Executive Families | | Blue Collar Families | Professional Executive Families | |
| Chest | 83.9 | 99.5 | 19 | 78.5 | 84.1 | 7 |
| Extremities | 52.0 | 70.6 | 36 | 48.4 | 70.3 | 45 |
| Upper | 27.8 | 38.3 | 38 | 22.0 | 27.5 | 25 |
| Lower | 24.2 | 32.3 | 33 | 26.4 | 42.8 | 62 |
| Spine-Pelvis | 18.5 | 21.5 | 16 | 20.9 | 33.4 | 60 |
| Abdomen | 26.5 | 31.6 | 19 | 33.2 | 37.7 | 14 |
| Head-Neck | 10.4 | 5.4 | — | 8.6 | 14.5 | 69 |
| Kidney | 7.6 | 12.8 | 68 | 4.8 | 5.1 | 6 |
| Other and Unclassified | 6.6 | 5.4 | — | 12.4 | 23.2 | 87 |
| TOTAL | 205.5 | 246.8 | 20 | 206.8 | 268.3 | 30 |

# Chapter 13

# LABORATORY PROCEDURES

Nearly 700 laboratory tests per thousand members were recorded for the study year. This number excludes simple urinalyses and hemoglobin tests, for which no separate payment is made, as well as tests on hospitalized patients, which are billed to the hospitalization insurers.

Since the excluded routine office tests are undoubtedly the most frequent, their exclusion from the utilization rates presented below must be emphasized, to preclude comparison with other experience where the same exclusion is not feasible.

The proportion of the membership having laboratory tests was not much higher than the proportion x-rayed—165 vs. 133 per thousand members—but the number of laboratory tests recorded per patient was nearly triple the number of x-ray procedures—4.2 vs. 1.5. In general, variations in x-ray and laboratory use among different population segments tended to follow similar patterns.

The great majority of recorded laboratory procedures were blood tests of one kind or another. With the exclusion of simple urinalysis from the list of tests paid for separately, the category urinalysis accounted for less than one per cent of tabulated procedures.

## Variations in Overall Utilization

### VARIATIONS BY AGE AND SEX

The frequency of laboratory tests increased steadily throughout childhood and adulthood, reaching its peak at ages 55 to 64 among the men and after 65 among the women.

The rate for children advanced from 162 procedures per thousand before age 5, to 453 at ages 15 to 19, averaging 262. The rate for adults increased from 576 at ages 20–24 to a top of 1370 at ages 55 to 64, averaging 982 procedures per thousand adults of all ages.

The utilization rates for women past 20 were substantially higher than for men at all ages except 55 to 64, when they were the same. These higher female rates resulted from a much higher proportion of laboratory users—high enough to override the finding of substantially more procedures per male than female patient, particularly from ages 25 through 64. Males who used any laboratory service averaged 4.7 tests each, vs. 3.9 for female patients.

The number of tests per laboratory patient ranged from 2.0 at the youngest age level to 5.8 at ages 55 to 64 (Table 95).

### VARIATIONS ASSOCIATED WITH RELATIONSHIP AND SEX

This is the only instance of a service for which the utilization rate of female subscribers was lower than that of male subscribers (888 vs. 945 procedures per thousand). The proportion of users was considerably higher among these women, but they had only 3.8 procedures per user as against 5.4 for the men.

### VARIATIONS ASSOCIATED WITH MARITAL STATUS

As with other types of service such as preventive care and home calls, marital status was associated with major differences

TABLE 95.  Laboratory Procedures *: Proportion of Membership Using,
Utilization Rates, and Number of Procedures Per Patient,
by Age, Sex, Marital Status, Relationship
and Family Size

| MEMBER CATEGORY | PROPORTION OF MEMBERSHIP USING | | | PROCEDURES PER 1000 EXPOSURE YEARS | | | PROCEDURES PER PATIENT | |
|---|---|---|---|---|---|---|---|---|
| | All | Male | Female | All | Male | Female | Male | Female |
| | % | % | % | | | | | |
| *All* | 16.5 | 14.1 | 19.0 | 693 | 658 | 732 | 4.7 | 3.9 |
| Adults | 21.2 | 17.4 | 25.2 | 982 | 922 | 1046 | 5.3 | 4.2 |
| Children | 9.5 | 9.2 | 9.9 | 262 | 257 | 267 | 2.8 | 2.7 |
| *Age* | | | | | | | | |
| Under 5 | 8.0 | 8.1 | 7.9 | 162 | 162 | 162 | 2.0 | 2.1 |
| 5–9 | 9.9 | 9.6 | 10.2 | 243 | 230 | 256 | 2.4 | 2.5 |
| 10–14 | 8.9 | 8.1 | 9.7 | 270 | 255 | 285 | 3.1 | 3.0 |
| 15–19 | 12.5 | 12.4 | 12.6 | 453 | 480 | 427 | 3.9 | 3.4 |
| 20–24 | 19.1 | 10.1 | 24.6 | 576 | 316 | 739 | 3.1 | 3.0 |
| 25–34 | 17.9 | 10.8 | 24.2 | 707 | 553 | 845 | 5.1 | 3.5 |
| 35–44 | 20.9 | 15.7 | 26.1 | 860 | 786 | 936 | 5.0 | 3.6 |
| 45–54 | 21.7 | 18.8 | 24.6 | 1068 | 985 | 1153 | 5.2 | 4.7 |
| 55–64 | 23.6 | 22.5 | 25.2 | 1370 | 1370 | 1370 | 6.1 | 5.2 |
| 65 and Over | 25.8 | 24.7 | 27.9 | 1279 | 1197 | 1442 | 4.8 | 5.2 |
| *Marital Status* | | | | | | | | |
| Married | 22.0 | 18.1 | 26.0 | 1023 | 972 | 1076 | 5.4 | 4.2 |
| Single | 15.0 | 12.6 | 18.7 | 683 | 591 | 820 | 4.7 | 4.4 |
| Widowed, Divorced, Separated | 16.1 | 12.3 | 19.0 | 660 | 586 | 714 | 4.8 | 3.8 |
| *Relationship* | | | | | | | | |
| Subscriber | 18.5 | 17.5 | 23.6 | 937 | 945 | 888 | 5.4 | 3.8 |
| Spouse | 24.7 | 15.8 | 25.5 | 1043 | 596 | 1082 | 3.8 | 4.2 |
| *Family Size* | | | | | | | | |
| 2 | 22.7 | | | 1194 | | | 5.2 | |
| 3 | 19.4 | | | 801 | | | 4.1 | |
| 4 | 16.6 | | | 615 | | | 3.7 | |
| 5 | 13.4 | | | 460 | | | 3.4 | |
| 6 or More | 10.0 | | | 376 | | | 3.8 | |

* Out-of-hospital procedures except simple urinalysis and hemoglobin tests.

in use of laboratory services. The rates of use among the married, both males and females, were over 50 per cent higher than among the spouseless. Rates for single persons were consistent with expectations based on age, but this was not true of the widowed-divorced-separated category.

### VARIATIONS BY FAMILY SIZE

The usual pattern of decreasing per capita use with increasing family size was found, with the largest families using less service than expected based on family composition.

### GEOGRAPHIC VARIATIONS

The geographic pattern of laboratory procedure utilization was generally similar to that found for diagnostic x-rays; the same six areas showed the higher range of use rates, from 705 to 834 procedures per thousand members, while members residing in the other four areas listed had rates of 361 to 490. (Thus the disparities between the two ranges are much greater than for x-rays.)

Comparison of the several indices which contributed to the laboratory utilization rate revealed that the areas with above-average numbers of procedures per thousand members were usually (but not always) above average on other laboratory test indices. It is also observed that three of the four areas with low laboratory utilization showed higher-than-average proportions of their resident membership using some other type of service.

Richmond, with a utilization rate of 475 laboratory procedures per thousand residents vs. the overall average of 693, showed a higher-than-average proportion reporting for medical service of some kind (87 per cent vs. 80 per cent); but of these, the smallest proportion of any area was sent for ambulatory laboratory tests, and they had fewer tests each, both factors contributing to the low rate. As has been hypothesized in explanation of low service rates for other types of ambulatory service in Richmond, it may be that physicians there wait until the patient is hospitalized to have laboratory tests performed.

Manhattan experienced the lowest percentage of members seeking any medical service, but of those reporting, sent the highest proportion for laboratory tests, and averaged more tests per patient than any area except Brooklyn.

Westchester had the highest proportion of laboratory users per thousand members of any area, but they had fewer tests each, bringing the procedure utilization rate down below that of the five leading areas.

The low rates in Suffolk may be attributed partly to its youthful population; but the membership of its neighbor Nassau, with a rate over 50 per cent higher, is not much older.

The three areas with the highest proportions of practicing specialists—Manhattan, Westchester and Nassau—sent the highest proportions of patients for laboratory tests. But the hypothesis suggested by this observation is not supported in other areas (Table 96).

TABLE 96. Laboratory Procedures *: Utilization Rates and Component Indices, by Area of Subscriber Residence

| AREA | Procedures Per 1000 Member Years | Laboratory Users Per 1000 Member Years | Procedures Per Patient | Users of Any Service Per 1000 Member Years | Laboratory Users Per 1000 Users of Any Service |
|---|---|---|---|---|---|
| Queens | 834 | 183 | 4.6 | 844 | 217 |
| Brooklyn | 813 | 164 | 4.9 | 832 | 197 |
| Manhattan | 794 | 169 | 4.7 | 674 | 251 |
| Nassau | 767 | 193 | 4.0 | 827 | 233 |
| Bronx | 759 | 160 | 4.7 | 794 | 202 |
| Westchester | 705 | 204 | 3.5 | 863 | 236 |
| AVERAGE | 693 | 165 | 4.2 | 802 | 206 |
| Suffolk | 490 | 164 | 3.0 | 876 | 187 |
| Richmond | 475 | 127 | 3.7 | 866 | 147 |
| New Jersey | 440 | 128 | 3.4 | 672 | 190 |
| Other New York | 361 | 128 | 2.8 | 816 | 157 |

* Out-of-hospital procedures except simple urinalysis and hemoglobin tests.

# LABORATORY PROCEDURES:
## OUT-OF-HOSPITAL UTILIZATION RATES,
## BY AGE AND SEX, AND BY OCCUPATION CLASS

**(Excluding Simple Urinalysis and Hemoglobin Tests)**

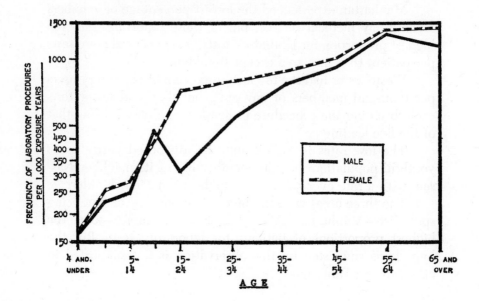

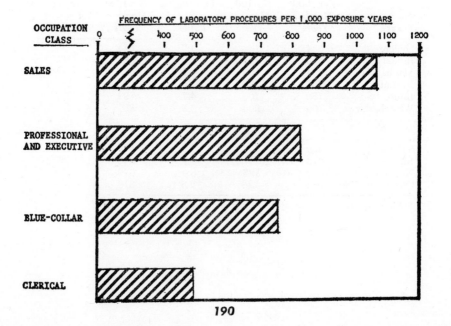

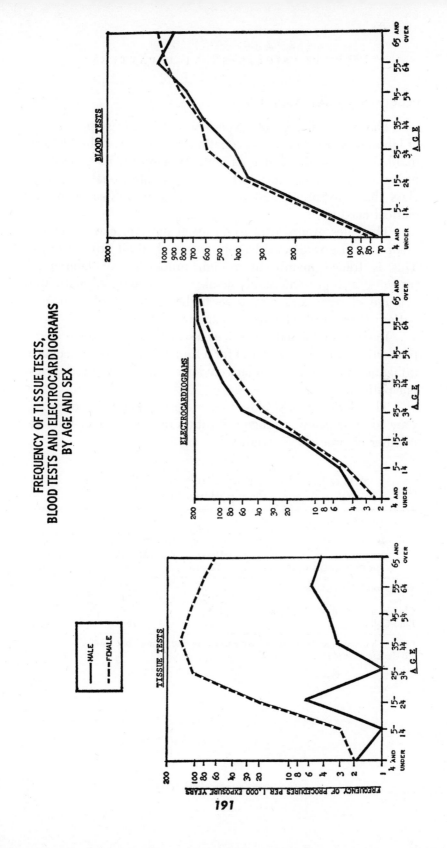

FREQUENCY OF TISSUE TESTS,
BLOOD TESTS AND ELECTROCARDIOGRAMS
BY AGE AND SEX

OCCUPATION CLASS VARIATIONS

The blue-collar group experienced the lowest proportion of laboratory users of any occupation category, but the highest number of procedures per patient. As a result, its procedure utilization rate was closer to that of the professional-executive class than any other, and over 50 per cent higher than the clerical class rate.

The sales group, true to its usual pattern, experienced a laboratory use rate considerably higher than all other groups. This is traced mainly to a high proportion of laboratory patients, 251 per thousand members, as compared with the average of 165; and also to a higher number of tests per patient than in other white-collar groups.

In the professional-executive class, the higher-than-average proportion of users accounted for a somewhat higher procedure utilization rate despite a relatively lower number of procedures per patient.

The clerical group, close to average on proportion of users, showed a far-below-average utilization rate because of the low number of procedures averaged per patient.

TABLE 97.  Laboratory Procedure Utilization,*
by Occupation Class

| OCCUPATION CLASS | Procedures Per 1000 Member Years † | Laboratory Users Per 1000 Member Years | Procedures Per Patient |
|---|---|---|---|
| Professional-Executive | 835 | 220 | 3.8 |
| Sales | 1073 | 251 | 4.3 |
| Clerical and White-Collar Unspecified | 496 | 159 | 3.1 |
| Blue-Collar | 761 | 158 | 4.8 |

* Out-of-hospital procedures except simple urinalysis and hemoglobin tests.
† Including dependents.

## Component Laboratory Procedures

### Distribution

With the exclusion of simple urinalyses, 74 per cent of all recorded laboratory procedures involved various types of blood tests. These accounted for 77 per cent of male and 71 per cent of female procedures. In second place among males were electrocardiograms, which were in third place for females, after tissue tests (mainly Pap smear). No other category accounted for as much as 5 per cent of all procedures (Table 98).

TABLE 98.  Distribution of Laboratory Procedures *
by Type of Test, by Sex

| TYPE OF TEST | Males and Females | Males | Females |
|---|---|---|---|
| | % | % | % |
| Blood | 73.9 | 77.0 | 71.1 |
| Electrocardiogram | 9.7 | 12.1 | 7.5 |
| Tissue | 5.0 | .5 | 9.3 |
| Feces | 3.9 | 4.2 | 3.5 |
| Skin | 1.3 | 1.3 | 1.3 |
| Sputum | .9 | .9 | 1.0 |
| Urine | .7 | .5 | .8 |
| Culture-Bacteria | .6 | .5 | .6 |
| Pregnancy | .4 | — | .8 |
| Basal Metabolism | .4 | .2 | .6 |
| Electroencephalogram | .3 | .3 | .2 |
| Audiogram | .3 | .3 | .4 |
| All Other | 2.6 | 2.2 | 2.9 |
| | 100.0 | 100.0 | 100.0 |

* Out-of-hospital procedures except simple urinalysis and hemoglobin tests.

The only age groups which differed significantly as to relative distribution of laboratory procedures among the various categories were the children, especially those under age 5. For the latter group the largest category remained blood tests, but it accounted for a much lower proportion (48 per cent) than among the rest of the population. Skin and culture tests with bacteria extracts, and sputum or urine tests, accounted for 36 per cent of the tests among children under 5, vs. 3.5 per cent for the membersihp as a whole (Tables 98 and 99).

TABLE 99.   Distribution of Laboratory Procedures * by Type
of Test: Population Under and Over Age 15

| TYPE OF TEST | Age Under 5 | Age 5–14 | Age 15 and Over |
|---|---|---|---|
| | % | % | % |
| Blood | 48.1 | 67.1 | 75.2 |
| Tissue | 1.3 | .5 | 5.5 |
| Feces | 2.7 | 8.3 | 3.5 |
| Skin | 18.6 | 7.7 | .3 |
| Sputum | 10.7 | 3.0 | .5 |
| Urine | 2.3 | 1.5 | .6 |
| Culture-Bacteria | 4.2 | 1.8 | .3 |
| Electrocardiogram | 2.0 | 2.2 | 10.6 |
| Electroencephalogram | .6 | 1.2 | .1 |
| Audiogram | .3 | 1.2 | .3 |
| All Other | 9.2 | 5.5 | 3.1 |
| | 100.0 | 100.0 | 100.0 |

* Out-of-hospital procedures except simple urinalysis and hemoglobin tests.

## Utilization Rates of Component Laboratory Procedures

Of the total utilization of 693 procedures per thousand
members, 502 were blood tests (Table 100). The next highest
rate, 66, occurred for electrocardiograms, followed by tests of
tissues, 34, and feces, 26. The incidence of other tests ranged
from 9 down to .1 or lower per thousand exposure years.

Within the blood-test category, the incidence of the twelve
leading procedures exceeded that of all types of non-blood
tests except electrocardiograms and tissue or feces tests. These
twelve leaders accounted for 83 per cent of all blood tests. The
next twelve in frequency order accounted for another 10 per
cent, and the remaining 7 per cent were distributed among
about seventy other procedures (Table 101).

*Age-Sex Variations.* In addition to higher rates for non-
blood tests such as tissue smears, basal metabolism, and
urinalysis, females experienced consistently higher rates than
males for such blood tests as complete blood count, red cell
count, white cell count, protein-bound iodine.

Male rates were most notably higher, as shown above, for
electrocardiogram; and, in the blood-test group, for cholesterol
level measurement, phosphatase, prothrombin time, and uric

TABLE 100.  Utilization Rates of Component Types
of Laboratory Procedures, by Sex

| TYPE OF TEST | NUMBER OF PROCEDURES * PER 1000 EXPOSURE YEARS | | |
|---|---|---|---|
| | All | Males | Females |
| Blood | 502.2 | 496.6 | 507.9 |
| Electrocardiogram | 66.1 | 78.2 | 53.4 |
| Tissue | 34.1 | 3.0 | 66.5 |
| Feces | 26.3 | 27.3 | 25.3 |
| Skin | 8.8 | 8.2 | 9.5 |
| Sputum | 6.1 | 5.6 | 6.7 |
| Urinalysis | 4.6 | 3.3 | 5.8 |
| Antibiotic Sensitivity | 4.6 | 3.6 | 5.6 |
| Pathology at Home | 3.7 | 2.3 | 5.1 |
| Culture for Bacteria | 3.7 | 3.0 | 4.4 |
| Basal Metabolism Rate | 2.8 | 1.4 | 4.3 |
| Biological Test for Pregnancy | 2.8 | — | 5.8 |
| Audiogram | 2.3 | 2.0 | 2.5 |
| Direct Smear | 2.0 | 1.2 | 2.9 |
| Allergy Patch Test | 1.9 | 1.8 | 2.1 |
| Electroencephalogram | 1.7 | 2.0 | 1.4 |
| Radioactive Iodine | 1.2 | .3 | 2.2 |
| All Other Known | 4.3 | 5.1 | 3.4 |
| Unclassified | 14.2 | 13.3 | 15.1 |
| TOTAL | 693.4 | 658.2 | 729.9 |

* Out-of-hospital procedures except simple urinalysis and hemoglobin tests.

acid tests. For these procedures, however, the women's rate at age 65 either closely approached (electrocardiogram, phosphatase), equalled (cholesterol) or greatly exceeded (prothrombin time) the male rate.

The general trend in utilization rates of most procedures was upward from early childhood through age 64 (Table 102), after which the rate sometimes continued upward (usually for women), sometimes fell off (usually for men). This pattern would be expected on inspection of overall utilization: the increase with each age increment was generally so large as to preclude a different pattern for the principal procedures, except of course those done mainly for women (e.g. cytological studies) or children (skin and sputum tests).

TABLE 101.  Utilization Rates of Component Procedures in Blood Test Category, by Age and Sex

| TYPE OF BLOOD TEST * | All | Male | Female | FREQUENCY PER 1000 EXPOSURE YEARS | | | | | | | |
| | | | | UNDER 14 | | 15–34 | | 35–54 | | 55 AND OVER | |
| | | | | Male | Female | Male | Female | Male | Female | Male | Female |
|---|---|---|---|---|---|---|---|---|---|---|---|
| All Blood Tests * | 502.2 | 496.6 | 507.9 | 131.7 | 147.6 | 390.8 | 487.0 | 679.2 | 721.4 | 1034.5 | 1004.8 |
| Complete Count | 98.2 | 86.0 | 110.8 | 45.0 | 48.5 | 77.3 | 111.7 | 104.9 | 149.6 | 145.9 | 178.7 |
| Sugar | 62.3 | 64.5 | 60.1 | 7.6 | 11.3 | 38.4 | 44.4 | 91.9 | 89.8 | 163.8 | 156.1 |
| Sedimentation Rate | 51.8 | 50.0 | 53.7 | 16.5 | 18.3 | 45.9 | 47.6 | 65.1 | 75.5 | 95.1 | 109.3 |
| Cholesterol | 35.4 | 40.0 | 30.6 | 3.2 | 1.8 | 28.0 | 21.8 | 57.8 | 50.6 | 97.3 | 78.0 |
| Hematocrit | 33.6 | 32.9 | 34.4 | 14.8 | 16.5 | 28.9 | 32.6 | 42.2 | 47.6 | 57.2 | 52.0 |
| Uric Acid | 25.3 | 29.8 | 20.7 | 1.0 | .9 | 23.1 | 14.0 | 47.6 | 36.8 | 62.4 | 47.2 |
| Complement Fixation | 23.6 | 23.9 | 23.2 | 5.2 | 7.0 | 24.7 | 27.5 | 33.5 | 32.2 | 42.7 | 35.2 |
| Phosphatase, Alkaline | 22.9 | 26.2 | 19.5 | 1.6 | .4 | 22.8 | 15.5 | 39.3 | 33.8 | 55.9 | 42.4 |
| Urea | 22.3 | 24.4 | 20.1 | 5.7 | 7.6 | 20.4 | 14.7 | 33.4 | 29.5 | 50.5 | 42.4 |
| Non-Protein Nitrogen | 17.1 | 17.6 | 16.5 | 2.1 | 2.1 | 10.0 | 10.6 | 22.9 | 28.2 | 50.5 | 38.0 |
| Prothrombin Time | 16.2 | 24.4 | 7.7 | .3 | .2 | 6.3 | 3.3 | 37.1 | 7.6 | 73.7 | 43.8 |
| Protein-Bound Iodine | 9.9 | 3.8 | 16.2 | .6 | 2.2 | 5.4 | 17.3 | 5.5 | 25.4 | 5.0 | 27.5 |
| White Cell Count | 6.6 | 5.9 | 7.3 | 4.9 | 5.5 | 5.0 | 8.1 | 6.9 | 7.0 | 7.2 | 12.5 |
| Cephalin Flocculation | 5.3 | 5.9 | 4.6 | 1.9 | .6 | 5.2 | 3.7 | 8.4 | 8.3 | 10.4 | 7.7 |
| Bilirubin | 4.6 | 5.1 | 4.0 | 1.0 | .2 | 6.3 | 6.3 | 6.6 | 5.4 | 8.8 | 6.3 |
| Red Cell Count | 4.3 | 2.3 | 6.4 | 2.0 | 1.9 | .9 | 10.6 | 2.7 | 8.1 | 3.8 | 4.8 |
| Thymol Turbidity | 3.9 | 4.0 | 3.8 | .7 | .4 | 3.4 | 3.7 | 5.9 | 6.6 | 7.9 | 5.8 |
| Total Protein | 3.8 | 3.8 | 3.9 | .3 | .7 | 2.7 | 3.9 | 6.2 | 6.6 | 7.6 | 5.3 |

196

| | | | | | | | | | | | |
|---|---|---|---|---|---|---|---|---|---|---|---|
| Heterophil Antibody | 3.8 | 3.2 | 4.4 | 3.3 | 4.0 | 6.3 | 8.4 | 2.5 | 1.8 | .3 | 5.3 |
| Flocculation Test | 3.6 | 3.3 | 3.9 | .4 | .4 | 4.3 | 6.7 | 5.0 | 4.8 | 4.1 | 4.8 |
| Albumin/Globulin Ratio | 3.6 | 3.3 | 4.0 | .3 | .7 | 2.0 | 4.1 | 5.3 | 6.4 | 6.9 | 6.3 |
| Platelet Count | 3.1 | 2.5 | 3.6 | 2.4 | 3.6 | 1.1 | 2.2 | 2.7 | 4.0 | 4.1 | 6.3 |
| Sugar Tolerance | 2.7 | 2.4 | 3.0 | .4 | 0 | 2.0 | 4.3 | 2.9 | 4.6 | 6.0 | 4.3 |
| Transaminase | 2.7 | 3.1 | 2.3 | .9 | .2 | 3.4 | 2.9 | 4.5 | 3.1 | 4.4 | 5.3 |
| Potassium | 2.5 | 2.3 | 2.7 | .1 | 0 | .2 | 1.8 | 3.4 | 3.3 | 7.5 | 12.0 |
| Calcium | 2.5 | 2.4 | 2.5 | 0 | .2 | 1.4 | 1.8 | 3.6 | 4.6 | 6.6 | 5.3 |
| RH Factor | 2.5 | .8 | 4.2 | .4 | .3 | 1.6 | 12.0 | 1.0 | 3.1 | .3 | 1.0 |
| Latex Fixation | 2.2 | 1.5 | 3.0 | .3 | .2 | .9 | 3.1 | 2.8 | 5.0 | 2.2 | 4.8 |
| Sodium | 2.2 | 1.9 | 2.4 | .1 | 0 | .2 | 1.6 | 2.4 | 2.7 | 7.2 | 11.1 |
| Phosphorus | 2.0 | 2.0 | 2.0 | 0 | .3 | .9 | 1.4 | 3.2 | 3.4 | 5.3 | 4.3 |
| Blood Typing | 1.9 | .8 | 3.0 | .3 | .2 | 1.4 | 8.6 | 1.1 | 2.3 | .3 | 1.4 |
| Creatinine | 1.4 | 1.5 | 1.2 | 0 | .2 | .7 | 2.0 | 2.7 | 1.7 | 3.4 | 1.4 |
| C-Reactive Protein | 1.3 | 1.0 | 1.6 | .6 | 1.8 | 1.4 | 1.6 | 1.1 | 1.6 | 1.3 | 1.0 |
| Phosphatase Acid | 1.3 | 2.2 | .4 | 0 | 0 | 0 | .8 | 2.8 | .4 | 9.4 | 1.0 |
| Antistreptolysin Titer | 1.2 | .8 | 1.6 | .7 | 1.8 | 1.6 | 2.8 | .8 | 1.1 | 0 | 0 |
| Differential Count | 1.1 | 1.1 | 1.2 | .7 | .4 | .7 | 2.0 | 1.7 | 1.3 | .9 | 1.9 |
| Chlorides | 1.1 | 1.0 | 1.3 | .1 | 0 | 0 | 1.2 | 1.3 | 1.0 | 3.8 | 6.7 |
| RH Titer | 1.1 | .2 | 2.0 | 0 | .1 | .5 | 6.7 | .1 | 1.0 | .3 | 0 |
| Reticulocyte Count | .9 | 1.0 | .9 | .3 | .9 | 0 | .8 | 1.8 | .7 | 1.9 | 1.9 |
| CO2 Combining Power | .9 | .7 | 1.1 | .1 | 0 | 0 | .2 | .8 | 1.3 | 2.5 | 6.3 |
| Coagulation Time | .8 | .5 | 1.1 | .9 | .7 | .5 | 1.2 | .1 | .6 | .3 | 3.4 |
| Bleeding Time | .8 | .6 | 1.1 | 1.4 | 1.8 | .5 | 1.2 | .1 | .3 | 0 | 1.0 |
| Basophilic Aggregates | .7 | .4 | 1.0 | .4 | 0 | .7 | 1.6 | .3 | 1.4 | .3 | 1.0 |
| All Other | 7.2 | 5.6 | 8.9 | 3.2 | 3.7 | 3.8 | 8.7 | 7.3 | 11.3 | 9.4 | 14.0 |

197

* Out-of-hospital, excluding hemoglobin tests.

TABLE 102.  Frequency of Laboratory Procedures by Type, by Age and Sex

NUMBER OF PROCEDURES PER 1000 EXPOSURE YEARS *

| TYPE OF PROCEDURE | UNDER 5 | | 5–14 | | 15–24 | | 25–34 | | 35–44 | | 45–54 | | 55–64 | | 65 AND OVER | |
|---|---|---|---|---|---|---|---|---|---|---|---|---|---|---|---|---|
| | M | F | M | F | M | F | M | F | M | F | M | F | M | F | M | F |
| Blood | 70.9 | 78.3 | 158.6 | 177.3 | 355.0 | 386.8 | 423.3 | 584.3 | 606.8 | 626.1 | 752.6 | 818.2 | 1069.7 | 991.9 | 903.8 | 1069.8 |
| Electrocardiogram | 3.8 | 2.5 | 5.8 | 5.1 | 16.1 | 14.0 | 63.9 | 38.7 | 104.0 | 66.5 | 141.1 | 110.0 | 188.4 | 154.7 | 199.7 | 194.8 |
| Tissue | 1.9 | 2.0 | 1.0 | 1.7 | 6.2 | 23.5 | .9 | 100.0 | 3.1 | 132.9 | 3.7 | 119.2 | 5.6 | 89.5 | 4.4 | 61.0 |
| Feces | 1.4 | 6.9 | 18.6 | 22.9 | 24.7 | 16.4 | 29.4 | 18.2 | 31.5 | 28.9 | 36.5 | 37.3 | 45.0 | 42.7 | 35.5 | 34.9 |
| Skin | 26.6 | 31.2 | 18.2 | 20.4 | 8.6 | 9.2 | 1.3 | 1.2 | 2.5 | 1.7 | .3 | 1.7 | 0 | 1.1 | 1.5 | 0 |
| Sputum | 21.0 | 11.9 | 6.4 | 8.9 | 4.3 | 4.8 | 3.9 | 13.9 | 3.1 | 5.1 | 1.1 | 2.0 | 4.4 | 1.1 | 1.5 | 0 |
| Urinalysis | 3.3 | 3.9 | 2.3 | 5.1 | 1.4 | 4.8 | 2.6 | 6.2 | 3.1 | 6.8 | 2.8 | 6.3 | 8.4 | 8.7 | 4.4 | 2.9 |
| Antibiotic Sensitivity | 8.8 | 8.4 | 5.2 | 5.3 | 2.3 | 4.0 | 3.0 | 10.8 | 1.1 | 4.8 | 2.0 | 4.6 | 4.0 | 2.4 | 0 | 0 |
| Pathology at Home | .9 | 1.5 | 1.5 | 2.4 | 2.4 | 4.7 | .5 | .8 | .6 | .8 | 5.4 | 5.2 | 4.7 | 25.5 | 1.5 | 40.7 |
| Culture for Bacteria | 6.5 | 6.4 | 4.6 | 4.7 | 2.8 | 5.2 | 3.0 | 2.7 | 1.4 | 6.2 | 1.1 | 4.3 | 2.8 | .6 | 0 | 0 |
| Basal Metabolism Rate | 0 | .5 | .2 | .6 | 2.4 | 7.2 | 0 | 7.0 | 1.9 | 5.4 | 3.4 | 6.0 | 1.6 | 4.6 | 3.0 | 2.9 |
| Biological Test for Pregnancy | — | 0 | — | .2 | — | 8.0 | — | 21.3 | — | 11.3 | — | 1.5 | — | 0 | — | 0 |
| Audiogram | .9 | 0 | 2.9 | 3.0 | 1.9 | 1.2 | 1.3 | 1.5 | 1.4 | 2.5 | 2.2 | 4.3 | 2.0 | 4.6 | 3.0 | 0 |
| Direct Smear | 1.9 | 2.5 | .6 | 1.7 | 2.4 | 2.8 | 1.7 | 4.6 | .6 | 4.0 | .8 | 3.2 | 1.2 | 1.7 | 2.9 | 0 |
| Allergy Patch Test | 1.4 | 1.0 | 3.1 | 2.8 | 1.9 | .8 | 2.2 | 4.2 | 1.7 | 1.9 | .6 | 2.5 | .8 | 0 | 1.5 | 0 |
| Unclassified | 1.4 | .5 | 3.7 | 2.1 | 2.8 | 1.6 | 0 | 1.2 | 1.7 | 1.4 | 1.1 | 1.2 | 2.0 | 1.1 | 1.5 | 0 |
| Electroencephalogram | 0 | 0 | .2 | .2 | .5 | 1.2 | .4 | 1.9 | .5 | 5.4 | .3 | 4.0 | .4 | 1.7 | 0 | 0 |
| Radioactive Iodine | 1.5 | 0 | 2.6 | .6 | 5.2 | 3.2 | 9.9 | 6.0 | 6.9 | 4.6 | 6.5 | 4.9 | 4.8 | 5.3 | 7.3 | 2.9 |
| All Other Known | 9.8 | 4.0 | 6.6 | 4.9 | 6.2 | 13.6 | 6.0 | 20.9 | 13.9 | 19.5 | 23.2 | 17.0 | 23.9 | 32.9 | 25.2 | 32.0 |
| TOTAL | 162.0 | 161.5 | 242.1 | 270.1 | 447.1 | 513.0 | 553.3 | 845.4 | 785.8 | 935.8 | 984.7 | 1153.4 | 1369.7 | 1370.1 | 1196.7 | 1441.9 |

* Out-of-hospital procedures except simple urinalysis and hemoglobin tests.

# Chapter 14

## AMBULATORY SURGERY

The term ambulatory surgery covers all surgery performed by a private physician for non-hospitalized patients (i.e. in office or outpatient departments). In addition to procedures involving cutting, or repairing of injuries, it includes certain diagnostic procedures such as sigmoidoscopy, proctoscopy, and other endoscopic examinations, as well as electro- or chemical cauterization.

In the present study, 104 different surgical procedures were found to have been performed for both ambulatory and hospitalized patients. Generally speaking, however, most types of surgery, including these 104, were typically done on one basis or the other and could thus be characterized as inpatient or outpatient procedures.

Hospital surgery is discussed in detail elsewhere. Appropriate references will also be introduced in the present section to permit comparison with ambulatory surgery.

Utilization indices available for surgery fall into two categories: demographic variations in overall use; and incidence by type of procedure.

### General Findings

The utilization rate for ambulatory surgery was 157 procedures per thousand members of the study population, as compared with 61 in-hospital procedures. The number of patients undergoing these procedures averaged 118 and 48 respectively per thousand eligibles; in other words, many patients underwent more than one procedure during the study year. Ambulatory surgical patients averaged one and one-third such procedures each. This ratio varied somewhat among various population subgroups, the oldest segment of patients having more (1.57) and the younger segment fewer (1.25) procedures per patient; but the two indices generally paralleled one another (Table 103).

TABLE 103. Comparison of Two Indices of Ambulatory Surgery Utilization Among Selected Membership Categories

| MEMBER CATEGORY | Proportion of Membership Having Ambulatory Surgery | Number of Procedures Per 1000 Exposure Years |
|---|---|---|
| | % | |
| All Members | 11.8 | 157 |
| Adults | 14.0 | 191 |
| Male | 13.0 | 175 |
| Female | 15.1 | 208 |
| Children | 8.5 | 107 |
| Male | 10.5 | 129 |
| Female | 6.6 | 85 |
| Under 65 | 11.7 | 156 |
| 65 and Over | 15.0 | 225 |
| Subscribers | 13.4 | 181 |
| Spouses | 14.8 | 204 |

As for the relationship between utilization patterns of ambulatory and hospital surgery, the questions posed parallel those asked in analyzing hospital vs. office consultations: Does one substitute for the other, i.e. if hospital surgery rates are higher than average for a given subgroup, are ambulatory surgery rates lower, or do the two indices move in the same direction?

There is occasional evidence, when the analysis focuses on variations by geographic area and occupation class, to suggest some basis for the first hypothesis of a high-low interrelated utilization pattern. But the predominating evidence supports the second hypothesis: generally both rates were either low or high; subgroups were likely to be high or low surgical utilizers irrespective of where the procedures were performed.

## Variations in Overall Utilization Rates Among Population Subgroups

VARIATIONS BY AGE AND SEX

Ambulatory surgery for both boys and girls occurred at increasing rates from early childhood to age 19, but at different levels of use, the boys averaging 53 per cent higher rates than the girls and reaching levels nearly 90 per cent higher at ages 15 to 19. The experience was in marked contrast to that of hospital surgery, where the rates of use tended to decline in adolescence rather than accelerate, and the rates for boys and girls aged 15 to 19 were identical.

During the adult years from 20 to 54, male ambulatory rates declined from their adolescent peak, leveled off until age

TABLE 104.  Surgical Utilization Rates, by Age and Sex

| | NUMBER OF PROCEDURES PER 1000 EXPOSURE YEARS | | | | | |
|---|---|---|---|---|---|---|
| | AMBULATORY | | | HOSPITAL | | |
| AGE | *All* | *Male* | *Female* | *All* | *Male* | *Female* |
| Under 5 | 84.8 | 99.0 | 69.9 | 52.4 | 62.6 | 41.6 |
| 5–9 | 92.3 | 106.2 | 78.1 | 56.4 | 62.3 | 50.5 |
| 10–14 | 101.4 | 123.9 | 77.8 | 29.0 | 38.0 | 19.7 |
| 15–19 | 169.9 | 223.5 | 120.5 | 34.7 | 34.7 | 34.8 |
| 20–24 | 210.1 | 152.0 | 246.4 | 55.9 | 32.3 | 70.6 |
| 25–34 | 175.2 | 161.1 | 187.9 | 54.9 | 38.9 | 69.4 |
| 35–44 | 187.6 | 155.9 | 219.7 | 72.6 | 45.7 | 99.8 |
| 45–54 | 200.2 | 182.9 | 217.8 | 80.8 | 58.2 | 103.7 |
| 55–64 | 181.1 | 182.9 | 178.4 | 77.1 | 76.9 | 77.4 |
| 65 and Over | 224.5 | 235.2 | 203.5 | 92.2 | 102.1 | 84.3 |
| Children | 107.1 | 129.4 | 84.5 | 43.1 | 49.8 | 36.3 |
| Adults | 190.9 | 175.1 | 207.5 | 72.5 | 56.6 | 89.1 |
| All Under 65 | 155.6 | 154.4 | 156.9 | 59.5 | 52.4 | 67.6 |
| ALL | 157.3 | 156.8 | 157.7 | 60.8 | 53.9 | 67.9 |

# AMBULATORY AND HOSPITAL SURGERY:
## UTILIZATION RATES,
### BY AGE AND SEX

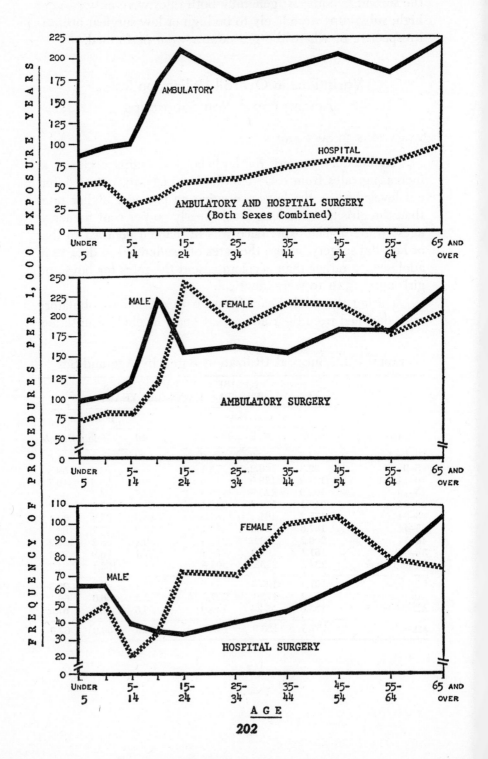

45, maintained a higher level for twenty years before reaching their highest point at 65-plus. The women's pattern was different, this rate reaching its high point at ages 20 to 24 and its low at ages 55 to 64, when it equalled the men's rate; at age 65 the female rate dipped below the male rate for the first time since the childhood years.

VARIATIONS ASSOCIATED WITH MARITAL STATUS AND
SUBSCRIBER RELATIONSHIP

Ambulatory surgical rates for the married were nearly 25 per cent higher than for the spouseless.

Of all marital and relationship categories, married women showed the highest surgical rates both in and out of the hospital.

The single women's rate for ambulatory surgery was about the same as for single men, although their hospital surgery rate was 27 per cent higher. In contrast, among the widowed-divorced-separated category, the women's rate of ambulatory procedures was 87 per cent higher than the men's (Table 105).

TABLE 105.  Surgical Utilization Rates, by Marital Status, Relationship and Family Size

| MEMBER CATEGORY | NUMBER OF PROCEDURES PER 1000 EXPOSURE YEARS | | | | | |
|---|---|---|---|---|---|---|
| | AMBULATORY | | | HOSPITAL | | |
| | All | Male | Female | All | Male | Female |
| *Marital Status* | | | | | | |
| Married | 195.7 | 182.8 | 212.6 | 75.4 | 58.1 | 93.0 |
| Single | 153.4 | 154.4 | 152.0 | 55.1 | 49.6 | 63.2 |
| Widowed, Divorced, | | | | | | |
| Separated | 159.7 | 106.5 | 198.8 | 34.7 | 28.7 | 39.1 |
| *Relationship* | | | | | | |
| Subscriber | 181.4 | 178.4 | 196.1 | 58.5 | 55.2 | 76.0 |
| Spouse | 203.5 | 128.4 | 210.0 | 90.9 | 76.6 | 92.1 |
| *Family Size* | | | | | | |
| 2 | 184.6 | | | 78.2 | | |
| 3 | 174.4 | | | 62.6 | | |
| 4 | 169.1 | | | 59.8 | | |
| 5 | 141.2 | | | 50.6 | | |
| 6 or More | 108.1 | | | 52.7 | | |

VARIATIONS BY FAMILY SIZE

Per capita use of ambulatory surgery decreased with increasing family size. As with other services, families of six or more experienced lower average rates per member than would have been expected from two adults and four children; their rates were at the average children's level.

OCCUPATION CLASS VARIATIONS

Analysis of surgical use among the various occupation classes provides an instance of the two component indices, ambulatory and hospital rates, behaving somewhat at variance with one another.

The hospital utilization rates of the different occupation classes showed small variations as compared with those found on analysis of other variables,—a 22 per cent difference between the highest users (clerical) and the lowest (executive). The other classes clustered within an even smaller range, 57.5 to 59.3 hospital procedures per thousand members.

But ambulatory surgery for the sales class, at 206 procedures per thousand members, was 37 per cent higher than for the blue-collar class, at 150, although both classes experienced identical rates of surgical utilization in the hospital. Under these circumstances, further detailed investigation would be required to determine whether the ambulatory rate for the sales class included procedures which might otherwise have taken place in the hospital, or is simply another example of the relatively high office-service demands which apparently are characteristic of this group.

If it can be assumed that ambulatory procedures are more likely to be of an elective or optional nature than hospital procedures, then the class cleavage in the ambulatory index acquires significance—the professional, executive and sales classes at one end, the clerical and blue-collar classes at the other. This is explored in more detail as part of the analysis of experience by type of procedure. In the meantime, Table 106

TABLE 106.   Surgical Utilization Rates, by Occupation Class
of Subscriber

| | NUMBER OF PROCEDURES PER 1000 EXPOSURE YEARS [*] | |
| OCCUPATION CLASS | Ambulatory | Hospital |
| --- | --- | --- |
| Professional | 199.4 | 57.5 |
| Executive | 196.7 | 52.1 |
| Sales | 206.4 | 59.3 |
| Clerical and White-Collar Unspecified | 158.5 | 63.8 |
| Blue-Collar | 150.4 | 59.3 |
| Student | 117.6 | 29.4 |
| Retired | 224.0 | 96.0 |

[*] Including dependents.

may be used to illustrate again the interpretive distortion which can occur when all white-collar segments, including clerical, are grouped together and their experience compared with that of the blue-collar segment.

GEOGRAPHIC VARIATIONS

The incidence of ambulatory surgery in the area with the highest rate (Nassau, 197) was double that of the area with the lowest rate (New Jersey, 99). Neither these extremes nor the broad scattering of intermediate rates occurring in the other areas studied could be explained by the age distribution of the membership residing in each area.

Nor did hospital surgery rates necessarily follow the ambulatory pattern. There was at least one instance, Richmond, where the high-low theory seemed to apply—hospital rates significantly higher than average, ambulatory rates significantly lower—indicating possible choice of hospital locale for some procedures customarily done in physicians' offices. The same type of balance, but less extreme than in Richmond, appeared for non-metropolitan New York areas, while the order was reversed in Brooklyn, with high-ambulatory, low-hospital surgical rates.

In seven of the ten areas listed, however, the pattern of the two surgical indices was consistent—high-high, or low-low, in relation to the overall average. But the degrees of variation are difficult to explain, both within each area and between almost any two areas.

Brooklyn, which might have been expected to have high rates of hospital surgery, had next to the lowest. The highest hospitalized surgical rates occurred mainly in the outlying areas—Westchester, Richmond, Suffolk, Nassau, "other" New York counties—although they have relatively more children, who should have brought down their average use rates. Three of these areas, Westchester, Nassau, and Suffolk, also showed the highest rates of ambulatory surgery—again unexpectedly.

It appears reasonable to conclude, tentatively at least, that local medical customs and facilities influenced the incidence of surgery in each area—a factor of some importance in attempts to define "norms."

TABLE 107.   Surgical Utilization Rates, by Area
of Subscriber Residence

| AREA | NUMBER OF PROCEDURES PER 1000 EXPOSURE YEARS | |
| --- | --- | --- |
| | *Ambulatory* | *Hospital* |
| New Jersey | 99.1 | 58.4 |
| Richmond | 123.3 | 80.9 |
| Manhattan | 135.1 | 49.1 |
| Bronx | 137.5 | 58.0 |
| Other New York | 145.9 | 69.0 |
| Brooklyn | 165.2 | 50.8 |
| Queens | 169.9 | 61.5 |
| Suffolk | 169.8 | 69.1 |
| Westchester | 183.0 | 87.1 |
| Nassau | 197.2 | 66.1 |
| AVERAGE, ALL AREAS | 157.3 | 60.8 |

VARIATIONS WITH DURATION OF ENROLLMENT

A positive correlation between years of coverage and increasing surgical utilization rates was found, but the pattern appears to have been more or less consistent with expectations based on the age distribution of the membership enrolled in various years. Further analysis would be required to ascertain whether duration of enrollment exerted any independent influence of its own.

TABLE 108. Surgical Utilization Rates, by Duration of Enrollment

| YEAR OF COVERAGE | NUMBER OF PROCEDURES PER 1000 EXPOSURE YEARS | |
|---|---|---|
| | *Ambulatory* | *Hospital* |
| 1st | 124 | 48.5 |
| 2nd | 112 | 38.7 |
| 3rd | 130 | 53.0 |
| 4th | 167 | 59.8 |
| 5th | 162 | 66.6 |
| 6th | 182 | 65.4 |
| 7th | 178 | 75.8 |
| 8th or Longer | 181 | 71.9 |

## Component Procedures

The following types of surgical procedures were generally performed on an ambulatory basis:

Diagnostic procedures: Sigmoidoscopy
                                   Proctoscopy
                                   Cystoscopy

Treatment of local infections or other aberrations:
    Incision and drainage of abscess, cyst, etc.
    Local excision or cauterization of small benign neoplasm, lesion, other tumor or cyst

Treatment of injuries:
    Fractures (closed reductions)
    Dislocations
    Epistaxis
    Suture of wounds
    Removal of foreign body
    Burns

Treatment of other musculoskeletal conditions

All together, about four out of five ambulatory procedures fell into one of these categories.

### Hospital vs. Office Procedures

The delineation between major and minor surgery is not always clear, and if it were, would not necessarily coincide with that between hospital and office surgery.

A total of 463 different procedures was performed. Of these, 266 were always in-hospital surgery, 93 were always ambulatory, and 104 were mixed. Of the mixed procedures, over half were characteristically ambulatory.

Examples of procedures about evenly divided between hospital and office include cystoscopy with fulguration of small tumor, closed reduction of jaw dislocations and fractures of radius and ulna, patella, and tibia.

### Most Frequent Procedures

When each surgical procedure was listed separately, in order of frequency, few hospital procedures were found among the leaders (six of the first twenty-five). The percentage of hospital procedures increased as the frequency of the individual procedure decreased. Thus, three-fourths of the fifty leading procedures were generally ambulatory, vs. 58 per cent of the next fifty.

As shown in Table 109, only four procedures, usually ambulatory, were reported with an incidence as high as 10 per thousand members. For the majority of the hundred leading procedures, the incidence was below one procedure per thousand members.

TABLE 109.   Incidence of Most Frequent Surgical Procedures
(In Order of Frequency)

| FREQUENCY RANK | PROCEDURE | Incidence Per 100,000 Exposure Years | Per Cent Ambulatory |
|---|---|---|---|
| 1 | Sigmoidoscopy, Diagnostic, Initial | 2715.2 | 97 |
| 2 | Primary, Secondary, or Delayed Suture of Wounds | 1415.1 | 97 |
| 3 | Local Excision of Small Benign Lesion | 1171.0 | 91 |
| 4 | Electro-Cauterization or Fulguration of Local Lesion, Small | 1002.1 | 99.5 |
| 5 | Tonsillectomy and/or Adenoidectomy | 915.2 | 9 |
| 6 | Drainage of Small Subcutaneous Abscess | 812.0 | 99.7 |
| 7 | Electro-Cauterization of Cervix | 617.2 | 100 |
| 8 | Dilation of Urethral Stricture by Passage of Sound | 445.9 | 98 |
| 9 | Drainage of Onychia or Paronychia | 441.2 | 99.5 |
| 10 | Drainage of Sebaceous Cyst | 436.5 | 98 |
| 11 | Dilation and Curettage (D & C) | 401.3 | 0 |
| 12 | Proctoscopy, Diagnostic without Biopsy | 340.3 | 99.3 |
| 13 | Epistaxis (Cauterization) | 302.7 | 98.5 |
| 14 | Incision and Removal of Foreign Body | 286.3 | 98 |
| 15 | Cystoscopy, Diagnostic, Subsequent | 274.6 | 68 |
| 16 | Chemical Cauterization of Cervix | 274.6 | 100 |
| 17 | Panhysterectomy | 253.5 | 0 |
| 18 | Chemical Cauterization of Local Lesion | 248.8 | 100 |
| 19 | Cystoscopy with Ureteral Cauterization | 220.6 | 23 |
| 20 | Hernioplasty, Herniorraphy, Herniotomy, Inguinal | 213.6 | 0 |
| 21 | Excision of Meibomian Glands | 190.1 | 96 |
| 22 | Arthrocentesis | 176.0 | 99 |
| 23 | Drainage of Furuncle | 176.0 | 99 |
| 24 | Acne Surgery—Marsupialization Opening | 171.3 | 100 |
| 25 | Appendectomy | 171.3 | 0 |
| 26 | Puncture for Aspiration of Bursa | 161.9 | 100 |
| 27 | Cholecystectomy | 157.2 | 0 |
| 28 | Fracture—Finger (Closed) | 147.8 | 89 |
| 29 | Electro-Cauterization of Local Lesion, Large | 145.5 | 100 |
| 30 | Intra-Auricular Injection into Joint | 140.8 | 100 |
| 31 | Excision of Cyst, Fibroadenoma of Other Benign Tumors | 133.7 | 5 |
| 32 | Irrigation of Antrum | 126.7 | 98 |
| 33 | Drainage of Large Subcutaneous Abscess | 124.4 | 96 |
| 34 | Drainage of Carbuncle | 115.0 | 98 |
| 35 | Puncture Aspiration of Abscess or Hematoma | 115.0 | 100 |
| 36 | Excision of Nail, Partial | 100.9 | 95 |
| 37 | Excision of Nail Bed or Nail Fold, Complete | 98.5 | 93 |
| 38 | Needling of Bursa | 93.8 | 97 |

TABLE 109. *(Cont'd)*

| FREQUENCY RANK | PROCEDURE | Incidence Per 100,000 Exposure Years | Per Cent Ambulatory |
|---|---|---|---|
| 39 | Wide Excision of Lesion, without Graft or Plastic Closure | 91.5 | 38 |
| 40 | Fracture—Radius (Closed) | 91.5 | 50 |
| 41 | Abscess, I and D, Including Ischiorectal | 86.8 | 68 |
| 42 | Hemorrhoidectomy, Internal | 86.8 | 0 |
| 43 | Removal of Foreign Body, Imbedded in Cornea | 86.8 | 100 |
| 44 | Resection of Malignant Lesion of Skin | 79.7 | 71 |
| 45 | Removal of Foreign Body from Surface of Cornea | 77.4 | 100 |
| 46 | Injection (Veins) | 75.1 | 100 |
| 47 | Enucleation of External Thrombotic Hemorrhoid | 75.1 | 100 |
| 48 | Myringotomy: Tympanotomy: Plicotomy of Middle Ear | 72.7 | 61 |
| 49 | Local Excision of Lesion of Cervix | 70.4 | 93 |
| 50 | Extraction of Lens, Combined Cataract Extraction | 65.7 | 0 |
| 51 | Fracture—Radius and Ulna (Closed) | 63.3 | 48 |
| 52 | Post-Nasal Pack for Epistaxis | 63.4 | 100 |
| 53 | Lipectomy | 61.0 | 23 |
| 54 | Fracture—Metatarsal Bone (Closed) | 61.0 | 92 |
| 55 | Submucous Resection | 61.0 | 0 |
| 56 | Blepharotomy with Drainage of Meibomian Glands | 61.0 | 100 |
| 57 | Biopsy of Skin or Subcutaneous Tissue | 61.0 | 96 |
| 58 | Hemorrhoids, Injection of | 58.7 | 100 |
| 59 | Excision of Carbuncle | 56.3 | 100 |
| 60 | Fracture—Clavicle (Closed) | 56.3 | 91 |
| 61 | Drainage of Abscess of External Auditory Canal | 56.3 | 100 |
| 62 | Fracture—Toe (Closed) | 54.0 | 100 |
| 63 | Drainage of Pilonidal Cyst | 51.6 | 100 |
| 64 | Fracture—Nasal Bones (Closed Reduction) | 51.6 | 68 |
| 65 | Hemorrhoidectomy with Fissurectomy | 51.6 | 0 |
| 66 | Colpoplasty: Posterior Vaginal Wall, Repair of Rectocele | 51.6 | 0 |
| 67 | Vein: Long Incision, Ligation and Excision, One Leg | 49.2 | 5 |
| 68 | Circumcision | 49.2 | 21 |
| 69 | Fracture—Metacarpal (Closed) | 46.9 | 100 |
| 70 | Antrum Puncture, Bilateral | 46.9 | 100 |
| 71 | Bronchoscopy (Diagnostic) | 46.9 | 0 |
| 72 | Excision of Eyelid, Multiple | 46.9 | 100 |
| 73 | Fistulotomy or Fistulectomy | 44.6 | 0 |
| 74 | Probing of Lacrimonasal Duct | 44.6 | 95 |

TABLE 109. (Concluded)

| FREQUENCY RANK | PROCEDURE | Incidence Per 100,000 Exposure Years | Per Cent Ambulatory |
|---|---|---|---|
| 75 | Strabismus, Unilateral | 44.6 | 0 |
| 76 | Hammer Toe Operation | 44.5 | 68 |
| 77 | Plaster Cast of Ankle | 44.5 | 95 |
| 78 | Subtotal Gastrectomy, Partial | 42.2 | 0 |
| 79 | Excision of Lesion of Tendon or Fibrous Sheath, In Other Locations | 39.8 | 6 |
| 80 | Antrum Puncture, Unilateral | 37.6 | 100 |
| 81 | Incision and Drainage—Bartholin's Abscess | 37.6 | 100 |
| 82 | Removal of Foreign Body from Surface of Conjunctiva | 37.6 | 100 |
| 83 | Fracture—Ribs (Closed) | 35.2 | 100 |
| 84 | Fracture—Colles (Closed) | 35.2 | 80 |
| 85 | Salpingo-Oophorectomy, Complete or Partial | 35.2 | 0 |
| 86 | Insufflation of Uterus and Tubes with Air or $CO_2$ | 35.2 | 100 |
| 87 | Radical Mastectomy, Unilateral | 32.9 | 0 |
| 88 | Veins: Long Incision, Ligation and Excision, Both Legs | 32.9 | 0 |
| 89 | Excision of Pilonidal Cyst or Sinus | 32.8 | 7 |
| 90 | Fracture—Humerus (Closed) | 32.8 | 57 |
| 91 | Fracture—Tibia and Fibula (Closed) | 32.8 | 57 |
| 92 | Excision of Nasal Polyp—Single I.P. | 32.8 | 57 |
| 93 | Sigmoidoscopy with Removal of Papillomas or Polyps | 32.8 | 57 |
| 94 | Puncture Aspiration of Cyst | 30.5 | 100 |
| 95 | Fracture—Fibula (Closed) | 30.5 | 85 |
| 96 | Arteriography | 30.5 | 0 |
| 97 | Large Bowel Resection | 30.5 | 0 |
| 98 | Gall Bladder Surgery with Choledochostomy | 30.5 | 0 |
| 99 | Transurethral Electrosection of Prostate | 30.5 | 0 |
| | TOTAL | 18,470.0 * | 78 |

* This total represents 87 per cent of all surgical procedures (excluding unclassified): 93 per cent of ambulatory procedures and 71 per cent of hospital procedures.

## Ambulatory Surgery Components:
## Variations by Age and Sex

Demographic variations in overall incidence of ambulatory surgery have been presented above. Analysis of the types of procedures which comprised the bulk of incidence at various age-sex levels reveals variations as follows:

### Diagnostic Procedures (21 per cent of Ambulatory Surgery)

Incidence was positively related to increasing age, among both males and females.

Diagnostic procedures accounted for over 30 per cent of all ambulatory surgery among those past 35.

The rate among women aged 25 to 64, while steadily increasing, remained below that of men of comparable age. At 65, the female rate jumped 38 per cent beyond its previous level and at this point slightly exceeded the male rate.

Sigmoidoscopy, the single most frequent ambulatory procedure, accounted for 81 per cent of the procedures in the diagnostic procedure category, and rates followed the overall age pattern just described. The average was 26.6 such procedures per thousand members.

Proctoscopy was relatively infrequent, increased after age 35 for both sexes, reached its highest level among women 65 and over.

Out-of-hospital cystoscopy rates sustained their greatest rise at age 55. The rate for men past 65 was five times the average for all males.

Rhinoscopy, laryngoscopy, and gastroscopy combined accounted for only .5 ambulatory procedures per thousand members.

### Drainage of Abscess, Cyst, Onychia or Paronychia (14 per cent)

Incidence reached its highest point at ages 15 to 24 (50 per thousand males, 31 per thousand females), declined steadily thereafter to a low of 12 and 9 per thousand males and females past 65.

For one procedure in this category, drainage of sebaceous cyst, the incidence among males 15–24 was nearly six times the overall male average and for females, nearly four times.

Males 25–34 experienced the highest rate of ambulatory surgery for pilonidal cysts.

Among males and females aged 45–54, drainage of small abscesses occurred at rates 50 per cent higher than for the membership as a whole.

### *Excision or Cauterization of Local Tumor, Cyst, Benign Neoplasm, Small Lesion (17 per cent)*

As with the previous category, the 15-to-24-year-old group experienced the highest incidence rate—44 per thousand, compared with the overall rate of 27. Thirty per cent of all ambulatory surgery for females aged 15–24 fell into this category.

The incidence of such procedures among girls under the age of 5, while low compared with other age groups, was nearly four times the rate among boys of the same age. Female rates were also significantly higher than male rates from ages 35 to 54 and after 65. Male rates were higher only at ages 5 to 14.

### *Injuries (16 per cent)*

The general age curve of office-treated injuries was highest in youth, decreasing after the teen years to a more or less steady rate until the mid-fifties, when it declined again, reaching the lowest point at age 65.

Overall, 20 per cent of ambulatory surgery for males involved treatment of injuries, as against 12 per cent for females.

The highest injury rates occurred among boys under 15 and girls under 5, with suture of wounds the principal procedure.

The injury rate among girls aged 5 to 14 was less than half the boys' rate at that age, while at ages 15 to 24 it plummeted to a quarter of the male rate.

From age 25 on, male and female rates tended to converge, compared with previous ages, with the female rate overtaking the male rate at ages 45 through 64.

*Fractures.* Office-treated fractures reached their highest level among males aged 15 to 24, who sustained a rate almost as high as that for suturing procedures—in contrast to the younger boys, who had far fewer fractures and many more sutured wounds.

At all ages to 34, males sustained fractures at substantially higher rates than females.

At 35 the pendulum started to swing the other way and accelerated thereafter, until at ages 55 to 64 the female rate was nearly two and one half times the male rate. (The differences are even more pronounced for hospital-treated fractures.)

Women past 65 constituted the only membership segment to experience a higher rate of hospitalized than non-hospitalized fractures (Table 110).

The most frequent fracture sites among males treated out-of-hospital were the upper extremities: the rate at ages 15 to 24

TABLE 110.  Comparison of Out-of-Hospital and In-Hospital Fracture Treatment Rates, by Age and Sex

| | NUMBER OF FRACTURES PER 1000 EXPOSURE YEARS | | | |
| | OUT-OF-HOSPITAL | | IN-HOSPITAL | |
| AGE | *Male* | *Female* | *Male* | *Female* |
|---|---|---|---|---|
| Under 5 | 6.1 | 3.9 | 2.3 | 1.5 |
| 5–14 | 14.1 | 7.5 | 5.4 | 1.9 |
| 15–24 | 20.4 | 4.4 | 5.2 | 2.0 |
| 25–34 | 6.1 | 2.7 | 3.0 | 1.6 |
| 35–44 | 6.7 | 7.3 | 1.7 | 2.3 |
| 45–54 | 4.2 | 6.0 | .8 | 1.4 |
| 55–64 | 4.0 | 9.8 | .8 | 3.5 |
| 65 and Over | 1.5 | 2.9 | 0 | 5.8 |
| ALL | 8.6 | 6.0 | 2.8 | 2.0 |

was 11.4 as compared with 4.3 fractures of the lower extremities and 3.3 fractured facial bones.

For females, fractures of the upper extremities predominated only during childhood, after which the lower extremities were most commonly involved (Table 111).

TABLE 111.   Frequency of Office-Treated Fractures of Upper and Lower Extremities, by Age and Sex

| | NUMBER PER 1000 EXPOSURE YEARS | | | |
|---|---|---|---|---|
| | UPPER EXTREMITIES | | LOWER EXTREMITIES | |
| AGE | Male | Female | Male | Female |
| Under 5 | 3.7 | 2.4 | .5 | 0 |
| 5–14 | 8.9 | 4.5 | 3.5 | 1.9 |
| 15–24 | 11.4 | .8 | 4.3 | 2.4 |
| 25–34 | 1.7 | 1.2 | 2.2 | 1.5 |
| 35–44 | 3.9 | 2.8 | 1.7 | 3.9 |
| 45–54 | 1.7 | 2.3 | .8 | 3.1 |
| 55–64 | 2.4 | 4.0 | .4 | 5.2 |
| 65 and Over | 0 | 2.9 | 1.5 | 0 * |

* 5.8 in hospital.

*Other Injuries.*   In addition to the principal components described previously, other ambulatory procedures classified under general injuries include removal of foreign body, treatment of dislocations, and burns.

Their combined incidence accounted for 3.5 procedures per thousand members (vs. 21.2 fractures and wound sutures): 2.8, removal of foreign body; .5, dislocations; .2, burns.

The highest incidence of all three types was incurred by males 5–14, with a combined rate 2.3 times the overall average.

## Other Musculoskeletal Procedures   (5.5 per cent)

The pattern here showed a clear rise in surgical treatment with increasing age, the rate jumping markedly at age 35 and reaching its highest level for both sexes at 65-plus.

The female rate was lower than the male to age 35 and generally higher after that.

Among women over 65, this category ranked third in importance, following diagnostic procedures (41.5 per cent) and tumors or cysts (20 per cent), and accounting for 13 per cent of their ambulatory surgery.

The chief subdivisions within this category involved treatment of joints and bursae. With respect to the former, women past 65 far surpassed all other groups in frequency of procedures, reaching a level nearly seven times the average.

Treatment of bursae among adult males accelerated with increasing age; the rate at ages 55 to 64 was double that for all males, while the rate after age 65 quadrupled the average.

In contrast, surgical office treatment of joints among male adults and of bursae among female adults dropped off after age 54.

### Gynecological Treatment   (7.3 per cent)

This category of procedures accounted for a third of all ambulatory surgery among women 25 to 34, and 23 per cent in the 35-to-44 group. It occurred less frequently at prior and subsequent age levels and dwindled to comparative unimportance after age 54.

Most ambulatory gynecological surgery involved some type of cervical cauterization.

### Genitourinary Procedures   (3.1 per cent)

With cystoscopy classified elsewhere, under diagnostic procedures, the chief component procedure here was "dilation of urethral stricture by passage of sound".

By far the highest incidence of this procedure occurred among males 65 and over, whose rate was ten times the overall average, 44.4 vs. 4.4 per thousand members of all ages.

Males 55 to 64 incurred the next highest rate, 17 procedures per thousand. Males younger than 45 averaged less than one such procedure per thousand.

Female rates of urethral stricture treatment during childhood (to age 14) and from 25 to 44 were six to ten times as high as male rates at comparable ages. The highest rate for women, however, 10 per thousand, occurred at ages 55 to 64.

### Eye Procedures   (4.1 per cent)

After age 15, the trend was slightly and irregularly upward through age 64, then downward.

Over half the procedures classified as ambulatory eye surgery involved the eyelid. The age groups 45 to 64, both male and female, incurred the highest frequencies of such surgery.

Men and women past 65 incurred identical rates of surgery of the lacrimal tract—2.9 procedures per thousand; this rate was nearly five times the overall male rate and nearly three times the overall female rate.

### Ear Procedures   (1 per cent)

This was one of the smallest categories, with the rate only a quarter of that for eye procedures, and with no discernible age pattern of frequency variations.

Men past 65 incurred more ear than eye procedures, at a rate nearly four times the average; while women of the same age incurred no ear procedures, but had a somewhat higher rate of eye surgery than the men.

### Nose and Throat Procedures   (4.8 per cent)

*Tonsillectomy.* Ambulatory tonsillectomies were performed most frequently for children under age 5—and within that group, about 50 per cent more frequently for girls than boys. (In the hospital the boys' rate was a third higher than the girls' at this age.)

Overall, this procedure accounted for one half of one per cent of all ambulatory surgery.

## TABLE 112. Incidence of Ambulatory Surgery, by Type of Surgery, by Age and Sex

Part I: to Age 24

| TYPE OR SITE OF PROCEDURE | All Members | NUMBER OF PROCEDURES PER 1000 EXPOSURE YEARS | | | | | | | |
|---|---|---|---|---|---|---|---|---|---|
| | | ALL | | UNDER 5 | | 5-14 | | 15-24 | |
| | | Male | Female | Male | Female | Male | Female | Male | Female |
| All Procedures * | 157.3 | 156.8 | 157.7 | 99.0 | 69.9 | 115.0 | 78.0 | 208.8 | 155.3 |
| *Diagnostic* | 33.0 | 36.2 | 29.8 | 2.3 | 2.5 | 1.3 | .8 | 8.1 | 13.6 |
| Sigmoidoscopy | 26.6 | 30.0 | 23.2 | 1.4 | 0 | .8 | .4 | 5.7 | 8.0 |
| Proctoscopy | 3.4 | 3.5 | 3.3 | 0 | .5 | .5 | .4 | 1.9 | 2.4 |
| Cystoscopy | 2.5 | 2.4 | 2.6 | 0 | 0 | 0 | 0 | .5 | 3.2 |
| *Drainage: Abscess, Cyst, etc.* | 21.4 | 22.8 | 19.8 | 9.8 | 5.9 | 15.5 | 14.2 | 50.3 | 30.7 |
| Small Abscess | 8.1 | 8.3 | 7.9 | 6.5 | 2.9 | 8.7 | 7.0 | 9.0 | 6.4 |
| Onychia or Paronychia | 4.4 | 4.5 | 4.3 | 2.3 | 1.5 | 3.1 | 3.0 | 8.1 | 4.4 |
| Sebaceous Cyst | 4.3 | 4.5 | 4.1 | 0 | 0 | .6 | 1.0 | 24.7 | 17.1 |
| *Excision or Cauterization* | 26.5 | 24.4 | 28.7 | 2.8 | 10.9 | 20.5 | 17.0 | 42.7 | 45.1 |
| Small Benign Neoplasm | 10.2 | 9.7 | 10.8 | 1.9 | 1.0 | 4.8 | 5.9 | 16.6 | 13.2 |
| Local Small Lesion | 10.0 | 9.0 | 11.0 | .9 | 6.9 | 11.0 | 6.0 | 14.3 | 20.3 |
| Other Tumor, Cyst, Lesion | 6.3 | 5.7 | 6.9 | 0 | 3.0 | 4.7 | 5.1 | 11.8 | 11.6 |
| *Other Infection or Skin Repair* | 4.8 | 5.2 | 4.5 | 4.6 | 4.0 | 1.9 | 2.8 | 21.3 | 9.6 |
| *Injuries* | 24.7 | 30.9 | 18.3 | 56.0 | 31.2 | 56.9 | 26.4 | 48.4 | 12.0 |
| Suture of Wounds | 13.8 | 17.9 | 9.6 | 44.8 | 23.8 | 34.7 | 15.5 | 22.3 | 5.6 |
| Fracture Reduction | 7.4 | 8.6 | 6.0 | 6.1 | 3.9 | 14.1 | 7.5 | 20.4 | 4.4 |
| *Other Musculoskeletal Treatment* | 8.5 | 9.0 | 7.9 | 3.7 | 1.5 | 3.1 | 1.3 | 5.7 | 4.0 |
| Joints | 3.6 | 3.7 | 3.4 | .9 | 1.0 | 1.3 | 0 | 1.0 | 1.2 |
| Bursae | 2.7 | 3.3 | 2.1 | 0 | 0 | .2 | 0 | 1.4 | 0 |

Table (procedure categories, percentages — column headings not printed on page):

| | 1 | 2 | 3 | 4 | 5 | 6 | 7 | 8 | 9 |
|---|---|---|---|---|---|---|---|---|---|
| *Eye* | 6.3 | 6.1 | 6.6 | 4.2 | 2.5 | 3.5 | 2.5 | 6.6 | 6.4 |
| Eyelid | 3.4 | 3.2 | 3.6 | 1.9 | 0 | 1.7 | .6 | 2.8 | 4.0 |
| Cornea | 1.8 | 1.7 | 1.8 | .9 | 1.5 | 1.0 | 1.7 | 3.3 | 1.6 |
| Lacrimal Tract | .7 | .6 | 1.0 | .5 | 1.0 | .2 | 0 | .5 | .4 |
| *Ear* | 1.6 | 1.5 | 1.6 | 1.4 | 1.0 | 1.0 | 2.6 | 1.0 | 1.6 |
| *Nose and Throat* | 7.3 | 9.1 | 5.6 | 8.4 | 8.4 | 9.1 | 6.2 | 17.1 | 4.4 |
| Epistaxis | 3.6 | 4.8 | 2.4 | 4.2 | 3.0 | 6.8 | 4.1 | 12.8 | 3.6 |
| Tonsillectomy | .8 | .8 | .9 | 3.3 | 4.9 | 1.9 | 1.7 | .5 | 0 |
| Antrum Irrigation | 1.2 | 1.2 | 1.3 | 0 | 0 | 0 | .4 | .9 | .8 |
| Nasal Polyp | .2 | .3 | .1 | 0 | 0 | 0 | 0 | 0 | 0 |
| Antrum Puncture | .9 | 1.1 | .5 | 0 | 0 | 0 | 0 | .5 | 0 |
| *Heart and Blood Vessels* | 1.0 | .6 | 1.3 | 0 | 0 | 0 | 0 | 0 | 0 |
| "Cut-down" | .2 | .3 | 0 | 0 | 0 | 0 | 0 | 0 | 0 |
| Leg-vein Injection | .8 | .3 | 1.3 | 0 | 0 | .6 | .2 | 0 | 0 |
| *Glands* | .6 | .1 | 1.1 | 0 | .5 | 0 | 0 | 0 | .4 |
| *Gastrointestinal-Abdominal System* | 2.7 | 3.1 | 2.3 | 1.9 | .5 | 0 | .2 | .9 | 1.6 |
| Hemorrhoid Treatment | 1.6 | 1.8 | 1.2 | 0 | 0 | .4 | 2.1 | .9 | .8 |
| Abscess, Incision and Drainage | .6 | .6 | .6 | 0 | 0 | .2 | 2.1 | 0 | .8 |
| *Genitourinary System* | 4.8 | 5.2 | 4.3 | 2.4 | .5 | 0 | .4 | .9 | .4 |
| Dilation, Urethral Stricture | 4.4 | 4.6 | 4.1 | 0 | .5 | 0 | .2 | .5 | .4 |
| *Gynecological Surgery* | 11.3 | — | 23.0 | — | 0 | — | — | — | 22.3 |
| Cauterization, Cervix | 8.9 | — | 18.2 | — | 0 | — | — | — | 17.1 |
| *Neurosurgery* | .2 | .2 | .2 | 0 | 0 | 0 | 0 | 0 | 0 |
| *Unclassified* | 2.6 | 2.4 | 2.7 | 1.4 | .4 | 1.3 | 1.5 | 5.7 | 3.2 |

* Procedures listed within categories do not include all components of those categories.

TABLE 112. (Cont'd)  Incidence of Ambulatory Surgery, by Type of Surgery, by Age and Sex

Part II: Ages 25 and Over

| | NUMBER OF PROCEDURES PER 1000 EXPOSURE YEARS | | | | | | | | | |
| | 25–34 | | 35–44 | | 45–54 | | 55–64 | | 65 AND OVER | |
| TYPE OR SITE OF PROCEDURE | Male | Female | Male | Female | Male | Female | Male | Female | Male | Female |
|---|---|---|---|---|---|---|---|---|---|---|
| All Procedures * | 161.1 | 187.9 | 155.9 | 219.7 | 182.9 | 217.8 | 182.9 | 178.4 | 235.2 | 203.5 |
| *Diagnostic* | 44.9 | 29.4 | 53.8 | 50.1 | 60.2 | 54.9 | 76.5 | 61.2 | 81.3 | 84.3 |
| Sigmoidoscopy | 40.6 | 22.8 | 45.2 | 38.8 | 50.9 | 46.0 | 61.7 | 49.1 | 60.6 | 61.1 |
| Proctoscopy | 3.4 | 3.5 | 6.7 | 6.2 | 5.4 | 4.3 | 6.0 | 5.8 | 4.4 | 11.6 |
| Cystoscopy | .9 | 2.3 | 1.9 | 5.1 | 3.9 | 3.2 | 8.4 | 5.7 | 11.8 | 5.8 |
| *Drainage: Abscess, Cyst, etc.* | 37.6 | 23.2 | 21.5 | 22.9 | 26.0 | 24.1 | 11.9 | 17.3 | 11.8 | 8.7 |
| Small Abscess | 9.9 | 5.4 | 7.0 | 9.9 | 12.1 | 12.9 | 4.7 | 8.1 | 2.9 | 5.8 |
| Onychia or Paronychia | 6.5 | 7.8 | 5.0 | 5.4 | 5.4 | 4.3 | 2.8 | 4.0 | 1.5 | 2.9 |
| Sebaceous Cyst | 9.1 | 5.4 | 3.4 | 2.5 | 1.1 | 2.9 | 1.6 | 2.3 | 3.0 | 0 |
| *Excision or Cauterization* | 24.2 | 26.4 | 23.7 | 31.9 | 32.0 | 40.2 | 25.1 | 28.9 | 25.2 | 40.7 |
| Small Benign Neoplasm | 11.7 | 11.6 | 11.7 | 14.1 | 12.7 | 16.9 | 10.7 | 10.4 | 10.4 | 17.5 |
| Local Small Lesion | 9.5 | 10.1 | 7.8 | 12.4 | 10.8 | 12.4 | 6.8 | 11.0 | 7.4 | 14.5 |
| Other Tumor, Cyst, Lesion | 3.0 | 4.7 | 4.2 | 6.4 | 8.5 | 10.9 | 7.6 | 7.5 | 7.4 | 8.7 |
| *Other Infection or Skin Repair* | 9.0 | 3.9 | 3.3 | 5.1 | 3.1 | 4.9 | 2.0 | 1.2 | 1.5 | 2.9 |
| *Injuries* | 15.6 | 11.2 | 17.9 | 15.6 | 12.4 | 16.1 | 9.2 | 13.3 | 8.9 | 5.8 |
| Suture of Wounds | 7.3 | 6.2 | 7.2 | 5.7 | 5.6 | 7.2 | 4.4 | 1.7 | 4.4 | 2.9 |
| Fracture Reduction | 6.1 | 2.7 | 6.7 | 7.3 | 4.2 | 6.0 | 4.0 | 9.8 | 1.5 | 2.9 |
| *Other Musculoskeletal Treatment* | 7.3 | 5.8 | 10.6 | 13.0 | 15.2 | 18.4 | 14.7 | 6.9 | 20.7 | 26.2 |
| Joints | 3.4 | 1.6 | 4.5 | 5.1 | 8.5 | 7.5 | 5.2 | 5.2 | 5.9 | 23.3 |
| Bursae | 2.6 | 1.9 | 4.4 | 5.1 | 5.6 | 5.2 | 6.7 | 1.7 | 13.3 | 0 |

| | | | | | | | | | | |
|---|---|---|---|---|---|---|---|---|---|---|
| *Eye* | 5.2 | 5.8 | 6.4 | 7.4 | 9.3 | 11.5 | 8.8 | 12.1 | 4.4 | 5.8 |
| Eyelid | 2.2 | 2.7 | 2.2 | 4.5 | 5.7 | 7.5 | 6.8 | 6.9 | 1.5 | 2.9 |
| Cornea | 2.1 | 1.6 | 3.1 | 1.7 | 2.0 | 2.0 | .4 | 2.9 | 0 | 0 |
| Lacrimal Tract | 0 | 1.5 | .3 | 1.2 | .8 | 1.1 | 1.2 | 2.3 | 2.9 | 2.9 |
| *Ear* | 2.6 | .8 | 1.4 | 1.1 | 2.0 | 2.3 | .4 | 1.2 | 5.9 | 0 |
| *Nose and Throat* | 5.6 | 3.1 | 8.1 | 4.8 | 7.6 | 4.6 | 7.2 | 9.8 | 16.3 | 5.8 |
| Epistaxis | 3.0 | 1.2 | 1.7 | .6 | 3.1 | 1.7 | 2.4 | 2.9 | 5.9 | 2.9 |
| Tonsillectomy | 0 | 0 | 0 | | 0 | 0 | 0 | 0 | 0 | 0 |
| Antrum Irrigation | .5 | .7 | 1.9 | 3.1 | 2.0 | .3 | 2.0 | 5.2 | 4.4 | 2.9 |
| Nasal Polyp | 0 | 0 | .5 | 0 | 0 | .3 | 1.2 | 0 | 3.0 | 0 |
| Antrum Puncture | 1.7 | .4 | 3.1 | 0 | 1.9 | .8 | 0 | 0 | 3.0 | 0 |
| *Heart and Blood Vessels* | .9 | 3.1 | .5 | 1.1 | .6 | 2.9 | .8 | 2.3 | 8.9 | 2.9 |
| "Cut-down" | .4 | 0 | 0 | 0 | 0 | 0 | .8 | 0 | 5.9 | 0 |
| Leg-vein Injection | .5 | 3.1 | .5 | 1.1 | .6 | 2.3 | 0 | 2.3 | 3.0 | 2.9 |
| *Glands* | 0 | .8 | 0 | 2.5 | .3 | 2.6 | 0 | .6 | 0 | 0 |
| *Gastrointestinal-Abdominal System* | 5.2 | 2.7 | 4.7 | 3.4 | 4.0 | 3.2 | 6.4 | 4.6 | 0 | 11.7 |
| Hemorrhoid Treatment | 3.5 | 1.2 | 2.8 | 1.7 | 2.2 | 2.0 | 4.8 | 2.9 | 0 | 8.7 |
| Abscess, Incision and Drainage | 1.7 | 1.5 | .8 | .8 | .8 | .6 | 1.2 | 0 | 0 | 0 |
| *Genitourinary System* | 1.3 | 8.1 | 1.7 | 7.1 | 6.5 | 4.0 | 17.1 | 11.0 | 44.4 | 0 |
| Dilation, Urethral Stricture | 1.3 | 8.1 | .6 | 6.5 | 5.7 | 3.7 | 17.1 | 9.8 | 44.4 | 0 |
| *Gynecological Surgery* | — | 62.4 | — | 49.2 | — | 21.6 | — | 5.8 | — | 8.7 |
| Cauterization, Cervix | — | 50.8 | — | 41.3 | — | 14.7 | — | 2.9 | — | 8.7 |
| *Neurosurgery* | .4 | 0 | .3 | 0 | .6 | 1.4 | 0 | 0 | 0 | 0 |
| *Unclassified* | 1.3 | 1.2 | 2.0 | 4.5 | 3.1 | 5.2 | 2.8 | 2.3 | 5.9 | 0 |

* Procedures listed within categories do not include all components of those categories.

*Treatment of Epistaxis.* As with fractures, treated nose-bleeds occurred most frequently among males aged 15 to 24 (12.8 per thousand). This type of treatment was also of more than average consequence to the younger boys.

Frequency among males dropped to a fraction of its earlier level from ages 25 through 64, ranging from 1.7 to 3.1, then spurted at age 65 to a rate of 5.9.

The female rate averaged half that of males, never exceeded the 4.1 per thousand incurred at ages 5 to 14.

*Antrum Irrigation or Puncture.* These procedures, with an overall incidence of 2.1, showed an erratic but generally upward curve, reaching a rate of 7.4 among males aged 65 and over.

### Treatment of Heart and Blood Vessels  *(.6 per cent)*

From ages 25 through 64, women incurred substantially higher rates than men, producing an overall rate for this category which more than doubled the male rate. This was accounted for almost entirely by leg vein injections.

At age 65, the male rate leaped upward, to three times the female rate (8.9 vs. 2.9) and fifteen times the overall male average (.6). Two procedures comprised the sudden spurt—exposure of an incision into vein ("cut-down"), and injection of leg vein.

### Gastrointestinal-Abdominal Procedures  *(1.7 per cent)*

In this category, the men generally showed substantially higher rates than the women to age 65, at which point the women's rate increased to 11.7 per thousand, i.e. five times the female average. The increase resulted from procedures involving enucleation or injection of external hemorrhoids.

*Ambulatory Components: Possible Implications of*
*Occupation Class Variations*

The incidence of ambulatory surgery was a third higher among the professional-executive than among the blue-collar class (200 vs. 150 procedures per thousand members).

Variations in the types of surgery undergone by the two groups have been analyzed in an attempt to learn whether the higher overall rate shown for the professional-executive category harbors social connotations.

The evidence in Table 113 suggests some basis for this hypothesis, particularly with respect to what might be classified as preventive surgery, i.e. treatment of local tumors and cysts. The overall rate in professional-executive families was more than double the rate in blue-collar families. The greatest differences occurred with respect to treatment of sebaceous cysts, but the rates of excisions of benign neoplasms for both sexes, and of cauterization of local lesions among females, were also substantially higher among the professional-executive groups. Since members of blue-collar families were not remiss about seeking medical care in general, and since there is no reason to suspect a lower incidence of the above conditions based on class, the data may suggest either a lesser consciousness of important symptoms among the blue-collar families or a difference in the quality of their office care.

While the data in Table 113 are not conclusive, they certainly suggest avenues of further investigation relevant to defining quantitative or qualitative adequacy of ambulatory medical care.

TABLE 113.  Comparison of Incidence of Leading Ambulatory
Surgical Procedures, Blue-Collar vs. Professional-Executive
Families, by Sex

| | NUMBER OF PROCEDURES PER 1000 EXPOSURE YEARS * | | | |
| | MALES | | FEMALES | |
| TYPE OF PROCEDURE | Blue Collar | Professional Executive | Blue Collar | Professional Executive |
|---|---|---|---|---|
| Tumor, Cyst | 26.0 | 51.8 | 27.3 | 59.5 |
| Benign Neoplasm (Excision) | 8.7 | 16.1 | 8.7 | 14.5 |
| Sebaceous Cyst (I and D) | 4.1 | 12.1 | 3.6 | 11.6 |
| Pilonidal Cyst (I and D) | .8 | 1.4 | .3 | 0 |
| Local Lesion (Cauterization) | 10.4 | 17.5 | 12.7 | 30.5 |
| Other | 2.0 | 4.7 | 2.0 | 2.9 |
| Abscess, Boil, Onychia, etc. (I and D) | 18.5 | 18.2 | 15.0 | 13.1 |
| Other Infection or Skin Repair | 4.5 | 10.1 | 3.9 | 8.0 |
| Injuries | 24.7 | 36.3 | 17.3 | 18.2 |
| Fracture: Closed Reduction | 6.6 | 13.5 | 5.9 | 8.0 |
| Suture of Wounds | 15.6 | 18.8 | 9.0 | 8.0 |
| Foreign Body Removal | 2.5 | 4.0 | 2.4 | 2.2 |
| Joints, Bursae Treatment | 8.1 | 1.4 | 4.6 | 13.8 |
| Eye Treatment | 4.8 | 10.1 | 6.3 | 7.3 |
| Eyelid | 2.3 | 8.1 | 3.4 | 2.2 |
| Urethral Stricture (Dilation) | 4.7 | 2.7 | 3.8 | 11.6 |
| Cervix (Cauterization) | — | — | 18.6 | 18.2 |
| Proctoscopy | 3.1 | 8.1 | 3.2 | 2.9 |
| Sigmoidoscopy | 33.4 | 31.6 | 25.9 | 23.9 |
| Cystoscopy | 3.1 | 1.3 | 2.2 | 2.2 |

* Including dependents.

# Chapter 15

# HOSPITAL SURGERY

Certain aspects of hospital surgery have been examined in previous sections: who performed, in what types of hospitals (Chapter 6), and relative incidence as compared with ambulatory surgery (Chapter 14). The most frequent types of hospital surgery were also shown, as part of the combined list of the hundred leading procedures.

The present chapter reviews total incidence variations among member subgroups as shown by a number of indices, introduces detailed incidence data for individual procedures, and compares procedure rates, by type of procedure, for age-sex subgroups. Further data on hospital surgery are included in the chapter on hospitalization studies. Obstetrical services are not included as surgical procedures.

## Frequency

The indices developed to describe the incidence of hospital surgery include the number of surgical procedures, the number of surgical admissions, and the number of individual surgical patients per thousand eligible persons per year. From these indices, others of interest from a medical care standpoint may be derived—admissions per patient, procedures per patient, procedures per admission.

Of each thousand comprehensive plan members insured

for the full study year, 48 individuals incurred 55 surgical admissions and underwent 61 surgical procedures. They accounted for nearly half of all hospital admissions.

Demographic variations in these overall averages have already been touched on in discussion of ambulatory surgery, to permit comparison of the two categories of surgical service. The emphasis changes in the following analysis, but a certain amount of repetition is unavoidable.

## Variations in Overall Utilization Rates Among Population Subgroups

The tested factors found to be associated with the widest variations in surgical-frequency rates were age, sex, and area of residence.

There were also demonstrable variations among adults in the different marital and subscriber-relationship categories. The experience in terms of duration of enrollment and family size, while showing a positive relationship, is explained primarily on the basis of age distribution.

Occupation class appeared to be of very little consequence with respect to total rates; incidence of hospital surgery among the different classes varied within a relatively narrow range. A hint of a challenge to quality researchers emerged, however, in certain class differences found among females, on analysis of types of surgery performed.

### VARIATIONS BY AGE AND SEX

Both the proportion of patients undergoing surgery in hospitals and the number of procedures performed per patient tended to rise with increasing age, except for the younger contingent. Any generalization about tendencies at various age levels, however, must be qualified by observation of the different patterns shown for males and females.

Male rates were lowest (32–39 procedures per thousand) from the ages of 10 through 34. They were higher before age 10 than at any time up to age 54. As a result, the average rate for boys (50) was not much lower than the average rate for men (57). In contrast, the rate for adult women was nearly two and one half times that of girls—89 vs. 36 procedures per thousand exposure years.

The female rate of procedures at ages 20 to 24 was twice that of the previous age span (71 vs. 35 at ages 15 to 19). It rose again, and peaked, at ages 35 to 54, when one hospital surgical procedure was recorded for every ten women.

Rates for women were thus dramatically and consistently higher (averaging about double) than male rates at all ages from 20 through 54, at which point the men's rate, continuing its rise, and the female rate, dropping suddenly, were at the same level for the first time since ages 15 to 19.

At age 65 the male rate exceeded the female rate by 41 per cent (compared with 15 per cent found for ambulatory surgery). Female rates at ages 45 to 54 were about on a par with male rates past 65.

The number of surgical procedures per admission and per patient had some effect on the age curve of utilization, since each index tended to rise. For example, among females aged 10 to 14, 19 per thousand became hospital surgical patients who averaged 1.023 procedures each, producing a procedure utilization rate of 19.7; while among females aged 35 to 44 there were four times as many surgical patients (76 per thousand) who averaged 1.307 procedures each, to produce a utilization rate of 99.8, or five times as high as the younger group. The same type of difference accounts for the finding that utilization rates were slightly higher for men than boys although surgical admission rates were practically the same (Table 114).

VARIATIONS ASSOCIATED WITH MARITAL STATUS,
RELATIONSHIP TO SUBSCRIBER, AND FAMILY SIZE

Married females experienced the highest rate, followed by single females, married males, single males, widowed-divorced-

TABLE 114. Hospital Surgery: Primary Utilization Indices, by Age and Sex

| | NUMBER PER 1000 EXPOSURE YEARS | | | | | | | | |
| | SURGICAL PROCEDURES | | | SURGICAL ADMISSIONS | | | DIFFERENT PATIENTS | | |
| AGE | Total | Male | Female | Total | Male | Female | Total | Male | Female |
|---|---|---|---|---|---|---|---|---|---|
| All | 60.8 | 53.9 | 67.9 | 55 | 48 | 61 | 48 | 43 | 54 |
| Adults | 72.5 | 56.6 | 89.1 | 63 | 49 | 79 | 54 | 41 | 67 |
| Children | 43.1 | 49.8 | 36.3 | 42 | 48 | 36 | 39 | 45 | 34 |
| Under 5 | 52.4 | 62.6 | 41.6 | 49 | 58 | 40 | 47 | 54 | 39 |
| 5– 9 | 56.4 | 62.3 | 50.5 | 55 | 61 | 50 | 52 | 57 | 47 |
| 10–14 | 29.0 | 38.0 | 19.7 | 29 | 38 | 20 | 27 | 34 | 19 |
| 15–19 | 34.7 | 34.7 | 34.8 | 34 | 34 | 34 | 32 | 32 | 32 |
| 20–24 | 55.9 | 32.3 | 70.6 | 50 | 28 | 63 | 45 | 25 | 58 |
| 25–34 | 54.9 | 38.9 | 69.4 | 50 | 36 | 63 | 44 | 28 | 58 |
| 35–44 | 72.6 | 45.7 | 99.8 | 64 | 39 | 89 | 56 | 35 | 76 |
| 45–54 | 80.8 | 58.2 | 103.7 | 69 | 50 | 89 | 57 | 41 | 73 |
| 55–64 | 77.1 | 76.9 | 77.4 | 66 | 64 | 69 | 56 | 54 | 58 |
| 65 and Over | 92.2 | 102.1 | 84.3 | 79 | 89 | 61 | 67 | 75 | 49 |

separated females and males. The rate for married females was 60 per cent higher than that for married males, 47 per cent higher than for single females. The latter rate in turn was 27 per cent higher than for single males.

Of all the various types of service for which they were eligible, hospital surgery stands out as the least used by the widowed-divorced-separated category, in comparison with use rates of other marital categories. Their rate was extraordinarily low—even lower than that of children. As will be seen later, their medical admissions were the highest. Moreover, their ambulatory surgery rates, while lower, were in the case of females well within sight of the married female rate, and higher than that for married males. But their hospital surgery rate was less than half the overall married rate; and even the married male rate, which was so much lower than that of married females, was nearly 50 per cent higher than the rate for widowed-divorced-separated women.

Both male and female spouses experienced considerably higher rates of hospital surgery than the corresponding classes of subscribers. In the case of male spouses, this was contrary to the pattern shown for office care, where they generally used fewer services than male subscribers. The ambulatory surgical rate among male spouses was 128, compared with 178 for male subscribers. The corresponding hospital rates for the two groups were 77 and 55. (This apparent instance of low-high surgical indices in a very small population segment, however, cannot be cited in support of hypotheses about unnecessary use of hospitalization without further refinement of the data.)

Hospital rates for families of different size followed the usual pattern with one exception. Although, as with ambulatory surgery, the per capita rates declined with increasing family size, the incidence of hospital surgery among the largest families was, for once, close to expectations based on family composition instead of lower, as for other services.

Whether this experience among families with four or more children stemmed from simultaneous tonsillectomies performed for the brood would require additional investigation.

TABLE 115.   Hospital Surgery: Primary Utilization Indices, by Marital Status, Relationship, and Family Size

| | NUMBER PER 1000 EXPOSURE YEARS | | | | | | | | |
|---|---|---|---|---|---|---|---|---|---|
| | SURGICAL PROCEDURES | | | SURGICAL ADMISSIONS | | | DIFFERENT PATIENTS | | |
| MEMBER CATEGORY | Total | Male | Female | Total | Male | Female | Total | Male | Female |
| *Adults* | | | | | | | | | |
| Married | 75.4 | 58.1 | 93.0 | 66 | 50 | 82 | 56 | 42 | 70 |
| Single | 55.1 | 49.6 | 63.2 | 47 | 42 | 54 | 41 | 36 | 49 |
| Widowed, Divorced, | | | | | | | | | |
| Separated | 34.7 | 28.7 | 39.1 | 31 | 29 | 33 | 31 | 29 | 33 |
| Subscriber | 58.5 | 55.2 | 76.0 | 50 | 47 | 66 | 43 | 40 | 57 |
| Spouse | 90.9 | 76.6 | 92.1 | 81 | 73 | 81 | 69 | 56 | 70 |
| *Family Size* | | | | | | | | | |
| 2 | 78.2 | | | 65 | | | 57 | | |
| 3 | 62.6 | | | 56 | | | 50 | | |
| 4 | 59.8 | | | 55 | | | 49 | | |
| 5 | 50.6 | | | 47 | | | 43 | | |
| 6 or More | 52.7 | | | 48 | | | 43 | | |

OCCUPATION CLASS VARIATIONS

Of all demographic variables considered, occupation class revealed the smallest range of variations with respect to hospital surgical rates (Table 116), in contrast to experience with out-of-hospital surgery where a wide range was found.

TABLE 116. Hospital Surgery: Primary Utilization Indices, by Occupation Class of Subscriber

| OCCUPATION CLASS | NUMBER PER 1000 EXPOSURE YEARS * | | |
|---|---|---|---|
| | Surgical Procedures | Surgical Admissions | Different Patients |
| Professional | 57.5 | 47.8 | 42 |
| Executive | 52.1 | 47.2 | 45 |
| Sales | 59.3 | 57.0 | 47 |
| Clerical and White-Collar Unspecified | 63.8 | 57.7 | 51 |
| Blue-Collar | 59.3 | 53.2 | 47 |
| Retired | 96.0 | 88.0 | 72 |
| Student | 29.4 | 29.4 | 29 |

* Including dependents.

The lowest utilization rate among employed classes (52 procedures per thousand) was found in the executive group, which was among the highest in incidence of office surgery. The highest rate (64) occurred in the clerical category, which experienced the next-to-lowest office surgery rate. Professional, sales, and blue-collar classes had almost identical rates of hospital surgery (58–59).

As will be shown in discussion of hospitalization use, the surgical indices for a given class are not necessarily indicative of the relative number of hospital days used by that class for surgical care. The clerical class, for example, despite highest surgical admission and procedure rates, was next to lowest on the hospitalization index because of relatively short stays.

The number of procedures per surgical admission ranged from 1.00 for students and 1.04 for the sales class to 1.203 in the professional category.

GEOGRAPHIC VARIATIONS

Wide variations in hospital surgical rates among different areas have already been discussed in the section on ambulatory surgery. The analysis attempted to determine whether high hospital surgical rates in an area might be offset by low ambulatory rates, and vice versa.

Aside from Manhattan, the highest rates of hospital surgery were found in the areas with the highest proportions of private voluntary or proprietary general care beds to population—Richmond and Westchester. In Richmond, the high rate (81 procedures per thousand) was partly attributable to an exceptionally high number of procedures per patient—1.444, vs. the average 1.263. Westchester was average as to this last index, but had more surgical patients and admissions than any other area, to account for its utilization rate of 87.

New Jersey, which recorded far-below-average use of all ambulatory services, was almost average with respect to hospital surgery and in fact slightly exceeded the average rate for the five-county area of New York City.

The broad range of experience shown in Table 117 indi-

TABLE 117. Hospital Surgery: Primary Utilization Indices, by Area of Subscriber Residence

| AREA | NUMBER PER 1000 EXPOSURE YEARS | | |
| --- | --- | --- | --- |
| | Surgical Procedures | Surgical Admissions | Different Patients |
| Manhattan | 49.1 | 45 | 40 |
| Bronx | 58.0 | 52 | 45 |
| Brooklyn | 50.8 | 47 | 42 |
| Queens | 61.5 | 55 | 48 |
| Richmond | 80.9 | 69 | 56 |
| Nassau | 66.1 | 59 | 51 |
| Suffolk | 69.1 | 64 | 59 |
| Westchester | 87.1 | 79 | 69 |
| Other New York | 69.0 | 62 | 53 |
| New Jersey | 58.4 | 51 | 46 |

cates the geographic variable as a probably fruitful avenue of further investigation for those interested in both quality and quantity of medical care.

## Component Procedures

### Distribution and Frequency, by Procedure Category

Although the ambulatory surgical rate was two and one half times that of hospital surgery, 370 different procedures were performed for in-patients as against 197 different ambulatory procedures. The concentration as to type of procedure was of course entirely different. As shown in Table 118, three

TABLE 118.  Comparison of Leading Categories of Surgery Performed on Ambulatory and In-Hospital Basis

| PER CENT OF ALL PROCEDURES * | | | |
|---|---|---|---|
| *Ambulatory* | | *In-Hospital* | |
| *Category* | % | *Category* | % |
| Drainage, Excision, or | | Gastrointestinal-Abdominal | 19.8 |
| Cauterization of Abscess, | | Gynecological and Breast | 19.5 |
| Cyst, Lesion, Tumor | | Nose and Throat | 16.7 |
| (excluding Gynecology) | 30.9 | Musculoskeletal Conditions | 9.9 |
| Diagnostic Procedures | 21.4 | Fractures | (4.1) |
| Other Skin Repairs | | Other | (5.8) |
| (Sutures or Infection) | 12.1 | Diagnostic Procedures | 8.8 |
| Musculoskeletal Conditions | 10.2 | | |
| Fractures | (4.8) | | |
| Other | (5.4) | | |
| | 74.6 | | 74.7 |

* Excluding unclassified.

fourths of ambulatory surgery involved local aberrations and repairs, diagnostic procedures, or musculoskeletal conditions. The largest categories in the hospital were gastrointestinal-abdominal, gynecological-breast, and nose-throat surgery. Diagnostic surgery accounted for more than one of every five ambulatory procedures, less than 10 per cent of hospital procedures.

Of passing interest is the coincidentally similar proportion of ambulatory and hospital procedures accounted for by musculoskeletal conditions, including fractures—in each case, 10 per cent of the total.

The diagnostic category, accounting for 8.8 per cent of in-hospital procedures, was comprised chiefly of cystoscopy (4.7 per cent of all procedures), sigmoidoscopy (1.7 per cent), bronchoscopy (1.2 per cent), laryngoscopy (.5 per cent) and esophagoscopy (.4 per cent). In contrast, one procedure, sigmoidoscopy, accounted for 17 per cent of all ambulatory surgery.

In the utilization rate tables which follow, diagnostic procedures have been classified according to system—e.g. cystoscopy is included with urinary tract surgery (and accounts for most of it).

TABLE 119.  Frequency of Hospital Surgery, by Category

| TYPE OF SURGERY | Number of Procedures Per 1000 Exposure Years |
|---|---|
| Gastrointestinal-Abdominal Tract | 12.7 |
| Gynecological System and Breast | 11.3 |
| Nose and Throat | 9.9 |
| Musculoskeletal System | 5.7 |
| Urinary Tract | 3.6 |
| Tumors, Cysts NEC | 3.0 |
| Heart or Blood Vessels | 2.2 |
| Eye | 2.1 |
| Male Genital Organs | 2.0 |
| Neurological NEC | 1.2 |
| Glands NEC | 1.1 |
| Bronchial-Thoracic | 1.0 |
| Skin | .9 |
| Ear | .8 |
| Unclassified | 3.3 |
| TOTAL | 60.8 |

NEC = Not elsewhere classified.

The hospital surgery categories listed in Table 118 are those showing an incidence of more than five procedures per 1000 members. The frequencies of procedures in the remaining categories ranged from .8 to 3.6 (Table 119).

TABLE 120. Most Frequent Hospital Procedures, Ranked According to Two Methods

| | METHOD 1 | | | | METHOD 2 | | |
|---|---|---|---|---|---|---|---|
| | INDIVIDUAL PROCEDURES | | | | SIMILAR PROCEDURES GROUPED | | |
| RANK | Procedure | Hospital Frequency Per 1000 Exposure Years | Per Cent of All Hospital Surgery | RANK | Procedure(s) | Hospital Frequency Per 1000 Exposure Years | Per Cent of All Hospital Surgery |
| 1. | Tonsillectomy-Adenoidectomy | 8.33 | 14.4 | 1. | Tonsillectomy-Adenoidectomy | 8.33 | 14.4 |
| 2. | Dilatation and Curettage | 4.01 | 6.9 | 2. | Dilatation and Curettage | 4.18 | 7.2 |
| 3. | Panhysterectomy | 2.21 | 3.8 | 3. | Hernioplasty | 2.96 | 5.1 |
| 4. | Hernioplasty, Inguinal, Uni-lateral | 1.81 | 3.1 | 4. | Cystoscopy | 2.72 | 4.7 |
| 5. | Appendectomy | 1.71 | 3.0 | 5. | Hysterectomy | 2.68 | 4.6 |
| 6. | Cystoscopy with Ureteral Catheterization | 1.69 | 2.9 | 6. | Tumors—Not Elsewhere Classified | 2.18 | 3.8 |
| 7. | Cholecystectomy | 1.57 | 2.7 | 7. | Appendectomy | 1.71 | 3.0 |
| 8. | Excision of Cyst, Fibroadenoma or Other Benign Tumor, Unilateral | 1.29 | 2.2 | 8. | Hemorrhoidectomy | 1.71 | 3.0 |

234

| | | | |
|---|---|---|---|
| 9. | Local Excision of Small Benign Lesion | 1.01 | 1.8 |
| 10. | Cystoscopy, Diagnostic | .89 | 1.5 |
| 11. | Hemorrhoidectomy, Internal | .87 | 1.5 |
| 12. | Sigmoidoscopy, Diagnostic | .75 | 1.3 |
| 13. | Cataract Removal | .66 | 1.1 |
| 14. | Submucous Resection | .61 | 1.1 |
| 15. | Wide Excision of Lesion, without Graft or Plastic Closure | .56 | 1.0 |
| 16. | Posterior Vaginal Wall, Repair of Rectocele | .52 | .9 |
| 17. | Hemorrhoidectomy with Fissurectomy | .52 | .9 |
| 18. | Varicose Veins, Repair, One Leg | .47 | .8 |
| 19. | Lipectomy | .47 | .8 |
| 20. | Bronchoscopy, Diagnostic | .47 | .8 |
| 21. | Fistulotomy or Fistulectomy | .45 | .8 |
| 22. | Strabismus Correction | .45 | .8 |
| 23. | Subtotal Gastrectomy | .42 | .7 |
| 24. | Excision of Lesion of Tendons or Fibrous Sheath in Other Locations | .38 | .7 |
| 25. | Salpingo-Oophorectomy | .35 | .6 |
| TOTAL | | 32.47 | 56.1 |

| | | | |
|---|---|---|---|
| 9. | Cholecystectomy | 1.57 | 2.7 |
| 10. | Excision of Breast Cyst | 1.29 | 2.4 |
| 11. | Sigmoidoscopy | .99 | 1.7 |
| 12. | Varicose Veins, Repair | .99 | 1.7 |
| 13. | Colpoplasty | .87 | 1.5 |
| 14. | Cataract Removal | .73 | 1.3 |
| 15. | Bronchoscopy | .66 | 1.2 |
| 16. | Prostatectomy | .66 | 1.2 |
| 17. | Salpingo-Oophorectomy | .63 | 1.1 |
| 18. | Submucous Resection | .61 | 1.1 |
| 19. | Fracture of Radius, Ulna | .59 | 1.0 |
| 20. | Strabismus Correction | .59 | 1.0 |
| 21. | Lipectomy | .52 | .8 |
| 22. | Fistulotomy or Fistulectomy | .45 | .8 |
| 23. | Gastrectomy | .45 | .8 |
| 24. | Thyroidectomy | .40 | .7 |
| 25. | Circumcision | .40 | .7 |
| TOTAL | | 38.87 | 67.5 |

## Leading Procedures

When procedure frequencies are listed individually, instead of in categories as on page 233, it becomes apparent that the strength of the leading categories depends, to a large extent, on relatively few procedures.

Gastrointestinal-abdominal surgery was the leading hospital category because it included a number of the most frequent procedures such as hernioplasty, appendectomy, cholecystectomy, hemorrhoidectomy, sigmoidoscopy. Similarly, gynecology was in second place mainly because of two procedures —dilatation-curettage ("D&C") and hysterectomy; while the category of nose and throat surgery ranked third on the basis of one operation—tonsillectomy.

The ranking of procedures in order of frequency introduces problems because of the number of variations involved for many operations. Eight different procedure descriptions are possible for the various types of hernia operations, of which one was among the twenty-five leading individual procedures performed in the hospital, accounting for 3 per cent of hospital surgery; all eight types combined comprised 5 per cent of the total. Two types of hemorrhoidectomy were among the leading operations, accounting for 2.4 per cent of all hospital surgery; when the other hospital variations of this procedure are added, the total becomes 3 per cent. The rank in frequency order changes, too, under the alternative methods of listing: panhysterectomy, for example, was third on the list of single procedures, but is outranked by hernioplasty and cystoscopy when all types of the latter two are combined. The differences produced by the two methods of selecting most frequent procedures are shown in Table 120.

## All Procedures

The incidence of all procedures performed for in-patients from the GHI comprehensive plan sample is given in a detailed listing in Table 121.

TABLE 121.   Incidence of All Surgical Procedures
Performed for In-Patients

| PROCEDURE NAME | Incidence Per 100,000 Exposure Years |
|---|---|
| Drainage of Sebaceous Cyst | 7.0 |
| Drainage of Furuncle | 2.3 |
| Drainage of Small Subcutaneous Abscess | 2.4 |
| Drainage of Carbuncle | 2.4 |
| Drainage of Large Subcutaneous Abscess | 4.7 |
| Drainage of Onychia or Paronychia | 2.3 |
| Incision and Removal of Foreign Body | 7.0 |
| Biopsy of Skin or Subcutaneous Tissue | 2.3 |
| Local Excision of Small Benign Neoplasm | 100.9 |
| Wide Excision of Lesion, without Graft or Plastic Closure | 56.3 |
| Wide Excision of Lesion, with Graft or Plastic Closure | 11.7 |
| Excision of Lesion of Unusual Size or Number | 18.7 |
| Lipectomy | 46.9 |
| Excision of Nail, Partial | 4.7 |
| Excision of Nail Bed or Nail Fold, Complete | 7.0 |
| Excision of Pilonidal Cyst or Sinus | 30.5 |
| Resection of Malignant Lesion of Skin | 23.4 |
| Plastic Operation of Skin | 14.1 |
| Skin Grafts | 14.0 |
| Treatment of Burns | 2.3 |
| Suture of Wounds | 35.2 |
| Electro-Cauterization or Fulguration of Local Small Lesions | 4.7 |
| Breast—Mastotomy with Exploration, Drainage of Abscess or Foreign Body Removal | 7.0 |
| Incision—Biopsy of Breast | 7.1 |
| Excision of Cyst or Benign Tumor, Breast, Unilateral | 129.3 |
| Excision of Cyst or Benign Tumor, Breast, Bilateral | 7.1 |
| Breast Excision—Complete (Simple) Mastectomy, Unilateral | 7.1 |
| Breast—Radical Mastectomy | 32.9 |
| Bones—Aspiration Biopsy of Bone Marrow | 4.7 |
| Bones—Incision of Periosteum | 2.4 |
| Bones—Sequestrectomy for Osteomyelitis | 2.4 |
| Bones—Incision—Removal of Metal Band, Plate Screws, or Nail | 4.7 |
| Bones—Incision—Femur, Subtrochanteric | 2.4 |
| Bones—Excision—Biopsy of Bone | 2.4 |
| Bones—Excision—Coccygectomy | 4.7 |
| Excision of Bone Cyst, Large Bones | 14.1 |
| Excision of Bone Cyst, Small Bones | 14.0 |
| Bones—Excision—Femur, Tibia, Humerus, Radius, Fibula, etc. | 4.7 |
| Bones—Repair—Spinal Fusion | 2.4 |
| Bones—Repair—Pectus Excavation | 2.4 |
| Bones—Repair—Femur | 2.4 |
| Fracture—Nasal Bone—Closed Reduction | 16.4 |
| Fracture—Nasal Bone—Open Reduction | 9.4 |
| Fracture—Malar Bone—Simple or Compound, Depressed, Open Reduction | 4.7 |

TABLE 121. *(Cont'd)* Incidence of All Surgical Procedures
Performed for In-Patients

| PROCEDURE NAME | Incidence Per 100,000 Exposure Years |
|---|---|
| Fracture—Maxilla—Closed Reduction | 2.4 |
| Fracture—Mandible—Simple or Compound, Closed Reduction | 4.7 |
| Fracture—Mandible—Simple or Compound, with Wiring of Teeth | 2.4 |
| Fracture—Zygoma—Open | 4.7 |
| Fracture—Vertebra—Closed | 4.7 |
| Fracture—Clavicle—Closed | 4.7 |
| Fracture—Humerus—Closed | 14.1 |
| Fracture—Humerus—Open | 4.7 |
| Fracture—Elbow—Open | 2.4 |
| Fracture—Radius—Closed | 18.8 |
| Fracture—Radius—Open | 4.7 |
| Fracture—Colles—Closed | 7.0 |
| Fracture—Radius and Ulna—Closed | 32.8 |
| Fracture—Radius and Ulna—Open | 2.4 |
| Fracture—Finger—Closed | 16.4 |
| Fracture—Finger—Open | 4.7 |
| Fracture—Femur, Hip or Shaft—Closed | 2.4 |
| Fracture—Femur, Hip or Shaft—Open | 11.7 |
| Fracture—Patella—Closed | 2.4 |
| Fracture—Tibia—Closed | 11.7 |
| Fracture—Fibula—Closed | 4.7 |
| Fracture—Tibia and Fibula—Closed | 14.1 |
| Fracture—Tibia and Fibula—Open | 4.7 |
| Fracture—Bimalleolar (Ankle)—Closed | 7.0 |
| Fracture—Trimalleolar (Ankle)—Closed | 9.4 |
| Fracture—Tarsal—Closed | 2.3 |
| Fracture—Os Calcis—Closed | 2.3 |
| Fracture—Metatarsal Bone—Closed | 4.7 |
| Joints—Incision—Knee | 2.4 |
| Joints—Arthrocentesis | 2.3 |
| Joints—Excision of Intervertebral Disc | 4.7 |
| Joints—Excision of Intervertebral Disc with Spinal Fusion— One Surgeon | 9.4 |
| Joints—Excision of Intervertebral Disc with Spinal Fusion— Two Surgeons | 2.4 |
| Joints—Meniscectomy—Excision of Semilunar Cartilege of Knee Joint | 16.4 |
| Joints—Excision—Ankle | 2.4 |
| Joints—Bunion Operation, Unilateral | 4.7 |
| Joints—Bunion Operation, Bilateral | 7.1 |
| Joints—Repair—Ankle | 2.4 |
| Joints—Hammer Toe Operation—Complete Chondolectomy, One Toe | 14.0 |
| Joints—Repair—Foot, Triple Arthrodesis, Unilateral | 2.4 |
| Joints—Manipulation—Shoulder | 2.4 |
| Joints—Club Foot and Application Cast—Unilateral | 2.3 |

TABLE 121. *(Cont'd)*

| PROCEDURE NAME | Incidence Per 100,000 Exposure Years |
|---|---|
| Dislocation—Jaw—Closed | 2.4 |
| Dislocation—Finger—Open | 4.7 |
| Dislocation—Hip—Closed | 7.1 |
| Drainage of Infected Bursa | 2.3 |
| Bursae—Incision—Removal of Subdeltoid Calcareous Deposits | 4.7 |
| Needling of Bursa | 2.3 |
| Bursae—Excision of Bursa, Olecranon | 2.4 |
| Bursae—Excision of Bursa, Other | 2.4 |
| Muscles—Incision—Removal of Foreign Body in Muscle | 2.4 |
| Muscles—Incision—Division of Scalenus Anticus | 2.4 |
| Muscles—Incision—Muscle Biopsy, Superficial | 4.7 |
| Muscles—Excision—Myectomy | 2.4 |
| Muscles—Repair of Diaphragmatic Hernia | 11.7 |
| Drainage of Tendon Sheath Infection for Tenosynovitis | 4.7 |
| Tendons, Tendon Sheaths and Fascia—Incision of Fibrous Sheath | 4.7 |
| Tendons, Tendon Sheaths—Removal of Foreign Body | 2.4 |
| Excision of Lesion of Tendon or Fibrous Sheath, including Ganglion, Digits Only | 9.4 |
| Excision of Lesion of Tendon or Fibrous Sheath, including Ganglion, in Other Locations | 37.5 |
| Tendons, Tendon Sheaths and Fascia—Incision—Excision of Baker's Cyst | 2.4 |
| Repair—Lengthening of Tendon, without Graft | 4.7 |
| Tendons, Tendon Sheaths and Fascia—Repair—Suture of Ruptured Tendon | 2.4 |
| Tendons, Tendon Sheaths and Fascia—Suture—Achilles Tenorrhaphy | 2.4 |
| Tendons, Tendon Sheaths and Fascia—Primary Suture— One Tendon | 14.1 |
| Extremities—Drainage of Single Infected Space of Hand | 4.7 |
| Amputation—Single Finger | 7.1 |
| Amputation—Thigh | 4.7 |
| Amputation—Leg | 4.7 |
| Amputation—Foot | 4.7 |
| Amputation—Single Toe | 7.1 |
| Plaster Cast—Shoulder to Hand | 2.3 |
| Plaster Cast—Ankle (Foot to Mid-Leg) | 2.3 |
| Nose—Excision of Nasal Polyp—Single I.P. | 14.1 |
| Nose—Excision—Submucous Resection | 61.0 |
| Nose—Repair—Rhinoplasty (Non-Cosmetic) | 4.7 |
| Epistaxis (Cauterization) | 4.7 |
| Accessory Sinuses—Antrum Window—Incision | 4.7 |
| Accessory Sinuses—Incision—Radical Antrum | 9.4 |
| Accessory Sinuses—Incision—Sphenoid Sinusotomy | 2.4 |
| Accessory Sinuses—Excision—Intranasal Radical Ethmoid | 4.7 |
| Accessory Sinuses—Excision—Intranasal Radical Ethmoid, Bilateral | 2.4 |
| Accessory Sinuses—Introduction—Irrigation of Antrum | 2.3 |
| Larynx—Incision—Laryngofissure of Tissue with Removal of Tumor | 2.4 |

TABLE 121. *(Cont'd)* Incidence of All Surgical Procedures
Performed for In-Patients

| PROCEDURE NAME | *Incidence Per 100,000 Exposure Years* |
|---|---|
| Larynx—Excision—Laryngectomy | 4.7 |
| Larynx—Introduction—Injection of Radiopaque Substance into Larynx for Bronchography | 2.4 |
| Larynx—Laryngoscopy—Diagnostic | 2.4 |
| Larynx—Endoscopy—Laryngoscopy (with Biopsy) | 2.4 |
| Larynx—Endoscopy—Laryngoscopy with Removal of Foreign Body | 4.7 |
| Larynx—Endoscopy—Laryngoscopy with Removal of Tumor from Vocal Chord | 18.8 |
| Trachea and Bronchi—Incision—Tracheotomy | 7.1 |
| Trachea and Bronchi—Endoscopy—Bronchoscopy (Diagnostic) | 46.9 |
| Trachea and Bronchi—Endoscopy—Bronchoscopy (with Biopsy) | 9.4 |
| Trachea and Bronchi—Endoscopy—Bronchoscopy with Lipiodol | 9.4 |
| Lungs and Pleura—Incision—Exploratory Thoracotomy with or without Biopsy | 2.4 |
| Lungs and Pleura—Incision—Closed Thoracotomy for Drainage | 4.7 |
| Lungs and Pleura—Incision—Pulmonary Decortication | 2.4 |
| Lungs and Pleura—Incision—Thoracentesis | 4.7 |
| Lungs and Pleura—Excision—Total Pneumonectomy | 2.4 |
| Lungs and Pleura—Excision—Lobectomy or Segmental Resection | 11.7 |
| Lungs and Pleura—Surgical Collapse, Therapy—Thoracoplasty | 2.4 |
| Heart and Pericardium—Incision—Cardiotomy with Exploration or Removal of Foreign Body | 2.4 |
| Heart and Pericardium—Incision—Mitral Valvulotomy or Commissurotomy | 2.4 |
| Heart and Pericardium—Introduction—Right Heart Catheterization | 14.1 |
| Heart and Pericardium—Introduction—Right Heart Catheterization—with Selective Angiocardiogram or Aortagram | 7.1 |
| Heart and Pericardium—Introduction—Left Heart Catheterization | 4.7 |
| Heart and Pericardium—Introduction—Left Heart Catheterization—with Selective Angiocardiogram or Aortagram | 7.1 |
| Heart and Pericardium—Repair—Open Heart Surgery (Operator) | 9.4 |
| Heart and Pericardium—Repair—Open Heart Surgery (Assistants, Pump, Monitor, etc.) | 2.4 |
| Heart and Pericardium—Arrhythmia Conversion—Cardioversion | 2.4 |
| Arteries and Veins—Incision—Arteriotomy with Exploration | 7.1 |
| Arteries and Veins—Introduction into Arteries and Veins | 4.7 |
| Arteries and Veins—Introduction—Arteriography | 30.5 |
| Arteries and Veins—Introduction—Translumbar Aortagram | 4.7 |
| Arteries and Veins—Introduction—Angiocardiography | 9.4 |
| Arteries and Veins—Introduction—Exposure of an Incision into Vein ("Cut-down") | 2.3 |
| Arteries and Veins—Introduction—Blood Transfusion | 7.1 |
| Arteries and Veins—Introduction—Repair of Aneurysm of Aorta | 2.4 |
| Arteries and Veins—Suture—Ligation or Section of Patent Ductus | 2.4 |
| Arteries and Veins—Suture—Ligation and Division—One Leg | 7.1 |

TABLE 121. *(Cont'd)*

| PROCEDURE NAME | *Incidence Per 100,000 Exposure Years* |
|---|---|
| Arteries and Veins—Suture—Ligation and Division—Both Legs | 4.7 |
| Arteries and Veins—Long Incision—Ligation and Excision— One Leg | 46.9 |
| Arteries and Veins—Long Incision—Ligation and Excision— Both Legs | 32.9 |
| Arteries and Veins—Ligation and Division, Short Saphenous Veins | 2.4 |
| Spleen—Excision—Spleenectomy | 7.1 |
| Incision—Drainage of Lymph Node Abscess or Lymphadenitis | 2.4 |
| Excision—Biopsy, Lymph Node, Superficial | 11.7 |
| Excision—Biopsy of Anterior Scalene Lymph Node | 18.8 |
| Lymph Nodes and Lymphatic Channels—Excision—Radical Axillary Dissection, Unilateral | 4.7 |
| Lymph Nodes and Lymphatic Channels—Excision—Radical Cervical Dissection, Bilateral | 2.4 |
| Mediastinum—Incision—Mediastinotomy with Exploration | 2.4 |
| Mouth—Excision of Benign Lesion of Buccal Mucosa | 2.4 |
| Mouth—Excision—Including Radical Neck Resection | 2.4 |
| V-Excision of Lesion of Lip | 2.3 |
| Lips—Repair—Cheiloplasty | 2.3 |
| Lips—Repair—Cheilostomatoplasty | 4.7 |
| Tongue—Excision—Partial Glossectomy | 2.4 |
| Palate and Uvula—Repair—Palatoplasty | 7.1 |
| Palate and Uvula—Repair—Palatoplasty with Pharyngoplasty | 2.4 |
| Palate and Uvula—Suture of Palate Wound or Injury | 2.4 |
| Salivary Glands and Ducts—Excision of Parotid Tumor | 11.7 |
| Pharynx, Adenoids and Tonsils—I and D Retropharyngeal Abscess | 2.4 |
| Tonsillectomy and/or Adenoidectomy | 833.1 |
| Resection of the Esophagus | 2.4 |
| Endoscopy—Esophagoscopy, Diagnostic | 14.1 |
| Endoscopy—Esophagoscopy,with Biopsy | 7.1 |
| Endoscopy—Esophagoscopy with Foreign Body | 2.4 |
| Stomach—Incision—Gastrotomy with Exploration or Foreign Body Removal | 2.4 |
| Stomach—Incision—Pyloric Stenosis | 4.7 |
| Stomach—Excision—Total Gastrectomy, Complete | 2.4 |
| Stomach—Excision—Subtotal Gastrectomy, Partial | 42.2 |
| Stomach—Endoscopy—Gastroscopy—Diagnostic | 7.1 |
| Stomach—Endoscopy—Gastroscopy—with Biopsy | 2.4 |
| Stomach—Repair—Pyloroplasty | 7.1 |
| Stomach—Repair—Gastroenterostomy . | 2.4 |
| Stomach—Repair—Gastrojejunostomy | 4.7 |
| Stomach Repair—Gastrostomy for Feeding | 2.4 |
| Intestines—Incision, except Rectum | 2.4 |
| Intestines—Excision, Small Bowel Resection, except Rectum | 2.4 |
| Intestines—Excision—Ileostomy, except Rectum | 2.4 |
| Intestines—Excision—Large Bowel Resection, except Rectum | 30.5 |

TABLE 121. *(Cont'd)*  Incidence of All Surgical Procedures
Performed for In-Patients

| PROCEDURE NAME | *Incidence Per 100,000 Exposure Years* |
|---|---|
| Intestines—Excision—Total Colectomy, except Rectum | 2.4 |
| Intestines—Repair—Colostomy, except Rectum | 4.7 |
| Intestines—Repair—Revision of Colostomy, except Rectum | 2.4 |
| Intestines—Destruction—Enterolysis, except Rectum | 11.7 |
| Intestines—Suture—Closure of Colostomy, except Rectum | 2.4 |
| Excision of Meckel's Diverticulum | 2.4 |
| Appendectomy | 171.3 |
| Appendicostomy | 4.7 |
| Rectum—Abdomino-perineal, Resection | 9.4 |
| Rectum—Proctoscopy—Diagnostic—without Biopsy | 2.4 |
| Rectum—Sigmoidoscopy—Diagnostic | 75.1 |
| Rectum—Sigmoidoscopy—with Biopsy | 9.4 |
| Rectum—Sigmoidoscopy—with Removal of Papillomas or Polyps | 14.1 |
| Rectum—Repair—Prolapse and Procidentia | 9.4 |
| Anus—Incision—Fistulotomy or Fistulectomy | 44.6 |
| Anus—Incision—Abscess, I and D, including Ischiorectal | 28.1 |
| Anus—Excision—Cutting Operation for Fissure | 4.7 |
| Anus—Excision—Cryptectomy, Papillectomy | 2.4 |
| Anus—Excision—Hemorrhoidectomy, Internal with or without External | 86.8 |
| Anus—Excision—Hemorrhoidectomy, External Only | 2.3 |
| Anus—Excision—Hemorrhoidectomy with Fissurectomy | 51.6 |
| Anus—Excision—Complicated and Multiple Fistulae | 2.4 |
| Anus—Repair—Proctoplasty | 2.4 |
| Anus—Repair—Anorectal Plastic Procedure for Incontinence | 2.4 |
| Biliary Tract—Incision—Gall Bladder Surgery with Choledochostomy | 30.5 |
| Biliary Tract—Incision—Cholecystotomy or Cholecystostomy | 9.4 |
| Biliary Tract—Excision—Cholecystectomy | 157.2 |
| Biliary Tract—Suture—Cholecystorrhaphy | 2.4 |
| Pancreas—Incision—Pancreatotomy | 2.4 |
| Incision into Abdomen, Peritoneum and Omentum | 2.4 |
| Abdomen, Peritoneum and Omentum—Incision—Exploratory Laparotomy | 11.7 |
| Abdomen, Peritoneum and Omentum—Incision—Drainage of Peritoneal Abscess | 2.4 |
| Abdomen, Peritoneum and Omentum—Incision—Paracentesis, Abdominal | 4.7 |
| Abdomen, Peritoneum and Omentum—Excision—Omentectomy, Epiploectomy | 2.4 |
| Abdomen, Peritoneum and Omentum—Repair—Hernioplasty—Inguinal, Unilateral | 180.7 |
| Abdomen, Peritoneum and Omentum—Repair—Hernioplasty—Recurrent | 7.0 |
| Abdomen, Peritoneum and Omentum—Repair—Hernioplasty—Inguinal, Bilateral | 25.8 |

TABLE 121. *(Cont'd)*

| PROCEDURE NAME | Incidence Per 100,000 Exposure Years |
|---|---|
| Abdomen, Peritoneum and Omentum—Repair—Hernioplasty—Femoral, Unilateral | 11.7 |
| Abdomen, Peritoneum and Omentum—Repair—Hernioplasty—Ventral, Incisional | 32.9 |
| Abdomen, Peritoneum and Omentum—Repair—Hernioplasty—Epigastric | 9.4 |
| Abdomen, Peritoneum and Omentum—Repair—Hernioplasty—Umbilical | 28.2 |
| Kidney—Nephrolithotomy with Removal of Calculus | 2.4 |
| Kidney—Nephrectomy | 7.0 |
| Kidney—Excision of Cyst of Kidney | 4.7 |
| Kidney—Pyeloplasty | 2.4 |
| Kidney—Extracorporeal Renal Dialysis | 2.4 |
| Ureter—Ureterotomy with or without Lithotomy | 18.8 |
| Ureter—Ureteroplasty | 2.4 |
| Ureter—Ureterocystostomy | 2.4 |
| Bladder—Cystectomy | 2.4 |
| Bladder—Transurethral Electro-Resection of Vesical Neck, Female | 2.4 |
| Bladder—Transurethral Resection of Bladder Tumors with or without Radium Insertion | 9.4 |
| Bladder—Cystoscopy—Diagnostic | 89.2 |
| Bladder—Cystoscopy with Biopsy | 2.4 |
| Bladder—Cystoscopy with Ureteral Catheterization | 169.0 |
| Bladder—Cystoscopy with Stone Removal, Ureteral Dilation | 7.0 |
| Bladder—Cystoscopy with Fulguration of Small Bladder Tumor | 4.7 |
| Bladder—Closure of Cystostomy of External Fistula of Bladder | 2.4 |
| Bladder—Closure of Vesicovaginal, Vesicouterine, or Vesicorectal Fistula | 4.7 |
| Urethra—Meatotomy: Cutting of Meatus and Suturing | 9.4 |
| Urethra—Urethroplasty | 2.4 |
| Urethra—Dilation of of Urethral Stricture by Passage of Sound | 9.4 |
| Penis—Circumcision | 39.9 |
| Penis—Repair—Hypospadias, 2nd Degree | 2.4 |
| Testis—Biopsy, Unilateral | 2.4 |
| Testis—Orchiectomy, Unilateral | 9.4 |
| Testis—Orchiectomy, Bilateral | 4.7 |
| Testis—Orchiopexy, Unilateral | 21.1 |
| Testis—Orchiopexy, Bilateral | 2.4 |
| Epididymis—Epididymectomy, Unilateral | 2.4 |
| Tunica Vaginalis—Puncture Aspiration of Hydrocele | 2.3 |
| Tunica Vaginalis—Excision of Hydrocele, Unilateral | 28.2 |
| Scrotum—Scrotoplasty | 2.4 |
| Vas Deferens—Vasectomy, Unilateral | 2.4 |
| Vas Deferens—Vasectomy, Bilateral | 2.4 |
| Spermatic Cord—Excision of Hydrocele, Unilateral | 2.4 |
| Spermatic Cord—Excision of Varicocele, Unilateral | 2.4 |

TABLE 121. *(Cont'd)* Incidence of All Surgical Procedures
Performed for In-Patients

| PROCEDURE NAME | *Incidence Per 100,000 Exposure Years* |
|---|---|
| Prostate—Incision—Biopsy | 11.7 |
| Prostate—Excision—Prostatectomy | 2.4 |
| Prostate—Prostatectomy, Perineal and Retropubic Radical | 2.4 |
| Prostate—Prostatectomy—Suprapubic | 25.8 |
| Prostate—Prostatectomy—Retropubic | 4.7 |
| Prostate—Transurethral—Electrosection of Prostate | 30.5 |
| Vulva—Vulvectomy, Partial | 2.4 |
| Vulva—Hymenectomy | 2.4 |
| Vulva—Bartholin Cyst—Excision, One Side | 18.8 |
| Vagina—Colpectomy or Colpocleisis, Complete | 2.4 |
| Vagina—Excision of Vaginal Cyst | 2.4 |
| Vagina—Repair of Cystocele—Anterior Vaginal Wall | 2.4 |
| Vagina—Repair of Cystocele with Repair of Urethrocele— Anterior Vaginal Wall | 4.7 |
| Vagina—Repair of Rectocele—Posterior Vaginal Wall | 51.6 |
| Vagina—Repair of Cystocele and Rectocele—Anterior and Posterior Vaginal Walls | 28.2 |
| Vagina—Repair of Rectocele and Perineoplasty—Posterior Vaginal Wall | 7.0 |
| Vagina—Repair of Cystocele, Rectocele, and Perineoplasty— Anterior and Posterior Vaginal Walls | 11.7 |
| Vagina—Reconstruction of Congenital Deformities of the Vagina | 2.4 |
| Vagina—Culdoscopy | 4.7 |
| Oviduct, Ovary and Uterus—Tubal Ligation | 11.7 |
| Oviduct, Ovary and Uterus—Salpingo-Oophorectomy, Complete or Partial | 35.2 |
| Oviduct, Ovary and Uterus—Oophorectomy—Complete or Partial | 28.2 |
| Oviduct, Ovary and Uterus—Myomectomy: Excision of Fibroid Tumor | 14.1 |
| Oviduct, Ovary and Uterus—Panhysterectomy, Abdominal or Vaginal | 220.6 |
| Oviduct, Ovary and Uterus—Subtotal Hysterectomy | 11.7 |
| Oviduct, Ovary and Uterus—Radical Hysterectomy | 2.4 |
| Oviduct, Ovary and Uterus—Vaginal Hysterectomy | 32.9 |
| Oviduct, Ovary and Uterus—Removal of Cervical Stump | 2.4 |
| Oviduct, Ovary and Uterus—Dilatation and Curettage with Amputation of Cervix | 21.1 |
| Oviduct, Ovary and Uterus—Local Excision of Lesion of Cervix | 4.7 |
| Oviduct, Ovary and Uterus—Dilatation and Curettage | 401.3 |
| Oviduct, Ovary and Uterus—Insertion of Radioactive Substance into Cervix | 2.4 |
| Oviduct, Ovary and Uterus—Hysteropexy (Manchester) | 7.0 |
| Oviduct, Ovary and Uterus—Tracheloplasty | 4.7 |
| Thyroid Gland—Thyroidectomy | 11.7 |
| Thyroid Gland—Hemithyroidectomy: Lobectomy | 30.5 |
| Thyroid Gland—Thyroglossal Cyst | 9.4 |

TABLE 121. *(Cont'd)*

| PROCEDURE NAME | *Incidence Per 100,000 Exposure Years* |
|---|---|
| Parathyroid, Thymus, Pineal and Adrenal Glands—<br>Adrenalectomy | 2.4 |
| Structures Overlying the Meninges, Brain and Spinal Cord—<br>Exploratory Burr Holes, Per Trephine, Bilateral | 2.4 |
| Structures Overlying the Meninges, Brain and Spinal Cord—<br>Laminectomy, Exploratory | 23.5 |
| Structures Overlying the Meninges, Brain and Spinal Cord—<br>Cranioplasty | 2.4 |
| Meninges and Meningeal Vessels—Drainage of Subdural Hematoma | 2.4 |
| Meninges and Meningeal Vessels—Lumbar Puncture | 9.4 |
| Meninges and Meningeal Vessels—Pneumoencephalogram | 11.7 |
| Meninges and Meningeal Vessels—Myelogram | 14.1 |
| Brain—Excision of Brain Cyst, Neoplasm or Abscess | 2.4 |
| Brain—Ventriculocisternostomy | 7.0 |
| Brain—Ventriculogram | 14.1 |
| Brain—Chemopallidectomy | 2.4 |
| Peripheral Nerves, Cerebral Nerves and Ganglia—Transection<br>of Vagus Nerve | 7.0 |
| Peripheral Nerves, Cerebral Nerves and Ganglia—Excision<br>of Peripheral Neuromata | 2.4 |
| Peripheral Nerves, Cerebral Nerves and Ganglia—Injection<br>of Alcohol, Intraspinal, Paravertebral or Paracranial | 4.7 |
| Peripheral Nerves, Cerebral Nerves and Ganglia—Paravertebral<br>Block | 2.4 |
| Major Nerve—Suture of Nerve, Recent Injury | 2.4 |
| Vegetative Nervous System—Sympathectomy: Lumbar,<br>Unilateral | 11.7 |
| Vegetative Nervous System—Sympathectomy: Lumbar,<br>Bilateral | 2.4 |
| Enucleation of Eyeball, Bulb or Globe | 2.4 |
| Sclera—Sclerotomy, with Removal of Intra-Ocular Foreign Body | 2.4 |
| Sclera—Sclerotomy for Glaucoma | 4.7 |
| Iris and Ciliary Body—Complete Iridectomy | 2.4 |
| Iris and Ciliary Body—Peripheral Iridectomy | 2.4 |
| Iris and Ciliary Body—Diathermy of the Ciliary Body | 2.4 |
| Iris and Ciliary Body—Iridotasis | 2.4 |
| Crystalline Lens—Discission: Needling of Lens | 4.7 |
| Crystalline Lens—Extraction of Lens after Preliminary Iridectomy,<br>Unilateral | 7.0 |
| Crystalline Lens—Extraction of Lens, Combined Cataract<br>Extraction, Unilateral | 65.7 |
| Retina—Reattachment of Retina, Electrocoagulation, Initial | 7.0 |
| Retina—Reattachment of Retina, Electrocoagulation, Subsequent | 2.4 |
| Ocular Muscles—Strabismus Correction, Unilateral | 44.6 |
| Ocular Muscles—Strabismus Correction, Bilateral | 14.1 |
| Eyelids—Excision of Meibomian Glands (Chalazion), Single | 7.0 |
| Eyelids—Blepharoplasty | 4.7 |

TABLE 121. *(Concluded)*

| PROCEDURE NAME | *Incidence Per 100,000 Exposure Years* |
|---|---|
| Eyelids—Blepharorrhaphy: Suture of Eyelid | 4.7 |
| Conjunctiva—Excision—Pterygium | 9.4 |
| Conjunctiva—Repair—Conjunctivoplasty: Free Graft of Conjunctiva | 4.7 |
| Lacrimal Tract—Dacryocystorrhinostomy | 4.7 |
| Lacrimal Tract—Probing of Lacrimonasal Duct | 2.4 |
| Lacrimal Tract—Probing of Lacrimonasal Duct under General Anesthesia | 11.7 |
| External Ear—Otoplasty | 4.7 |
| Middle Ear—Myringotomy: Tympanotomy: Plicotomy | 28.2 |
| Middle Ear—Mobilization of the Stapes | 2.4 |
| Middle Ear—Mastoidectomy, Simple, Unilateral | 7.0 |
| Middle Ear—Mastoidectomy, Radical, Unilateral | 2.4 |
| Middle Ear—Tympanoplasty (Type 1), with or without Graft | 4.7 |
| Middle Ear—Tympanoplasty (Type 2–4), with or without Graft | 2.4 |
| Middle Ear—Stapedectomy, with or without Graft | 21.1 |
| Internal Ear—Fenestration of Semicircular Canals | 2.4 |

## Monthly Variations in Volume

Since the twenty-five leading individual procedures accounted for over half the total volume of hospital surgery, their distribution over the months of the study year might be expected to parallel that of all procedures combined, and with minor deviations this did occur (Table 122). The lightest volume months were August and February, followed by December, while April and May were the heaviest. Varying obvious explanations lend authenticity to such findings—vacation time, short month, Christmas season, tonsillectomy season—and emphasize the elective nature of much of the surgery.

When the leading procedures are considered separately (Table 123), broad variations in monthly volume emerge. Certain procedures seem weighted in favor of certain months for which the total volume was otherwise generally light, and vice versa, but such findings may or may not be of any significance; for most procedures, the small number of cases, when further subdivided by months, provide statistically unreliable results. Eventually it may be feasible and useful to determine whether

TABLE 122.  Distribution of All Hospital Surgery, and 25
Leading Procedures Combined, by Month Performed

| MONTH PERFORMED | Per Cent of All Procedures | Per Cent of 25 Leading Procedures |
|---|---|---|
| | % | % |
| January | 8.6 | 8.7 |
| February | 7.1 | 6.9 |
| March | 8.5 | 9.6 |
| April | 9.5 | 10.3 |
| May | 10.0 | 10.3 |
| June | 9.2 | 9.4 |
| July | 8.0 | 7.4 |
| August | 6.1 | 5.0 |
| September | 7.6 | 7.5 |
| October | 8.8 | 9.0 |
| November | 9.0 | 8.7 |
| December | 7.6 | 7.2 |
| TOTAL | 100.0 | 100.0 |

outstanding variations are traceable to the nature of the illness, to pyschological or personal considerations affecting decisions by patient and surgeon, to varying hospital-bed availability or occupancy pressures, or to chance. For the present, the data may be observed with interest and as a starting point for further studies, but no conclusions are warranted.

## Hospital Surgery Components:
## Variations by Age and Sex

The list of *predominating* types of surgery for the GHI population is probably indicative of overall community practice as of the period studied. By the same token, it provides a base for trend analysis in future years, which would be expected to reflect any major surgical discoveries or changes in surgical practice—as for example if the popularity of tonsillectomies were to decline.

In addition to data on the study population as a whole, variations in type-of-procedure utilization among population subgroups have been derived in order to clarify differences or similarities in total utilization rates by subgroups and to render the findings comparable with experience of other populations.

TABLE 123.  Distribution of 25 Leading Hospital Surgical Procedures, by Month Performed

*(All figures are percentages; each procedure row totals 100.0%)*

| PROCEDURE DESCRIPTION | TOTAL | January | February | March | April | May | June | July | August | September | October | November | December |
|---|---|---|---|---|---|---|---|---|---|---|---|---|---|
| Tonsillectomy and/or Adenoidectomy | 100.0 | 8.7 | 7.6 | 14.5 | 12.3 | 15.0 | 8.7 | 1.6 | .8 | 6.0 | 9.5 | 9.8 | 5.5 |
| Dilatation and Curettage | 100.0 | 10.2 | 6.2 | 11.4 | 9.1 | 11.9 | 7.9 | 5.1 | 7.4 | 4.0 | 9.7 | 9.1 | 8.0 |
| Panhysterectomy | 100.0 | 5.1 | 4.1 | 10.2 | 14.3 | 7.1 | 12.3 | 12.2 | 2.0 | 8.2 | 10.2 | 4.1 | 10.2 |
| Hernioplasty | 100.0 | 12.9 | 7.8 | 6.5 | 7.8 | 5.2 | 10.4 | 11.7 | 7.8 | 9.1 | 6.5 | 6.5 | 7.8 |
| Appendectomy | 100.0 | 9.3 | 6.7 | 6.7 | 10.7 | 8.0 | 4.0 | 5.3 | 12.0 | 8.0 | 12.0 | 9.3 | 8.0 |
| Cystoscopy with Ureteral Catheterization | 100.0 | 5.9 | 0 | 11.7 | 11.8 | 4.2 | 9.9 | 7.0 | 7.0 | 9.9 | 11.3 | 9.9 | 11.3 |
| Cholecystectomy | 100.0 | 7.3 | 10.1 | 10.1 | 11.6 | 11.6 | 15.9 | 7.3 | 0 | 10.1 | 7.3 | 7.3 | 1.4 |
| Excision of Cyst Fibroadenoma or Other Benign Tumor, Unilateral | 100.0 | 6.8 | 6.8 | 13.5 | 6.8 | 6.8 | 6.8 | 13.5 | 8.5 | 6.8 | 6.8 | 10.1 | 6.8 |
| Local Excision of Small Benign Lesion | 100.0 | 9.8 | 9.7 | 7.3 | 9.8 | 9.8 | 4.9 | 14.6 | 9.8 | 0 | 14.6 | 2.4 | 7.3 |
| Hemorrhoidectomy, Internal, with or without External | 100.0 | 2.6 | 7.7 | 0 | 12.8 | 15.4 | 12.8 | 12.8 | 5.1 | 10.3 | 15.4 | 5.1 | 0 |
| Cystoscopy, Diagnostic, Subsequent | 100.0 | 13.1 | 5.3 | 2.6 | 13.1 | 13.1 | 7.9 | 7.9 | 5.3 | 5.3 | 13.2 | 5.3 | 7.9 |
| Sigmoidoscopy, Diagnostic, Initial | 100.0 | 9.7 | 0 | 0 | 9.7 | 3.2 | 22.6 | 16.1 | 0 | 12.9 | 6.4 | 9.7 | 9.7 |
| Cataract Removal | 100.0 | 8.8 | 0 | 11.8 | 11.8 | 2.9 | 8.8 | 11.8 | 0 | 11.8 | 8.8 | 5.9 | 17.6 |
| Submucous Resection | 100.0 | 14.8 | 11.1 | 7.4 | 7.4 | 0 | 3.7 | 7.4 | 3.7 | 11.1 | 7.4 | 14.9 | 11.1 |
| Wide Excision of Lesion, without Graft or Plastic Closure | 100.0 | 8.0 | 12.0 | 8.0 | 8.0 | 12.0 | 8.0 | 12.0 | 4.0 | 8.0 | 0 | 8.0 | 12.0 |
| Posterior Vaginal Wall, Repair of Rectocele | 100.0 | 8.7 | 4.4 | 4.4 | 4.4 | 4.3 | 21.7 | 17.4 | 4.3 | 17.4 | 8.7 | 4.3 | 0 |
| Hemorrhoidectomy with Fissurectomy | 100.0 | 13.6 | 18.2 | 0 | 13.6 | 9.1 | 4.6 | 4.6 | 0 | 18.2 | 0 | 13.6 | 4.5 |
| Long Incision, Ligation and Excision, One Leg | 100.0 | 18.2 | 13.6 | 4.6 | 4.6 | 0 | 4.5 | 9.1 | 13.6 | 0 | 9.1 | 18.2 | 4.5 |
| Lipectomy | 100.0 | 4.6 | 9.1 | 0 | 13.6 | 13.6 | 22.7 | 18.2 | 4.5 | 4.5 | 0 | 4.6 | 4.6 |
| Bronchoscopy, Diagnostic | 100.0 | 10.0 | 0 | 0 | 0 | 20.0 | 5.0 | 5.0 | 10.0 | 20.0 | 0 | 10.0 | 20.0 |
| Fistulotomy or Fistulectomy (I.P.) | 100.0 | 0 | 9.1 | 4.6 | 0 | 22.7 | 13.6 | 4.6 | 13.6 | 9.1 | 4.5 | 18.2 | 0 |
| Strabismus Correction | 100.0 | 5.3 | 0 | 15.8 | 21.0 | 0 | 0 | 15.8 | 10.5 | 10.5 | 5.3 | 15.8 | 0 |
| Subtotal Gastrectomy, Partial | 100.0 | 11.1 | 11.1 | 5.5 | 0 | 5.5 | 0 | 5.6 | 16.7 | 5.6 | 11.1 | 16.7 | 11.1 |
| Excision of Lesion of Tendon or Fibrous Sheath in Other Locations | 100.0 | 0 | 5.9 | 11.7 | 5.9 | 5.9 | 11.8 | 5.9 | 17.6 | 5.9 | 5.9 | 0 | 17.6 |
| Salpingo-Oophorectomy | 100.0 | 8.4 | 4.2 | 8.4 | 8.5 | 17.6 | 11.7 | 11.8 | 5.9 | 5.9 | 11.8 | 5.9 | 5.9 |
| **25 PROCEDURE TOTAL** | 100.0 | 8.7 | 6.9 | 9.6 | 10.3 | 10.3 | 9.4 | 7.4 | 5.0 | 7.5 | 9.0 | 8.7 | 7.2 |

(Since hospital surgery is the most widely insured physician's service, it is potentially the likeliest area for the production of comparable data from the experience of other insurance plans.)

The figures in Table 125 were derived from one year's experience of the study population, and because of the fineness of the data breakdown would undoubtedly vary for a different population or for the same population in a different year. It may be that over a period of years, relative stability will be established for some procedure rates among some subgroups, and even now certain age-sex trends for certain operations may be accepted as probably valid, on the basis of general knowledge; but detailed frequencies of individual operations for each age-sex subgroup must be viewed cautiously, since the smaller the subgroup and/or number of cases, the greater the likelihood of variance in studies of other experience. The following selective comments are made with this reservation in mind.

### Distribution of Procedures

The relative importance of different categories of hospital surgery to different age-sex groups is shown in Table 124.

For males, gastrointestinal-abdominal surgery comprised at least 20 per cent of total procedures at all ages except 5 to 14, rising to a peak of 42 per cent at ages 45 to 54 when it far outranked all other categories, decreasing proportionately thereafter and at age 65 taking second place to genitourinary surgery. The latter category accounted for a constantly increasing proportion of male surgery—8 to 10 per cent at ages under 35, 17 to 18 per cent from 35 to 54, 24 per cent from 55 to 64, 38 per cent at 65-plus. Orthopedic surgery including fractures was in first place for males aged 15 to 24, second place at ages 5 to 14 and 25 to 34, third place at 35 to 44, and of relatively little importance at other ages. Nose and throat surgery (mainly tonsillectomy) far outranked other types to age 14 (47 per cent of all procedures to age 5, 52 per cent from ages 5 to 14), and still accounted for every fourth operation among males aged

Part I: to Age 34

TABLE 124. Distribution of Hospital Surgery by Category, by Age and Sex

| TYPE OF SURGERY | UNDER 5 | | 5–14 | | 15–24 | | 25–34 | |
|---|---|---|---|---|---|---|---|---|
| | Male | Female | Male | Female | Male | Female | Male | Female |
| | % | % | % | % | % | % | % | % |
| Orthopedic Surgery | 7.1 | 7.7 | 16.5 | 8.1 | 30.3 | 15.7 | 20.8 | 4.7 |
| Eye | 3.1 | 11.5 | 2.1 | 4.4 | 3.0 | 3.9 | 3.9 | 1.2 |
| Ear | 3.2 | 1.3 | 2.1 | 2.5 | 0 | 1.0 | 2.6 | 1.8 |
| Nose and Throat | 46.5 | 52.6 | 51.7 | 65.8 | 24.3 | 15.7 | 6.5 | 5.9 |
| Gastrointestinal-Abdominal | 20.5 | 6.4 | 14.0 | 9.3 | 21.2 | 16.6 | 27.2 | 24.8 |
| Urinary and Male Genital | 8.6 | 2.6 | 8.1 | 3.7 | 9.0 | 3.9 | 10.4 | 5.3 |
| Gynecological-Breast | | 1.3 | | | | 24.5 | | 43.8 |
| Heart-Blood | 6.3 | 3.8 | .8 | 0 | 1.5 | 1.0 | 2.6 | 2.4 |
| Thoracic | | | 0 | .6 | 0 | 2.0 | 1.3 | .6 |
| Neurological | 3.1 | 2.5 | 0 | 0 | 0 | 3.9 | 9.1 | 1.8 |
| Glands | 0 | 1.3 | 1.3 | .6 | 0 | 3.9 | 0 | 1.2 |
| Tumors-Cysts | 1.6 | 3.8 | 1.7 | 3.1 | 4.6 | 9.8 | 13.0 | 5.3 |
| Skin | 0 | 5.2 | 1.7 | 1.9 | 6.1 | 2.0 | 2.6 | 1.2 |
| | 100.0 | 100.0 | 100.0 | 100.0 | 100.0 | 100.0 | 100.0 | 100.0 |

250

TABLE 124. (Cont'd)  Distribution of Hospital Surgery by Category, by Age and Sex

Part II: Ages 35 and Over

| TYPE OF SURGERY | 35–44 | | 45–54 | | 55–64 | | 65 AND OVER | |
|---|---|---|---|---|---|---|---|---|
| | Male | Female | Male | Female | Male | Female | Male | Female |
| | % | % | % | % | % | % | % | % |
| Orthopedic Surgery | 13.4 | 5.5 | 5.8 | 9.4 | 6.2 | 13.1 | 3.0 | 10.4 |
| Eye | 4.5 | .6 | 4.2 | 2.3 | 4.5 | 8.2 | 11.7 | 17.2 |
| Ear | 1.3 | .6 | .5 | 2.0 | 0 | 0 | 1.5 | 0 |
| Nose and Throat | 5.1 | 3.2 | 5.3 | 2.6 | 3.9 | .8 | 1.5 | 0 |
| Gastrointestinal-Abdominal | 32.7 | 14.6 | 42.1 | 21.5 | 30.7 | 25.4 | 27.9 | 27.6 |
| Urinary and Male Genital | 17.3 | 5.2 | 18.4 | 4.6 | 24.0 | 7.4 | 38.2 | 0 |
| Gynecological-Breast | | 55.7 | | 42.7 | | 22.9 | | 41.3 |
| Heart-Blood | 7.7 | 5.2 | 4.8 | 3.1 | 6.7 | 6.6 | 1.5 | 0 |
| Thoracic | 1.3 | .9 | 4.2 | .9 | 10.1 | 0 | 2.9 | 0 |
| Neurological | .7 | 0 | 5.3 | 2.0 | 4.4 | 6.6 | 4.4 | 0 |
| Glands | 1.3 | 3.2 | 4.2 | 2.3 | 1.1 | 1.6 | 1.5 | 3.5 |
| Tumors-Cysts | 12.1 | 4.4 | 4.2 | 5.4 | 6.7 | 5.7 | 4.4 | 0 |
| Skin | 2.6 | .9 | 1.0 | 1.2 | 1.7 | 1.7 | 1.5 | 0 |
| | 100.0 | 100.0 | 100.0 | 100.0 | 100.0 | 100.0 | 100.0 | 100.0 |

15 to 24, after which it dropped off. Bronchial-thoracic surgery (including bronchoscopy) was in third place for males at ages 55 to 64, accounting for 10 per cent of all procedures, but was relatively unimportant at other ages.

For females, gynecological and breast surgery accounted for every fourth procedure at ages 15 to 24, increased to a peak of 56 per cent of all hospital surgery at ages 35 to 44, dropped thereafter. At ages 55 to 64, this category was outranked by gastrointestinal-abdominal procedures, but returned to its leading position at age 65-plus, when, as at ages 25 to 34 and 45 to 54, it accounted for over two of every five procedures. Gastrointestinal-abdominal procedures were generally of less relative importance to females than males, at all age levels, but contributed an increasing proportion of female surgery from childhood through young adulthood; at ages 25 to 34 and after 55, every fourth operation was in this category. Eye surgery was the third largest category for women at 65-plus, accounting for 17 per cent of procedures, as compared with 4 per cent for all age-sex groups combined. The proportion of orthopedic surgery was much higher among males than females from ages 5 through 44, at which point a reversal occurred, with the percentage of procedures in this category dropping for men and rising for women. The predominance of nose-throat surgery among children was even more pronounced for girls than boys, accounting for 53 per cent of hospital surgery among girls under age 5, and 66 per cent among those aged 5 to 14.

## Procedure Utilization Rates

As shown previously (Table 114), boys' utilization of hospital surgery was over a third higher than girls', while the rate for women was 57 per cent higher than that for men. There were two age periods with equivalent rates for both sexes—15 to 19, and 55 to 64. At ages 10 to 14, the male rate was twice the female rate; at 20 to 54, the reverse occurred; and at 65-plus, the male rate again surpassed that of females. The combined age curve for both sexes showed a precipitous drop at age 10, a precipitous rise at age 20, another at 35, another at 65; but this was not characteristic of either sex separately. While the male rate was more or less stationary from 15 to 34, rising steadily thereafter, the female rate at 15 to 19 was doubled at 20 to 24 and tripled at ages 45 to 54.

Most of the excess in female surgical rates as compared with male rates is traceable to gynecological or breast surgery. The overall rate for this category, 23 procedures per thousand female years, compares with a rate of 4 male genital procedures per thousand males. The female rate reached its peak at ages 35 to 44, largely because of "D and C's" and hysterectomies. The sudden drop in overall surgical rates for women at age 55 reflects mainly a decrease in this category. At age 65, the rate rose again, because of hysteropexies, salpingo-oophorectomies and breast surgery.

The peak for male genital surgery occurred after age 65. The rate for prostatectomy was below one per thousand to age 54, rose to 5.5 at ages 55–64, and finally reached 16.3. Other procedures contributing to the tremendous increase in male surgical rates at age 65 (to the level reached by women aged 45 to 54) were cystoscopy, sigmoidoscopy, colon resection, cataract removal.

The rate of cystoscopy was nearly 40 per cent higher among males than females, for all ages combined, but was higher among females up to age 35; at ages 25 to 34 the female rate doubled the male rate, after which the male rate increased rapidly, finally reaching 14.8 per thousand.

In the gastrointestinal-abdominal category, the overall male rate was 19 per cent higher than that of females. The male hernioplasty rate was nearly two and one half times that of females, with the largest differences occurring in childhood and at ages 55 to 64. The highest rates for this procedure among males (7–8.3 per thousand) occurred before age 5 and after age 55; the peak for females (5.9) occurred after age 65. Male rates of colon resection and gastrectomy were also significantly higher. In contrast, the female rate of cholecystectomy was more than five times the male rate, when all ages are included, and eight and one half times at ages 45 to 54, when it reached 6.9 per thousand; the highest male rate (1.6) occurred after age 55.

The rates for appendectomy and hemorrhoidectomy were similar for the two sexes, overall, but not at each age level. Male rates for hemorrhoidectomy peaked at ages 45 to 54, reaching 4.2 procedures per thousand, while the female rate was highest, at 5.8, after age 65. For both males and females, highest appendectomy rates were recorded at ages 15 to 24.

Tonsillectomy rates were somewhat higher for males. The age curve was similar for both sexes, dropping off at age 15 and almost disappearing after age 25.

The rates of cataract removal were the same for males and females. They were higher for women aged 35 to 44 and nearly a third higher at ages 55 to 64. At age 65 the rate for both sexes jumped to nearly nine procedures per thousand persons.

Although the overall rate of hospital-treated fractures was higher among males, this is traceable entirely to the years before age 35, at which point the female rate increased as the male rate declined. By age 45, the men's rate was .8 hospitalized fractures per thousand, compared with a peak of 5.4 at ages 5 to 14. The women reached their peak rate of 5.8 at ages 65 and over—about the same as the rate for boys aged 5 to 14. The majority of the male fractures involved upper extremities, up to age 25, and their overall rate for such fractures was two and one half times the corresponding female rate. The majority of the female fractures involved the lower extremities, and the incidence of these was two-thirds higher than among males. On the other hand, the rate of amputations among males was double that among females, reaching a high of 1.5 per thousand males aged 65 or over.

For surgery involving joints, the overall female rate doubled the male incidence, but from ages 5 through 44 the male rate surpassed that of females. From ages 45 to 64 the female rate of 2.9 procedures per thousand was over three and one half times the combined rate for both sexes of all ages.

Tendon surgery was about evenly divided between the

sexes and showed a somewhat erratic age pattern, with females reaching their highest incidence at ages 45 to 54, males at ages 55 to 64.

Surgery involving glands (other than mammary) showed similar rates for both sexes at ages 45 to 54 (by far the highest point for male surgery of this kind), but the female rate overall was twice the male rate. The age curve of utilization peaked at 35 to 44, among women. Thyroid surgery accounted for the majority of procedures for females, reaching a rate of 1.7 per thousand at ages 35 to 54. The overall male rate of thyroid surgery was less than a quarter of the overall female rate.

Hospital surgery for tumors and cysts not elsewhere classified was generally much more frequent for girls and women to age 24 and at ages 45 to 54. At other ages, male frequencies were higher. The age curve reached its peak among men of 35 to 44, women 45 to 54, reversing the peaks shown for gland surgery.

Bronchoscopy, comprising seven out of ten procedures classified under bronchial-thoracic surgery, was performed over three times as frequently for males as for females, showing very low utilization before age 45 and a top rate of 4.8 per thousand males aged 55 to 64. The highest rate reached by females, .9, occurred at ages 45 to 54.

Neurosurgical procedures never reached a high rate, were generally higher for males except at ages 55 to 64, where the female rate peaked at 4.6 procedures per thousand, as compared with the overall female rate of 1.0. The peak male rate, 4.4, occurred after age 65, was three times the overall male rate.

For procedures involving heart and blood vessels, or skin infections and repairs, overall rates were similar for the two sexes, but the pattern varied at different ages. Heart and vein surgery rates were higher among the young (to age 24) and older (past 54) males. Skin procedures performed for in-patients, averaging one per thousand eligibles of each sex, reached their highest incidence (1.9) among girls under age 5 and males aged 15 to 24.

Ear surgery rates, at .8 per thousand overall, were some-

## TABLE 125. Incidence of Hospital Surgery by Type of Procedure, by Age and Sex

*Part I: to Age 24*

| PROCEDURE TYPE OR SITE | | NUMBER OF PROCEDURES PER 1,000 EXPOSURE YEARS | | | | | | | | |
|---|---|---|---|---|---|---|---|---|---|---|
| | | ALL | | UNDER 5 | | 5-14 | | 15-24 | | |
| | Total | M | F | M | F | M | F | M | F | |
| Grand Total | 60.8 | 53.9 | 67.9 | 62.6 | 41.6 | 50.2 | 35.5 | 34.2 | 44.7 | |
| Total Excluding Unclassified | 57.5 | 50.6 | 64.7 | 59.3 | 38.2 | 48.8 | 34.3 | 31.3 | 40.7 | |
| **I** | | | | | | | | | | |
| Gynecological and Breast | 11.3 | — | 22.9 | — | 0 | — | 0 | — | 9.9 | |
| Breast | 1.9 | — | 3.9 | — | 0 | — | 0 | — | 3.1 | |
| Dilatation and Curettage | 4.2 | — | 8.5 | — | 0 | — | 0 | — | 3.2 | |
| Hysterectomy | 2.7 | — | 5.4 | — | 0 | — | 0 | — | .8 | |
| Hysteropexy | .1 | — | .1 | — | 0 | — | 0 | — | 0 | |
| Colpoplasty | .9 | — | 1.8 | — | 0 | — | 0 | — | 0 | |
| Salpingectomy, Oophorectomy | .6 | — | 1.3 | — | 0 | — | 0 | — | 2.0 | |
| Culdoscopy | 0* | — | .1 | — | 0 | — | 0 | — | 0 | |
| Other | .9 | — | 1.8 | — | 0 | — | 0 | — | .8 | |
| **II** | | | | | | | | | | |
| Male Genital | 2.0 | 4.0 | — | 4.2 | — | 2.1 | — | 2.4 | — | |
| Prostatectomy | .6 | 1.3 | — | 0 | — | 0 | — | 0 | — | |
| Circumcision | .4 | .8 | — | 2.8 | — | .2 | — | .5 | — | |
| Other | 1.0 | 1.9 | — | 1.4 | — | 1.9 | — | 1.9 | — | |
| Total Excluding Categories I, II and Unclassified | 44.2 | 46.6 | 41.8 | 55.1 | 38.2 | 46.7 | 34.3 | 28.9 | 30.8 | |
| **III** | | | | | | | | | | |
| Urinary System | 3.6 | 4.1 | 3.1 | .9 | 1.0 | 1.8 | 1.3 | .5 | 1.6 | |
| Cystoscopy | 2.7 | 3.2 | 2.3 | .4 | .5 | 1.2 | 1.3 | .5 | .8 | |
| Other | .9 | .9 | .8 | .5 | .5 | .6 | 0 | 0 | .8 | |

256

| | | | | | | | | | |
|---|---|---|---|---|---|---|---|---|---|
| **IV** | | | | | | | | | |
| Gastrointestinal-Abdominal Tract | 12.7 | 13.8 | 11.6 | 12.2 | 2.5 | 6.8 | 3.2 | 6.6 | 6.8 |
| Hernioplasty | 3.0 | 4.1 | 1.7 | 7.0 | 1.0 | 3.5 | .4 | 1.9 | 0 |
| Appendectomy | 1.7 | 1.8 | 1.6 | .9 | 1.0 | 2.7 | 2.6 | 4.2 | 3.6 |
| Hemorrhoidectomy | 1.7 | 1.7 | 1.8 | .5 | 0 | 0 | 0 | .5 | .4 |
| Cholecystectomy | 1.6 | .5 | 2.7 | 0 | 0 | 0 | 0 | 0 | 1.6 |
| Sigmoidoscopy | 1.0 | 1.1 | .9 | 0 | 0 | .2 | 0 | 0 | .4 |
| Colon Resection | .3 | .5 | .2 | 0 | 0 | 0 | 0 | 0 | 0 |
| Gastrectomy | .5 | .6 | .3 | 0 | 0 | 0 | 0 | 0 | 0 |
| Esophagoscopy | .2 | .2 | .2 | .5 | 0 | 0 | 0 | 0 | 0 |
| Gastroscopy | .1 | .1 | .1 | 0 | 0 | 0 | 0 | 0 | 0 |
| Exploratory Laparotomy | .1 | .1 | .1 | 0 | 0 | 0 | 0 | 0 | .4 |
| Other | 2.5 | 3.1 | 2.0 | 3.3 | .5 | .4 | .2 | 0 | .4 |
| **V** | | | | | | | | | |
| Eye, Ear, Nose and Throat | 12.8 | 13.3 | 12.4 | 31.3 | 25.3 | 27.3 | 24.9 | 8.5 | 8.4 |
| Eye | 2.1 | 2.1 | 2.2 | 1.9 | 4.5 | 1.0 | 1.5 | .9 | 1.6 |
| Removal of Cataract | .7 | .7 | .7 | 0 | 0 | 0 | 0 | 0 | 0 |
| Strabismus Correction | .6 | .6 | .6 | 1.9 | 1.0 | .8 | 1.5 | .4 | 1.2 |
| Other | .8 | .8 | .9 | 0 | 3.5 | .2 | 0 | .5 | .4 |
| Ear | .8 | .7 | .9 | 1.9 | .5 | 1.1 | .9 | 0 | .4 |
| Nose and Throat | 9.9 | 10.5 | 9.3 | 27.5 | 20.3 | 25.2 | 22.5 | 7.6 | 6.4 |
| Tonsillectomy/Adenoidectomy | 8.3 | 9.0 | 7.7 | 27.5 | 20.3 | 24.8 | 21.9 | 4.7 | 4.0 |
| Submucous Resection | .6 | .6 | .6 | 0 | 0 | 0 | 0 | 1.9 | 1.6 |
| Laryngoscopy | .3 | .2 | .4 | 0 | 0 | 0 | .2 | 0 | 0 |
| Other | .7 | .7 | .6 | 0 | 0 | .4 | .4 | 1.0 | .8 |
| **VI** | | | | | | | | | |
| Musculoskeletal System | 5.7 | 5.9 | 5.5 | 4.2 | 3.0 | 8.1 | 2.8 | 9.5 | 6.4 |
| Fractures | 2.4 | 2.8 | 2.0 | 2.3 | 1.5 | 5.4 | 1.9 | 5.2 | 2.0 |
| Upper Extremities | 1.1 | 1.5 | .6 | 1.4 | 1.0 | 3.5 | 1.1 | 2.8 | .4 |
| Lower Extremities | .8 | .6 | 1.0 | .9 | 0 | .9 | .6 | 1.0 | 1.6 |
| Facial Bones | .4 | .5 | .4 | 0 | .5 | .6 | .2 | 1.4 | 0 |
| Spine and Trunk | .1 | .1 | 0* | 0 | 0 | .4 | 0 | 0 | 0 |
| Treatment of Joints | .8 | .6 | 1.0 | 0 | .5 | .4 | .2 | 1.9 | .8 |
| Treatment of Tendons | .8 | .8 | .9 | .5 | 0 | .4 | .5 | .5 | .8 |
| Treatment of Bone Disease | .6 | .6 | .6 | .5 | 0 | .8 | .2 | 0 | 1.2 |
| Amputations | .3 | .4 | .2 | 0 | 0 | 1.1 | 0 | .5 | 0 |
| Treatment of Bursae | .2 | .3 | .2 | 0 | 0 | .4 | 0 | .5 | .4 |
| Other | .6 | .5 | .6 | .9 | 1.0 | 0 | 0 | .9 | 1.2 |

TABLE 125. *(Cont'd)*   Incidence of Hospital Surgery by Type of Procedure, by Age and Sex

*Part I: to Age 24 (Concluded)*

| | NUMBER OF PROCEDURES PER 1,000 EXPOSURE YEARS | | | | | | | | | |
| PROCEDURE TYPE OR SITE | ALL | | | UNDER 5 | | 5-14 | | 15-24 | |
| | Total | M | F | M | F | M | F | M | F |
|---|---|---|---|---|---|---|---|---|---|
| **VII** | | | | | | | | | |
| Glands—NEC † | 1.1 | .7 | 1.4 | 0 | .5 | .6 | .2 | 0 | 1.6 |
| Lymph Glands or Nodes | .4 | .5 | .3 | 0 | .5 | .2 | 0 | 0 | 0 |
| Thyroid | .5 | .2 | .9 | 0 | 0 | .4 | 0 | 0 | 1.2 |
| Other | .2 | 0 | .2 | 0 | 0 | 0 | .2 | 0 | .4 |
| **VIII** | | | | | | | | | |
| Tumors—Cysts—NEC † | 3.0 | 2.8 | 3.2 | .9 | 1.5 | .8 | 1.1 | 1.4 | 4.0 |
| **IX** | | | | | | | | | |
| Heart and/or Vein Surgery | 2.2 | 2.2 | 2.1 | 3.7 | 1.5 | .4 | 0 | .5 | .4 |
| Venous Ligation | 1.0 | .8 | 1.1 | 0 | .5 | 0 | 0 | .5 | 0 |
| Other | 1.2 | 1.4 | 1.0 | 3.7 | 1.0 | .4 | 0 | 0 | .4 |
| **X** | | | | | | | | | |
| Bronchial-Thoracic Surgery | 1.0 | 1.4 | .5 | 0 | 0 | 0 | .2 | 0 | .8 |
| Bronchoscopy | .7 | 1.0 | .3 | 0 | 0 | 0 | .2 | 0 | 0 |
| Other | .3 | .4 | .2 | 0 | 0 | 0 | 0 | 0 | .8 |
| **XI** | | | | | | | | | |
| Neurosurgery | 1.2 | 1.5 | 1.0 | 1.9 | 1.0 | 0 | 0 | 0 | 0 |
| **XII** | | | | | | | | | |
| Skin Surgery | .9 | .9 | 1.0 | 0 | 1.9 | .9 | .6 | 1.9 | .8 |
| **XIII** | | | | | | | | | |
| Unclassified | 3.3 | 3.3 | 3.2 | 3.3 | 3.4 | 1.4 | 1.2 | 2.9 | 4.0 |

258

**TABLE 125.** (*Cont'd*) Incidence of Hospital Surgery by Type of Procedure, by Age and Sex

*Part II: Ages 25 and Over*

| PROCEDURE TYPE OR SITE | NUMBER OF PROCEDURES PER 1,000 EXPOSURE YEARS | | | | | | | | | |
|---|---|---|---|---|---|---|---|---|---|---|
| | 25–34 | | 35–44 | | 45–54 | | 55–64 | | 65 AND OVER | |
| | M | F | M | F | M | F | M | F | M | F |
| Grand Total | 38.9 | 69.4 | 45.7 | 99.8 | 58.2 | 103.7 | 76.9 | 77.4 | 102.1 | 84.3 |
| Total Excluding Unclassified | 33.3 | 65.5 | 43.5 | 97.0 | 53.7 | 100.3 | 71.3 | 70.5 | 100.6 | 84.3 |
| **I** | | | | | | | | | | |
| Gynecological and Breast | — | 28.7 | — | 54.0 | — | 42.9 | — | 16.2 | — | 34.9 |
| Breast | — | 3.5 | — | 7.3 | — | 8.7 | — | 2.9 | — | 8.7 |
| Dilatation and Curettage | — | 12.4 | — | 21.2 | — | 14.9 | — | 5.2 | — | 2.9 |
| Hysterectomy | — | 4.2 | — | 15.3 | — | 11.2 | — | 3.4 | — | 5.8 |
| Hysteropexy | — | 0 | — | .3 | — | 0 | — | 0 | — | 5.8 |
| Colpoplasty | — | 1.2 | — | 3.7 | — | 3.2 | — | 3.5 | — | 11.7 |
| Salpingectomy, Oophorectomy | — | 3.1 | — | 3.1 | — | .6 | — | .6 | — | 0 |
| Culdoscopy | — | .4 | — | .3 | — | 0 | — | 0 | — | 0 |
| Other | — | 3.9 | — | 2.8 | — | 4.3 | — | .6 | — | 0 |
| **II** | | | | | | | | | | |
| Male Genital | 1.7 | — | 2.8 | — | 3.7 | — | 8.3 | — | 22.2 | — |
| Prostatectomy | 0 | — | .3 | — | .6 | — | 5.5 | — | 16.3 | — |
| Circumcision | 1.7 | — | .8 | — | .3 | — | 0 | — | 1.5 | — |
| Other | 0 | — | 1.7 | — | 2.8 | — | 2.8 | — | 4.4 | — |
| Total Excluding Categories I, II and Unclassified | 31.6 | 36.8 | 40.7 | 43.0 | 50.0 | 57.4 | 63.0 | 54.3 | 78.4 | 49.4 |
| **III** | | | | | | | | | | |
| Urinary System | 1.7 | 3.5 | 4.7 | 5.1 | 6.2 | 4.6 | 8.7 | 5.2 | 16.3 | 0 |
| Cystoscopy | 1.3 | 2.7 | 3.9 | 3.7 | 4.5 | 3.2 | 7.1 | 4.0 | 14.8 | 0 |
| Other | .4 | .8 | .8 | 1.4 | 1.7 | 1.4 | 1.6 | 1.2 | 1.5 | 0 |

259

## TABLE 125. (Cont'd)  Incidence of Hospital Surgery by Type of Procedure, by Age and Sex

*Part II: Ages 25 and Over (Cont'd)*

| PROCEDURE TYPE OR SITE | NUMBER OF PROCEDURES PER 1,000 EXPOSURE YEARS | | | | | | | | | |
|---|---|---|---|---|---|---|---|---|---|---|
| | 25–34 | | 35–44 | | 45–54 | | 55–64 | | 65 AND OVER | |
| | M | F | M | F | M | F | M | F | M | F |
| **IV** | | | | | | | | | | |
| Gastrointestinal-Abdominal Tract | 9.1 | 16.3 | 14.2 | 14.1 | 22.6 | 21.5 | 21.9 | 17.9 | 28.1 | 23.3 |
| Hernioplasty | 1.7 | 2.0 | 3.0 | 2.0 | 3.7 | 4.0 | 8.3 | 2.3 | 7.4 | 5.9 |
| Appendectomy | 1.3 | 2.3 | .8 | .6 | 1.7 | .3 | 1.2 | 1.1 | 0 | 0 |
| Hemorrhoidectomy | 2.2 | 3.1 | 2.8 | 4.2 | 4.2 | 3.1 | 1.2 | 0 | 1.5 | 5.8 |
| Cholecystectomy | 0 | 3.5 | .8 | 2.5 | .8 | 6.9 | 1.6 | 5.2 | 1.5 | 2.9 |
| Sigmoidoscopy | .9 | 2.3 | 1.7 | 1.1 | 2.5 | 1.7 | .8 | 0 | 5.9 | 2.9 |
| Colon Resection | 0 | 0 | .3 | .3 | .3 | .6 | 2.0 | .6 | 4.4 | 0 |
| Gastrectomy | 0 | .8 | 1.1 | 0 | 1.1 | 1.1 | 1.2 | .6 | 1.5 | 0 |
| Esophagoscopy | 0 | 0 | .3 | 0 | .3 | .9 | .8 | 1.1 | 0 | 0 |
| Gastroscopy | 0 | 0 | 0 | .3 | .3 | .3 | .4 | 0 | 0 | 0 |
| Exploratory Laparotomy | 0 | 0 | 0 | 0 | 0 | 0 | .8 | 1.2 | 0 | 0 |
| Other | 3.0 | 2.3 | 3.4 | 3.1 | 7.7 | 2.6 | 3.6 | 5.8 | 5.9 | 5.8 |
| **V** | | | | | | | | | | |
| Eye, Ear, Nose and Throat | 4.3 | 5.8 | 4.7 | 4.3 | 5.4 | 6.9 | 6.0 | 6.4 | 14.8 | 14.5 |
| Eye | 1.3 | .8 | 1.9 | .6 | 2.3 | 2.3 | 3.2 | 5.8 | 11.8 | 14.5 |
| Removal of Cataract | 0 | 0 | 0 | .6 | 1.2 | 1.1 | 2.4 | 3.5 | 8.9 | 8.7 |
| Strabismus Correction | .4 | 0 | .5 | 0 | 0 | .3 | 0 | 0 | 0 | 0 |
| Other | .9 | .8 | 1.4 | 0 | 1.1 | .9 | .8 | 2.3 | 2.9 | 5.8 |
| Ear | .9 | 1.1 | .6 | .6 | .3 | 2.0 | 0 | 0 | 1.5 | 0 |
| Nose and Throat | 2.1 | 3.9 | 2.2 | 3.1 | 2.8 | 2.6 | 2.8 | 0 | 1.5 | 0 |
| Tonsillectomy/Adenoidectomy | .4 | 1.5 | .8 | .6 | .3 | .3 | 0 | .6 | 0 | 0 |
| Submucous Resection | 1.3 | 1.2 | 1.1 | .8 | .6 | .6 | 0 | 0 | 0 | 0 |
| Laryngoscopy | 0 | .4 | 0 | .8 | .8 | .6 | .8 | 0 | 0 | 0 |
| Other | .4 | .8 | .3 | .9 | 1.1 | 1.1 | 2.0 | 0 | 1.5 | 0 |

| | | | | | | | | | | |
|---|---|---|---|---|---|---|---|---|---|---|
| **VI** | | | | | | | | | | |
| Musculoskeletal System | 6.9 | 3.1 | 5.9 | 5.4 | 3.1 | 9.5 | 4.4 | 9.2 | 2.9 | 8.7 |
| Fractures | 3.0 | 1.5 | 1.7 | 2.3 | .8 | 1.4 | .8 | 3.4 | 0 | 5.8 |
| Upper Extremities | .9 | 0 | .6 | .3 | .3 | .3 | .8 | 1.7 | 0 | 0 |
| Lower Extremities | 1.7 | .4 | .3 | .9 | 0 | 1.1 | 0 | 1.7 | 0 | 5.8 |
| Facial Bones | .4 | 1.1 | .5 | .8 | .5 | 0 | 0 | 0 | 0 | 0 |
| Spine and Trunk | 0 | 0 | .3 | .3 | 0 | 0 | 0 | 0 | 0 | 0 |
| Treatment of Joints | .9 | .4 | .3 | 0 | .3 | 2.9 | .4 | 2.9 | 1.4 | 0 |
| Treatment of Tendons | .9 | .4 | 0 | 1.7 | .6 | 2.0 | 1.2 | .6 | 0 | 0 |
| Treatment of Bone Disease | .8 | .4 | .6 | 0 | .8 | 1.7 | .4 | .5 | 0 | 2.9 |
| Amputations | 0 | 0 | .6 | .3 | 0 | .6 | .8 | .6 | 1.5 | 0 |
| Treatment of Bursae | .4 | 0 | .8 | .5 | 0 | 0 | .4 | 0 | 0 | 0 |
| Other | .9 | .4 | 1.9 | .6 | .6 | .9 | .4 | 1.2 | 0 | 0 |
| **VII** | | | | | | | | | | |
| Glands—NEC † | 0 | .8 | .6 | 3.1 | 2.3 | 2.3 | .8 | 1.2 | 1.5 | 2.9 |
| Lymph Glands or Nodes | 0 | 0 | .6 | .8 | 1.7 | .6 | .8 | 0 | 1.5 | 0 |
| Thyroid | 0 | .8 | 0 | 1.7 | .6 | 1.7 | 0 | .5 | 0 | 0 |
| Other | 0 | 0 | 0 | .6 | 0 | 0 | 0 | .7 | 0 | 2.9 |
| **VIII** | | | | | | | | | | |
| Tumors—Cysts—NEC † | 4.3 | 3.5 | 5.3 | 4.2 | 2.2 | 5.4 | 4.8 | 4.0 | 4.4 | 0 |
| **IX** | | | | | | | | | | |
| Heart and/or Vein Surgery | .9 | 1.5 | 3.3 | 5.1 | 2.5 | 3.2 | 4.8 | 4.6 | 1.5 | 0 |
| Venous Ligation | .9 | 1.5 | 1.7 | 3.4 | .8 | .9 | 1.6 | 2.3 | 1.5 | 0 |
| Other | 0 | 0 | 1.6 | 1.7 | 1.7 | 2.3 | 3.2 | 2.3 | 0 | 0 |
| **X** | | | | | | | | | | |
| Bronchial-Thoracic Surgery | .5 | .4 | .6 | .8 | 2.3 | .9 | 7.2 | 0 | 3.0 | 0 |
| Bronchoscopy | .5 | 0 | .3 | .5 | 1.7 | .9 | 4.8 | 0 | 3.0 | 0 |
| Other | 0 | .4 | .3 | .3 | .6 | 0 | 2.4 | 0 | 0 | 0 |
| **XI** | | | | | | | | | | |
| Neurosurgery | 3.0 | 1.2 | .3 | 0 | 2.8 | 2.0 | 3.2 | 4.6 | 4.4 | 0 |
| **XII** | | | | | | | | | | |
| Skin Surgery | .9 | .7 | 1.1 | .9 | .6 | 1.1 | 1.2 | 1.2 | 1.5 | 0 |
| **XIII** | | | | | | | | | | |
| Unclassified | 5.6 | 3.9 | 2.2 | 2.8 | 4.5 | 3.4 | 5.6 | 6.9 | 1.5 | 0 |

* Less than .05.

† Not elsewhere classified.

what higher for females than males. The age curve showed no pattern for either sex. Among males, the highest rates occurred at the lowest (under 5) and highest (past 65) age levels; the female rate peaked at ages 45 to 54.

### Variations by Occupation Class

It has already been shown that, unlike ambulatory surgery, the total frequency of hospital surgery varied within a relatively narrow range among major occupation classes (Table 116).

The number of procedures per thousand male exposure years ranged from 52 in the blue-collar class and 53 in the professional-executive class to 56 in the clerical-sales class. Among females the range was broader, with the professional-executive class lowest (62), the blue-collar class next (66) and the clerical-sales class highest (71).

Further breakdown of experience into surgical categories showed generally similar patterns within occupation groupings; the same types of surgery tended to be relatively frequent or infrequent for each class.

Although actual frequency rates for different individual procedures varied, conclusions are not warranted because of the small number of cases involved. It is observed that the rate of breast surgery in females of the professional-executive class was 76 per cent higher than in the other classes, while the rates for hysterectomy and dilatation-curettage were significantly lower. It is also observed that females of the professional-executive class sustained a much higher rate of strabismus operations, submucous resections, cystoscopies, thyroid operations and venous ligations (for varicose veins), while females of the blue-collar class had more appendectomies, cholecystectomies, tonsillectomies than females of other classes. There may very well be social connotations associated with these differences—possible neglect of early or preventive care, on the one hand, possible unnecessary surgery on the other; but further sampling as well as more detailed analysis would be required to validate such inferences, particularly since the class observations made for females were generally inapplicable to males.

# MORBIDITY STUDIES

# Chapter 16

# DISTRIBUTION AND INCIDENCE
# OF ATTENDED ILLNESS

Diagnoses entered on claim forms by treating physicians have been analyzed in conjunction with demographic and treatment variables. The first type of analysis, relating illness data to the population at risk, results in the derivation of morbidity rates, discussed below. The second approach, coordinating treatment with diagnosis on a case basis, is presented in the following chapter.

The need for periodic, reasonably up-to-date indices of conditions for which demographically described populations receive physicians' services has long been recognized by medical care planners and epidemiologists. The ability to compare trends over time and in different geographic regions is clearly of importance in the assessment of problems and the evaluation of progress. Present methods of collecting and reporting morbidity data, however, have not solved problems associated with reliance on household respondents for medical information. In the search for alternatives, the growing body of medical insurance material which is potentially the richest source of population-related, physician-reported data on morbidity is a logical candidate for exploration.

As with data from any source, there are of course drawbacks attached to the use of insurance material from the standpoint of both completeness and accuracy; but its net advantages deserve recognition. The fact that insurance sources can refer only to *treated* morbidity need not inhibit production of valuable data so long as they are thus identified. The ability to relate data to a described population at risk is a major advantage over surveys of physician practices (which also, incidentally, are limited to treated morbidity).

Furthermore, as a regular source of data not requiring special collection efforts, insurance records have advantages with respect to lower costs, which should be a plus factor of some weight in arranging for eventual annual or biannual morbidity indices. As for accuracy of terminology, reliance on physicians for reports of diagnosis, whatever the shortcomings, is clearly preferable to consumer impressions of ailments as interpreted by household interviewers. Perfection of source material cannot be a prerequisite for compilation of needed data. In this connection it should be recalled that entries by physicians on death certificates are deemed the likeliest assurance of accuracy and are accepted for compilation of mortality statistics, even though some degree of incorrect, inconsistent, or unstandardized cause-of-death labeling, of unknown extent, must be assumed. The same will always be true of morbidity reporting.

In addition to its records of physician-reported diagnoses, population characteristics and treatment patterns, GHI's advantages as a collector of morbidity data stem from its type of organization and coverage: the fact that it operates within the still-predominating free-choice fee-per-service framework removes the need to consider the possible influence of this factor (except for special comparative studies); while its provision of comprehensive coverage permits an integrated presentation of combined ambulatory-hospital experience. Morbidity studies confined to hospitalized illness can be helpful in evaluating and comparing hospital utilization, but ambulatory patients' diagnoses comprise the bulk of conditions demanding physicians' services. (See Table 126 for diagnostic comparison of hospital illness and all illness.) Similarly, the inclusion of all reported incidence in one analysis (as opposed to the separation of

TABLE 126. All Diagnoses vs. Hospital Admissions:
Comparison of Diagnostic Distributions

| CATEGORY | PER CENT OF REPORTED DIAGNOSES | |
|---|---|---|
| | All Cases | Hospital Admissions |
| TOTAL | 100.0 | 100.0 |
| Infective and Parasitic Diseases | 5.8 | .8 |
| Neoplasms | 1.9 | 9.2 |
| Malignant Neoplasms | .4 | 2.8 |
| Allergic, Endocrine System, Metabolic and Nutritional Diseases | 5.0 | 2.7 |
| Diseases of Blood and Blood-Forming Organs | .7 | .5 |
| Mental, Psychoneurotic and Personality Disorders | .4 | .5 |
| Diseases of Nervous System | 1.2 | 1.9 |
| Diseases of the Eye | 2.6 | 2.0 |
| Diseases of the Ear | 3.8 | 1.1 |
| Diseases of the Circulatory System | 5.2 | 10.1 |
| Heart Diseases | 1.9 | 5.2 |
| Diseases of the Respiratory System | 29.4 | 13.1 |
| Diseases of the Digestive System | 7.0 | 14.8 |
| Diseases of the Urinary System | 1.5 | 3.6 |
| Diseases of the Male Genital Organs | .4 | 1.5 |
| Diseases of the Female Genital Organs and Breast | 3.2 | 5.2 |
| Deliveries and Complications of Pregnancy, Childbirth and Puerperium | 1.0 | 17.1 |
| Diseases of Skin and Subcutaneous Tissues | 6.0 | 1.9 |
| Diseases of Bones and Organs of Movement | 4.3 | 3.1 |
| Injuries and Adverse Effects of External Causes | 8.3 | 7.3 |
| Symptoms, Senility and Ill-Defined Conditions | 3.5 | 2.4 |
| Preventive Care | 8.6 | 0 |
| Other (Congenital Malformations and Certain Diseases of Early Infancy) | .2 | 1.2 |

"chronic" and "acute" conditions), together with subsequent analyses relating treatment to diagnosis, helps to develop an integrated picture of the "whys" of the medical care detailed in previous chapters.

## Notes on Methods of Classification and Analysis

In classifying physicians' diagnostic entries retrieved from claim forms, twenty-three categories have been used, including separate categories for eye conditions, ear conditions, one for "undetermined" and one for "supplementary"—the latter generally indicating preventive care rather than a diagnosis of illness. Except for these few modifications, the classification system follows that of the "International Classification of Diseases".

For those unfamiliar with its details, certain sources of confusion built into this system may be mentioned here. Most diseases are classified by systems or organs; but all disorders attributable to such systems or organs are not included, because of the special categories based on diseases. The categories "neoplasms," "infective and parasitic diseases," "other and ill-defined symptoms" each encompass disorders applicable to various parts of the body. Skin disorders may be classified not only in a category of their own but also under infective or parasitic disorders (dermatophytoses) or as neoplasms. The same is true of intestinal disorders: intestinal virus is an infective or parasitic disease, intestinal tumor is a neoplasm, symptoms referable to the gastrointestinal system are assigned to the symptoms category, while gastroenteritis is a disease of the digestive system. "Migraine" is a disease of the nervous system, "headache" is classified under "symptoms". Unless and until a better system is devised, however, the analytic problems implicit in such irregularities can be minimized if the system is applied consistently by different researchers and understood by data interpreters.

Rates of conditions reported for the full-year membership with comprehensive coverage have been calculated (a) for the study population as a whole, (b) for age-sex subgroups, (c) for occupation class subgroups; and have been adjusted to the age-sex composition of the general population in the study area.

In the process, diagnostic categories have been subdivided to show rates for their principal components. The technical problem raised by this procedure is one that is always faced in the calculation of illness rates: how to count frequencies of individual diseases if the same person sought care for two or more episodes of the same illness during the study year; and how to count overall frequencies in categories when the same person had more than one illness in the same category. The count can vary with the number and type of disorders selected for separate listing under each category.

No completely satisfactory solution to this problem exists. For acute illnesses, it might be advantageous in some respects to count each episode, rather than the number of persons attended for the illness during the year. For chronic illnesses, however, it is preferable to know the number of persons with the illness. Since both methods cannot be used simultaneously in one data retrieval program, and since in any event if they were the results would be difficult to interpret, the present study counts each illness only once per person. Where two separate illnesses within the same general category were experienced by the same person, a concession to both approaches is made by the use of "net" and "gross" totals for each category, with the net representing the number of persons having any disease within that category and the gross adding the number with more than one disease in that category. For example, the net rate of benign neoplasms was 26.6 per thousand persons, the gross rate 28.0, indicating up to 1.4 persons per thousand with more than one type of benign neoplasm.

This method reflects primary concern with the medically attended frequency of each disease and the number of persons treated; it does not identify the multiple conditions for which any one individual was treated. If the same person had heart disease and diabetes he would be counted under each listing. The fact that many patients were treated for multiple conditions is evident from a comparison of the number of persons treated with the number of conditions reported. The problem of identifying multiple diagnoses for individuals, however, involves an entirely different approach. (See Chapter 17.)

The morbidity data presented, like previous data on service utilization, are based on the experience of full-year members. The resulting problem is similar to that encountered in hospitalization studies based on discharges rather than admissions. The exclusion of members who died during the year of observed experience and of whose deaths GHI was notified, results in an unknown degree of understatement as to incidence of conditions associated with member deaths. The overall impact of this problem is probably minor; the age distribution of part-year members was generally younger than that of full-year members, and the reasons for their part-year membership were in most instances undoubtedly associated with joining or leaving a covered group because of employment changes, or being part of a whole group which joined or withdrew. Nevertheless, the subject merits a high priority for special study.

As with any statistical tabulation based on sampling, the smaller the size of the analytic cell, the greater the likelihood that results from another sample would deviate from the findings shown. In the present case, the detail of the individual diagnoses listed compounds the detail of the demographic subgroups to make such a likelihood almost a certainty, particularly for rare diseases. Thus, the study of one year's experience of one population realizes its greatest substantive value when supplemented by repeated studies in the same locale and by comparable studies conducted elsewhere.

It may also be observed, despite the reservations raised as to projectability of individual disease rates for population subgroups, that the data give a generally reassuring impression of plausibility. They may or may not be applicable to other populations; but for the study population, they appear to offer reasonable explanations of previously shown variations in demands for medical care. Moreover, for diagnostic categories susceptible to rough checking based on common knowledge, overall experience as well as age-sex trends are consistent with expectations. For example, respiratory disorders far outstripped all other categories; infective diseases were most frequent at ages 5 to 9, preventive care at ages under 5; the injury rate was highest among boys aged 15 to 19, as were skin disorders; the pregnancy rate was highest at ages 20 to 24; diseases of bones and joints, circulatory disorders, eye disorders, blood disorders, malignant neoplasms, male genitourinary disorders, all increased in frequency with age, reaching their peak after 65.

## Overall Findings

Overall rates have been calculated for the study population and adjusted to the age-sex composition of the general population in the area. Both sets of rates are presented.

The rates of many component disorders show substantial differences when adjusted to the composition of the general population, because the GHI study population was relatively underrepresented in some age-sex subgroups (e.g. ages 20 to 24 and 65-plus) and overrepresented in others (e.g. under 14) in which comparatively high (or low) frequencies of certain conditions were found. Thus, the under-representation of females in the highest child-bearing years, ages 20 to 24, produced a much lower birth rate per thousand GHI population (17) than would have accrued with a normal representation of this group (21). For conditions which occur mainly at older ages, such as heart disorders and cataracts, the overall rate found for the insured study population increased by 50 per cent or more when adjusted to the composition of the general population. The adjusted incidence of diabetes represents a one-third increase over the unadjusted.

Respiratory diseases of one type or another were reported for 40 per cent of the insured population (38 per cent, adjusted) during the course of the year. They contributed 29.4 per cent of all diagnoses listed for the study population, and far out-ranked the next most frequent category of positive diagnoses, injuries, reported for 14 per cent of the membership and accounting for 8.3 per cent of all diagnoses.

Half the respiratory conditions were designated as pharyngitis, bronchitis, or tonsillitis. The individuals treated for some type of respiratory illness included many with more than one type; the sum of the persons reported under the various components was 569 per thousand (532, adjusted) vs. a rate of 399 (377, adjusted) which would have been experienced if each patient had had only one of the listed types.

In addition to respiratory conditions and injuries, each of the following categories involved ten or more per cent of the membership: "supplementary" classifications (preventive and diagnostic service), 16 per cent *; diagnosis undetermined, 12.5 per cent; disorders of the digestive system, 12 per cent; infective and parasitic diseases, 10 per cent; and skin disorders, 10 per cent.

Five to nine per cent of the population sought medical care in seven more categories—allergic or metabolic conditions, 9 per cent; circulatory disorders, 8 per cent; disorders of bones, joints or muscles (other than injuries), 7 per cent; ear conditions, 7 per cent; symptoms and ill-defined conditions, 6 per cent; diseases of female sex organs, 5 per cent (11 per cent of females); eye disorders, 5 per cent.

In the nine remaining categories, reported incidence involved from one to 32 persons per thousand members.

The tendency for the same patients to have more than one disease in a category was highest in the respiratory category, where the overlap amounted to 43 per cent. It was next highest for circulatory conditions, with an overlap of 22 per cent. Overlaps ranging from 17 to 10 per cent were found for diseases of the digestive system, female sex organs, injuries, bone or joint disorders, skin conditions, neoplasms, allergic or metabolic disorders, and infective or parasitic diseases.

### Most and Least Frequent Entries

Inspection of incidence rates of individually listed disorders (as opposed to disease categories) brings into quick focus the relative infrequency of some of the more dramatic, disabling or lethal disorders and the comparatively routine

---

* This does not reflect the extent to which preventive services were sought; such an entry was likely to appear in the line for diagnosis only in the absence of a positive finding of some disorder.

nature of many of those most frequently reported—the latter reflecting, of course, the inclusion of diagnoses rendered in connection with office or home visits (Table 127).

Of the 38 diagnoses listed among the most frequent, 20 affected 2 or more per cent of the population, and 18 affected between 1.0 and 1.9 per cent. This list is dominated by acute conditions but includes exceptions such as arthritis, arterioscle-

TABLE 127.   Selected Incidence Rates, Most and Least
Frequent Diagnoses Listed

CASES REPORTED PER 1000 EXPOSURE YEARS
(ADJUSTED TO AGE-SEX COMPOSITION OF GENERAL POPULATION)

*Most Frequent* *

| | | | |
|---|---|---|---|
| Pharyngitis | 113.8 | Cellulitis | 20.3 |
| Bronchitis | 87.7 | German Measles | 19.1 |
| Gastroenteritis-Colitis | 54.7 | Myositis | 17.8 |
| Tonsillitis | 52.9 | Laryngitis | 17.7 |
| Sprain-Strain | 47.9 | Hay Fever | 16.7 |
| Otitis Media | 42.8 | Cystitis | 16.3 |
| Intestinal Virus | 40.4 | "Strep Throat" | 15.2 |
| Arthritis | 30.3 | Cervicitis | 15.2 |
| Dermatitis | 29.8 | Fracture | 14.3 |
| Influenza | 29.8 | Asthma | 14.1 |
| Laceration | 29.7 | Menstrual Disorder | 14.0 |
| Benign Neoplasm | 29.5 | Anemia | 13.8 |
| Synovitis-Bursitis | 28.2 | Arteriosclerotic Heart Disease | 13.2 |
| Obesity | 25.2 | Diabetes | 12.9 |
| Contusion(s) | 24.3 | Hemorrhoids | 11.9 |
| Sinusitis | 22.5 | Pneumonia | 11.6 |
| Conjunctivitis | 22.4 | Vaginitis | 11.3 |
| Gastritis-Duodenitis | 21.9 | Ulcers | 11.1 |
| Normal Delivery | 20.6 | Head Injury | 10.1 |

*Least Frequent* †

| | | | |
|---|---|---|---|
| Muscular Dystrophy | .1 | Nephritis-Nephrosis | .9 |
| Hodgkin's Disease | .1 | Scoliosis | 1.1 |
| Ectopic Pregnancy | .1 | General Arteriosclerosis | 2.3 |
| Leukemia | .2 | Abortion | 2.6 |
| Pulmonary Embolism | .2 | Cataract | 3.7 |
| Infectious Hepatitis | .3 | Glaucoma | 4.0 |
| Multiple Sclerosis | .3 | Acute Coronary Occlusion | 4.5 |
| Retinal Detachment | .3 | Malignant Neoplasm | 8.6 |
| Complicated Delivery | .4 | | |

* Ten or more cases per 1000 exposure years.

† Diseases occurring at a rate of less than 1 case per 10,000 exposure years were not tabulated separately.

rotic heart disease, diabetes, ulcer—each reported for 1 to 3 per cent of the population.

The rarest diseases listed separately, in the incidence tabulations presented, affected one tenth of one per cent of the population: approximately one case each of Hodgkin's disease and muscular dystrophy were reported per 10,000 persons (9.4 and 11.7 respectively, per 100,000). There were 2.35 persons reported with leukemia, 3 with multiple sclerosis, 3.29 with infectious hepatitis, 9.39 with nephritis or nephrosis, per 10,000 persons. Small as these rates appear, in contrast to those for the common disorders, they would indicate sizable problems if projected to the population as a whole—e.g. over 3,000 cases of multiple sclerosis in the New York metropolitan area, or over 55,000 in the United States.

Heart disease of some type was found at (adjusted) rates of 42 persons and 55 conditions reported per thousand persons. Cancer was listed at (adjusted) frequencies of 7.3 persons, 8.6 malignancies, per thousand.

### Seasonal Distribution

Annual analysis of diagnoses in terms of month treatment was sought could conceivably be of epidemiological interest, or, for certain categories, might indicate possible areas of changing needs for facilities or personnel during different periods of the year. For whatever they may be worth, Tables 128 and 129 demonstrate two approaches to such analysis. Disease categories are used in one instance, and most frequent individual diagnoses in the other. First month of treatment was the basis for classification.

Although there is little point in examining the findings for content until comparison can be made with data for at least one subsequent year, some of the initial observations demonstrate credibility based on common knowledge, others may suggest the possibility of seasonal patterns that are not generally recognized, while still others seem unlikely to withstand additional testing.

January was found to be the leading month for beginning treatment of emotional disorders—a post-Christmas phenomenon previously observed by psychiatrists.

Acute upper respiratory infections were highest from December through February, lowest from June through August. The season for acute bronchitis, however, started earlier, in October, and lasted until spring. For influenza, the peak month by far was January, but most of the fall and winter months were relatively high.

Another condition with highest incidence in January was asthma. This seems to tie in with findings as to emotional illness and etiological theories about asthma. Hay fever incidence was also high in January but higher in April and May. Sinusitis peaked in January-February, was lowest from May through August.

Treatment of obesity was characterized by highest initiation of treatment in April and June and fairly high rates from January through June, followed by a marked six-month lull beginning in July and lasting through December.

October and November were the peak months for diabetes, while January and July were lowest.

Arteriosclerotic heart disease treatment in the study year was initiated more often in April than in other months. December and January were relatively low months.

Cystitis was reported most frequently in October, followed by May and March. Low months were July, August, November.

Treatment of contusions was highest in early summer and fall—June, July, September, October—and lowest in January and February; sprains and strains were registered most frequently for March and May, with the low point coming in September; while the general category of "injuries and adverse effects of external causes," which also includes fractures, showed fairly consistent highs for the entire period May through October, balanced by lower levels from November through April. The pattern for "diseases of bones and organs of movement" was more erratic through the year—highest in October, April and May, lowest in June and December.

TABLE 128. Distribution of Attended Illness by First Month of Service, by Diagnostic Category

Part I: to June

| DIAGNOSTIC CATEGORY | Total | FIRST MONTH OF SERVICE | | | | | |
|---|---|---|---|---|---|---|---|
| | | January | February | March | April | May | June |
| | % | % | % | % | % | % | % |
| Infective and Parasitic Diseases | 100.0 | 10.5 | 10.7 | 14.0 | 11.5 | 9.2 | 6.0 |
| Neoplasms | 100.0 | 9.1 | 6.8 | 9.1 | 9.1 | 9.8 | 8.6 |
| Allergic, Endocrine System, Metabolic and Nutritional Diseases | 100.0 | 11.5 | 7.9 | 9.5 | 10.5 | 10.3 | 9.3 |
| Diseases of Blood and Blood-Forming Organs | 100.0 | 10.7 | 6.6 | 6.3 | 9.4 | 13.0 | 11.5 |
| Mental, Psychoneurotic and Personality Disorders | 100.0 | 13.9 | 7.0 | 7.2 | 9.4 | 4.9 | 9.7 |
| Diseases of Nervous System | 100.0 | 6.1 | 8.8 | 8.8 | 11.2 | 8.4 | 9.0 |
| Diseases of the Eye | 100.0 | 8.5 | 5.9 | 8.2 | 8.7 | 8.6 | 8.4 |
| Diseases of the Ear | 100.0 | 9.3 | 8.5 | 9.9 | 8.4 | 10.0 | 8.5 |
| Diseases of the Circulatory System | 100.0 | 8.8 | 8.9 | 8.9 | 9.2 | 8.9 | 8.4 |
| Diseases of the Respiratory System | 100.0 | 10.0 | 10.2 | 9.7 | 8.8 | 7.7 | 6.4 |
| Diseases of the Digestive System | 100.0 | 10.1 | 8.2 | 8.2 | 8.8 | 8.7 | 7.7 |
| Diseases of the Urinary System | 100.0 | 8.2 | 6.9 | 10.8 | 8.7 | 9.7 | 7.8 |
| Diseases of the Male Genital Organs | 100.0 | 11.6 | 4.9 | 9.2 | 10.1 | 8.5 | 7.2 |
| Diseases of the Female Genital Organs | 100.0 | 9.2 | 7.1 | 8.7 | 9.3 | 9.0 | 8.9 |
| Deliveries and Complications of Pregnancy, Childbirth and Puerperium | 100.0 | 9.1 | 7.7 | 7.5 | 8.6 | 6.5 | 8.0 |
| Diseases of Skin and Subcutaneous Tissues | 100.0 | 8.9 | 8.7 | 7.9 | 8.3 | 9.1 | 10.0 |
| Diseases of Bones and Organs of Movement | 100.0 | 7.7 | 8.5 | 8.5 | 9.5 | 9.9 | 6.7 |
| Congenital Malformations | 100.0 | 8.8 | 8.8 | 4.4 | 9.4 | 8.5 | 8.8 |
| Diseases of Early Infancy | 100.0 | 12.9 | 13.9 | 4.9 | 3.0 | 5.9 | 10.9 |
| Symptoms, Senility and Ill-Defined Conditions | 100.0 | 8.6 | 9.0 | 8.2 | 8.9 | 9.8 | 8.3 |
| Injuries and Adverse Effects of External Causes | 100.0 | 7.1 | 6.6 | 7.8 | 7.9 | 9.2 | 8.9 |
| Supplementary Classifications (General Medical Examination, Well Baby Care) | 100.0 | 7.0 | 7.6 | 6.8 | 8.8 | 8.0 | 9.4 |
| Undetermined Classifications | 100.0 | 10.4 | 8.8 | 10.4 | 8.5 | 8.6 | 8.1 |
| TOTAL | 100.0 | 9.3 | 8.6 | 9.1 | 9.1 | 8.8 | 8.0 |
| TOTAL EXCLUDING UNDETERMINED CLASSIFICATIONS | 100.0 | 9.2 | 8.6 | 9.0 | 9.1 | 8.8 | 8.0 |

*Part II: July to December*

## FIRST MONTH OF SERVICE

| DIAGNOSTIC CATEGORY | July | August | September | October | November | December |
|---|---|---|---|---|---|---|
| | % | % | % | % | % | % |
| Infective and Parasitic Diseases | 4.7 | 5.5 | 6.4 | 6.2 | 7.6 | 7.7 |
| Neoplasms | 7.2 | 7.3 | 8.6 | 8.2 | 7.2 | 9.0 |
| Allergic, Endocrine System, Metabolic and Nutritional Diseases | 6.3 | 6.8 | 7.2 | 7.9 | 6.8 | 6.0 |
| Diseases of Blood and Blood-Forming Organs | 5.9 | 5.1 | 8.4 | 9.6 | 7.6 | 5.9 |
| Mental, Psychoneurotic and Personality Disorders | 7.2 | 7.3 | 11.1 | 7.3 | 7.8 | 7.2 |
| Diseases of Nervous System | 10.0 | 7.2 | 7.5 | 8.1 | 8.3 | 6.6 |
| Diseases of the Eye | 8.2 | 6.6 | 9.4 | 10.2 | 8.3 | 9.0 |
| Diseases of the Ear | 9.4 | 7.2 | 7.3 | 7.7 | 7.2 | 6.6 |
| Diseases of the Circulatory System | 7.7 | 7.8 | 7.6 | 9.2 | 8.0 | 6.6 |
| Diseases of the Respiratory System | 4.8 | 6.2 | 7.8 | 9.8 | 9.2 | 9.4 |
| Diseases of the Digestive System | 7.7 | 7.8 | 8.4 | 8.7 | 8.5 | 7.2 |
| Diseases of the Urinary System | 6.2 | 7.6 | 8.3 | 11.7 | 6.8 | 7.3 |
| Diseases of the Male Genital Organs | 6.4 | 11.6 | 8.2 | 8.5 | 6.8 | 7.0 |
| Diseases of the Female Genital Organs | 7.8 | 7.3 | 8.1 | 9.6 | 8.8 | 6.2 |
| Deliveries and Complications of Pregnancy, Childbirth and Puerperium | 8.6 | 7.7 | 7.6 | 9.8 | 9.6 | 9.3 |
| Diseases of Skin and Subcutaneous Tissues | 8.5 | 8.8 | 8.8 | 7.9 | 6.9 | 6.2 |
| Diseases of Bones and Organs of Movement | 8.6 | 7.7 | 8.1 | 10.0 | 7.6 | 7.2 |
| Congenital Malformations | 8.2 | 4.1 | 11.8 | 13.3 | 6.5 | 7.4 |
| Diseases of Early Infancy | 3.9 | 7.9 | 7.9 | 13.9 | 4.0 | 10.9 |
| Symptoms, Senility and Ill-Defined Conditions | 7.4 | 6.6 | 7.0 | 9.4 | 9.2 | 7.6 |
| Injuries and Adverse Effects of External Causes | 9.7 | 8.9 | 9.3 | 9.1 | 7.9 | 7.6 |
| Supplementary Classifications (General Medical Examination, Well Baby Care) | 6.9 | 9.4 | 9.4 | 10.0 | 11.2 | 5.5 |
| Undetermined Classifications | 6.3 | 6.7 | 7.0 | 9.2 | 8.1 | 7.9 |
| TOTAL | 6.8 | 7.3 | 8.0 | 9.1 | 8.4 | 7.5 |
| TOTAL EXCLUDING UNDETERMINED CLASSIFICATIONS | 6.9 | 7.4 | 8.1 | 9.1 | 8.4 | 7.4 |

*Part I: to June*

TABLE 129.   Distribution of Leading Individual Diagnoses,
by First Month of Service

| DIAGNOSIS | Total | FIRST MONTH OF SERVICE | | | | | |
|---|---|---|---|---|---|---|---|
| | | January | February | March | April | May | June |
| | % | % | % | % | % | % | % |
| Acute Upper Respiratory Infection of Multiple or Unspecified Sites | 100.0 | 10.6 | 10.8 | 9.4 | 8.8 | 7.5 | 5.9 |
| Diagnostic Screening Without Physician Referral | 100.0 | 6.8 | 8.7 | 5.7 | 10.0 | 7.9 | 7.8 |
| Other Acute Pharyngitis | 100.0 | 9.2 | 9.5 | 9.7 | 8.6 | 8.5 | 7.7 |
| Other Hypertensive Diseases Without Mention of Heart | 100.0 | 9.7 | 8.8 | 9.1 | 9.1 | 9.0 | 8.0 |
| Well Baby and Child Care | 100.0 | 8.2 | 7.5 | 8.2 | 8.6 | 8.8 | 10.5 |
| Acute Bronchitis | 100.0 | 10.1 | 10.9 | 10.1 | 9.2 | 6.9 | 5.0 |
| Obesity | 100.0 | 9.7 | 9.0 | 10.0 | 11.0 | 9.6 | 11.0 |
| Acute Tonsillitis | 100.0 | 8.5 | 11.4 | 9.7 | 10.1 | 8.4 | 7.6 |
| General Medical Examination | 100.0 | 6.3 | 5.3 | 7.0 | 7.3 | 7.4 | 11.4 |
| Sprains and Strains | 100.0 | 8.3 | 8.2 | 9.3 | 8.7 | 9.1 | 8.4 |
| Otitis Media | 100.0 | 9.5 | 8.9 | 10.6 | 9.0 | 9.4 | 8.1 |
| Hay Fever | 100.0 | 12.9 | 8.0 | 10.2 | 14.0 | 14.3 | 10.0 |
| Gastroenteritis and Colitis | 100.0 | 10.5 | 9.0 | 9.4 | 8.2 | 8.1 | 7.9 |
| Other Diseases Attributable to Viruses | 100.0 | 10.2 | 8.9 | 10.5 | 7.4 | 7.5 | 5.7 |
| Bronchitis, Unqualified | 100.0 | 9.1 | 8.4 | 8.7 | 8.2 | 8.1 | 6.7 |
| Synovitis, Bursitis and Tenosynovitis | 100.0 | 7.2 | 7.5 | 9.1 | 9.3 | 9.4 | 7.6 |
| Asthma | 100.0 | 17.5 | 6.5 | 7.3 | 6.7 | 7.9 | 9.1 |
| Diabetes Mellitus | 100.0 | 6.8 | 7.8 | 7.6 | 8.0 | 9.2 | 8.5 |
| Influenza | 100.0 | 15.4 | 12.0 | 11.6 | 7.3 | 5.5 | 4.7 |
| Acute Nasopharyngitis | 100.0 | 10.7 | 10.5 | 8.5 | 8.1 | 8.5 | 6.6 |
| Contusion | 100.0 | 6.7 | 7.3 | 8.2 | 7.1 | 7.9 | 9.1 |
| Acute Sinusitis and Pansinusitis | 100.0 | 11.1 | 11.1 | 8.9 | 8.5 | 6.6 | 7.2 |
| Gastritis and Duodenitis | 100.0 | 9.6 | 7.3 | 9.7 | 10.5 | 10.3 | 7.7 |
| Arteriosclerotic Heart Disease | 100.0 | 6.9 | 8.5 | 7.4 | 11.4 | 8.4 | 9.0 |
| Cystitis | 100.0 | 8.7 | 7.6 | 10.3 | 9.7 | 11.4 | 7.0 |
| **TOTAL** | 100.0 | 9.5 | 9.0 | 9.0 | 9.1 | 8.5 | 7.8 |
| **GRAND TOTAL** | 100.0 | 9.2 | 8.6 | 9.0 | 9.1 | 8.8 | 8.0 |

*Part II: July to December*

| DIAGNOSIS | FIRST MONTH OF SERVICE | | | | | |
|---|---|---|---|---|---|---|
| | July | August | September | October | November | December |
| | % | % | % | % | % | % |
| Acute Upper Respiratory Infection of Multiple or Unspecified Sites | 4.5 | 5.8 | 7.6 | 9.4 | 9.5 | 10.2 |
| Diagnostic Screening Without Physician Referral | 6.9 | 11.2 | 5.9 | 8.6 | 15.7 | 4.8 |
| Other Acute Pharyngitis | 5.4 | 7.5 | 8.3 | 9.3 | 8.0 | 8.3 |
| Other Hypertensive Diseases Without Mention of Heart | 6.8 | 7.5 | 7.8 | 9.6 | 8.1 | 6.5 |
| Well Baby and Child Care | 7.4 | 7.4 | 11.0 | 9.2 | 6.9 | 6.3 |
| Acute Bronchitis | 3.9 | 5.9 | 7.6 | 10.9 | 10.2 | 9.3 |
| Obesity | 6.3 | 6.2 | 6.2 | 7.3 | 6.9 | 6.8 |
| Acute Tonsillitis | 7.0 | 6.4 | 7.7 | 7.6 | 7.4 | 8.2 |
| General Medical Examination | 6.6 | 8.3 | 13.6 | 13.2 | 7.6 | 6.0 |
| Sprains and Strains | 8.0 | 7.5 | 7.4 | 8.5 | 8.8 | 7.8 |
| Otitis Media | 8.6 | 6.6 | 7.1 | 7.4 | 7.6 | 7.2 |
| Hay Fever | 5.8 | 6.0 | 6.5 | 5.3 | 3.6 | 3.4 |
| Gastroenteritis and Colitis | 7.7 | 6.9 | 8.5 | 8.2 | 8.3 | 7.3 |
| Other Diseases Attributable to Viruses | 4.8 | 7.6 | 8.5 | 8.2 | 10.2 | 10.5 |
| Bronchitis, Unqualified | 4.7 | 7.3 | 8.5 | 10.9 | 10.4 | 9.0 |
| Synovitis, Bursitis and Tenosynovitis | 8.7 | 6.8 | 7.1 | 11.2 | 8.0 | 8.1 |
| Asthma | 6.6 | 6.7 | 7.1 | 9.6 | 8.0 | 7.0 |
| Diabetes Mellitus | 5.5 | 8.9 | 8.2 | 10.9 | 11.1 | 7.5 |
| Influenza | 3.6 | 5.2 | 5.1 | 11.1 | 7.4 | 11.1 |
| Acute Nasopharyngitis | 5.3 | 5.1 | 7.6 | 10.8 | 8.4 | 9.9 |
| Contusion | 9.3 | 8.2 | 9.4 | 9.9 | 8.5 | 8.4 |
| Acute Sinusitis and Pansinusitis | 4.4 | 5.5 | 7.7 | 10.1 | 9.9 | 9.0 |
| Gastritis and Duodenitis | 6.4 | 9.5 | 9.8 | 5.2 | 7.2 | 6.8 |
| Arteriosclerotic Heart Disease | 9.5 | 9.3 | 7.1 | 9.5 | 8.4 | 4.6 |
| Cystitis | 4.4 | 5.9 | 8.7 | 12.8 | 5.8 | 7.7 |
| TOTAL | 6.2 | 7.2 | 7.9 | 9.2 | 8.9 | 7.7 |
| GRAND TOTAL | 6.9 | 7.4 | 8.1 | 9.1 | 8.4 | 7.4 |

In the category of preventive care, diagnostic screening was highest in November, lowest in December; well-baby care was highest in June and September, lowest in November and December; general medical examination was far higher in September, October, June than in any of the other nine months.

The technique used for retrieval of data on seasonal patterns can of course be applied to any disease in which researchers might express particular interest.

## Analysis of Variations Among Population Subgroups

Two principal approaches to an examination of the tabulated data on membership subgroups are implied in the presentations: a (horizontal) comparison of the experience of subgroups as to relative frequency of various categories or diseases; and a (vertical) comparison of the experience *within* subgroups, to show which categories or diseases were relatively most significant to that subgroup. Generally, but not always, the types of illness which were relatively most significant within a subgroup were also likely to have occurred more frequently for that subgroup than for others, and vice versa.

For the sake of convenience, age-sex tabulations are presented in summary form by category (Table 131) as well as in more detailed form (Table 132) to provide figures on principal components of the categories. Even in the latter case, however, not every component is listed; although all that occurred can be found by reference to the retrieved source data, the classification "other" has been used at the end of most categories to lighten somewhat the unwieldiness of the detailed presentation.

### Variations in Incidence Among Males and Females

The comparative longevity of women raises speculation as to the possibly contributory role played by their greater inclination toward medical attention.

# INCIDENCE OF ATTENDED ILLNESS,
## BY DIAGNOSTIC CATEGORY
### (Comprehensive Plan Sample)

NUMBER OF PERSONS WITH ONE OR MORE DIAGNOSES IN INDICATED CATEGORY, PER 1,000 EXPOSURE YEARS

0    25    50    75    100    125    150    175    300    425

DISEASES OF RESPIRATORY SYSTEM

PREVENTIVE CARE

INJURIES AND ADVERSE EFFECTS OF EXTERNAL CAUSES

DISEASES OF THE DIGESTIVE SYSTEM

INFECTIVE AND PARASITIC DISEASES

DISEASES OF SKIN AND SUBCUTANEOUS TISSUES

ALLERGIC, ENDOCRINE SYSTEM, METABOLIC AND NUTRITIONAL DISEASES

DISEASES OF CIRCULATORY SYSTEM

DISEASES OF BONES AND ORGANS OF MOVEMENT

DISEASES OF EAR

SYMPTOMS, SENILITY AND ILL-DEFINED CONDITIONS

DISEASES OF FEMALE GENITAL ORGANS AND BREAST

DISEASES OF EYE

NEOPLASMS

DISEASES OF URINARY SYSTEM

DISEASES OF NERVOUS SYSTEM

DELIVERIES AND COMPLICATIONS OF PREGNANCY, CHILDBIRTH AND PUERPERIUM

DISEASES OF BLOOD AND BLOOD FORMING ORGANS

DISEASES OF MALE GENITAL ORGANS

MENTAL, PSYCHONEUROTIC AND PERSONALITY DISORDERS

CONGENITAL MALFORMATIONS

CERTAIN DISEASES OF EARLY INFANCY

281

# INCIDENCE OF ATTENDED ILLNESS, MALES,
## BY DIAGNOSTIC CATEGORY
### (Comprehensive Plan Sample)

NUMBER OF MALES WITH ONE OR MORE DIAGNOSES IN INDICATED CATEGORY, PER 1,000 EXPOSURE YEARS

```
0      25     50     75    100    125    150    175   300    425
```

DISEASES OF RESPIRATORY SYSTEM

PREVENTIVE CARE

INJURIES AND ADVERSE EFFECTS OF EXTERNAL CAUSES

DISEASES OF THE DIGESTIVE SYSTEM

DISEASES OF SKIN AND SUBCUTANEOUS TISSUES

INFECTIVE AND PARASITIC DISEASES

DISEASES OF CIRCULATORY SYSTEM

DISEASES OF BONES AND ORGANS OF MOVEMENT

ALLERGIC, ENDOCRINE SYSTEM, METABOLIC AND NUTRITIONAL DISEASES

DISEASES OF EAR

SYMPTOMS, SENILITY AND ILL-DEFINED CONDITIONS

DISEASES OF EYE

NEOPLASMS

DISEASES OF NERVOUS SYSTEM

DISEASES OF URINARY SYSTEM

DISEASES OF MALE GENITAL ORGANS

DISEASES OF BLOOD AND BLOOD FORMING ORGANS

MENTAL, PSYCHONEUROTIC AND PERSONALITY DISORDERS

CONGENITAL MALFORMATIONS

CERTAIN DISEASES OF EARLY INFANCY

282

# INCIDENCE OF ATTENDED ILLNESS,
## FEMALES, BY DIAGNOSTIC CATEGORY
### (Comprehensive Plan Sample)

NUMBER OF FEMALES WITH ONE OR MORE DIAGNOSES IN INDICATED CATEGORY, PER 1,000 EXPOSURE YEARS

0    25    50    75    100    125    150    175    300    425

DISEASES OF RESPIRATORY SYSTEM

PREVENTIVE CARE

INJURIES AND ADVERSE EFFECTS OF EXTERNAL CAUSES

DISEASES OF THE DIGESTIVE SYSTEM

INFECTIVE AND PARASITIC DISEASES

DISEASES OF FEMALE GENITAL ORGANS AND BREAST

ALLERGIC, ENDOCRINE SYSTEM, METABOLIC AND NUTRITIONAL DISEASES

DISEASES OF SKIN AND SUBCUTANEOUS TISSUES

DISEASES OF CIRCULATORY SYSTEM

DISEASES OF BONES AND ORGANS OF MOVEMENT

DISEASES OF EAR

SYMPTOMS, SENILITY AND ILL-DEFINED CONDITIONS

DISEASES OF EYE

NEOPLASMS

DELIVERIES AND COMPLICATIONS OF PREGNANCY, CHILDBIRTH AND PUERPERIUM

DISEASES OF URINARY SYSTEM

DISEASES OF NERVOUS SYSTEM

DISEASES OF BLOOD AND BLOOD FORMING ORGANS

MENTAL, PSYCHONEUROTIC AND PERSONALITY DISORDERS

CONGENITAL MALFORMATIONS

CERTAIN DISEASES OF EARLY INFANCY

283

At this stage of development, the data cannot be expected to answer epidemiological queries, nor even to posit a specific connection between early, frequent, or preventive attention and women's survival rates; but the results of the analysis do suggest the tentative hypothesis that men may shorten their life span by waiting until disorders become serious before seeking help.

Disorders for which male rates were significantly higher include many of the more serious conditions. Higher male rates were found for most types of heart disease—arteriosclerotic, acute coronary occlusion, coronary insufficiency, angina pectoris; for malignant neoplasms of the digestive system, respiratory system, urinary system, brain; for chronic brain disease and mental deficiency; for ulcers and abdominal hernias; for lung and liver disease; for fractures, other head injuries and lacerations.

Females had significantly higher rates of treatment for malignant neoplasms of endocrine glands, and benign neoplasms of the mouth; for multiple sclerosis; for arthritis; for scoliosis; for diseases of the thyroid gland and of the gall bladder; for obesity, anemia, migraine, headaches in general, varicose veins, gastroenteritis and colitis, nasopharyngitis, pharyngitis, sinusitis, cystitis; for most types of mental disorders; and for complications of surgical or medical procedures.

For a small number of diagnoses, the rate for males and females precisely coincided—e.g. appendicitis, lymphadenitis, diseases of pancreas, muscular dystrophy, internal injuries.

In another assortment of conditions, the male-female differences in rates were so small as to be attributable to chance—chickenpox, mumps, measles, mononucleosis, tonsillitis, pneumonia, benign skin neoplasms, asthma, hay fever, epilepsy, conjunctivitis, cataract, glaucoma, deafness and other ear conditions, skin disorders, hemorrhoids, general arteriosclerosis, infective myositis, osteomyelitis, superficial injuries, contusions.

## Age-Sex Trends

Differences in total treated incidence rates between males and females were minor to age 14, with boys' rates slightly higher; substantial at ages 15 to 19, with boys' rates 16 per cent higher; major from ages 20 through 64, with women always much higher; and again minor after 65.

*Ages to 19.* At ages to 19, most of the medical attention was for respiratory illness, well-baby or child care, injuries, infective diseases, ear conditions, intestinal tract complaints, or skin disorders.

Skin complaints were particularly heavy among boys aged 15 to 19, with rates of 176 persons treated, 197 conditions reported per thousand members—the highest of any age-sex subgroup.

Even more outstanding was the injury record of the 15-to-19-year-old boys—331 injuries reported for 274 boys, per thousand in this group, or about double the experience of the study population as a whole, and more than double the girls' rate at the same age (140 injuries per thousand). This category accounted for much of the wide discrepancy between total incidence rates of boys and girls aged 15 to 19.

Infective diseases reached their peak rate for both sexes at ages 5 to 9, with an incidence more than double the average for all ages. Boys' rates were slightly higher before age 5 and from 15 to 19.

Treatment of respiratory conditions was high at all ages and similar for both sexes. By far the highest rates occurred at ages before 5, with over two thirds of this population listed for this category and an incidence of 1,150 conditions per thousand member years. At age 5 a marked decrease in incidence rates was recorded, and the trend downward continued at ages 10 through 19, by which point only about two of five members reported treatment for respiratory illness.

Ear disorders, too, were far higher at ages under 5 than at any subsequent period, and somewhat more frequent among boys than girls. Rates decreased at each succeeding age interval throughout childhood; by the latter teens, incidence was less than a third of that found at the youngest ages.

Intestinal complaints, like respiratory and ear disorders, were most frequent before age 5.

Unlike ear disorders, eye conditions were treated at similar rates through age 19. These rates tended to approximate the average for all ages.

The neoplasm rate (mainly benign) was fairly constant to age 15, at which point it spurted ahead. The rate reached by males aged 15 to 19 was more or less maintained until age 45. The female pattern was entirely different after age 19 (see below).

There were six obstetrical cases per thousand girls aged 15 to 19 and fifty cases of disorders of female sex organs—mainly menstrual complaints.

*Adults (Aged 20 or more).* One of the most striking findings is the sudden change in incidence rates experienced by each sex at age 20. The change was in opposite directions, boys' rates dropping off and girls' rates rising precipitously. This was found both as to the proportion seeking medical attention and the number of diagnoses reported.

In the case of males, the drop in total reported diagnoses, from 2,070 to 1,385 per thousand, between the late teens and early twenties, was associated with decreases in almost all categories but particularly in injuries, preventive care, and respiratory conditions.

Among females, a good part of the sudden spurt in incidence at age 20 resulted from pregnancies and from disorders of female organs, but there were also substantial increases in the incidence of most other categories—benign neoplasms, infective diseases, disorders of blood, bones, joints, digestive and urinary tract, mental and neurological conditions, circulatory disorders. The highest rate of skin disorders among females was recorded for those aged 20 to 24.

At 20 to 24, total female incidence rates were nearly double the male rates. The gap narrowed with each succeeding age increment, but remained substantial up to age 65.

At no age level did the combined incidence of pregnancy and treatment of female sex organs account for most of the difference in incidence rates between men and women. Up to age 55, women showed higher rates in most categories, the principal exceptions being injuries and skin disorders; but even here, female rates were higher from age 35 on.

Certain disease categories showed a clear upward trend among adults with increasing age, for both sexes—malignant neoplasms, diseases of the nervous system, eye disorders, disorders of bones and joints, circulatory disorders. The latter category showed dramatic changes at every age level after 25; at ages past 65, circulatory diseases topped respiratory diseases as the leading diagnosis and involved well over a quarter of the population, but particularly women. Malignant neoplasms increased dramatically at age 55, doubling the rate found for the previous age interval.

For other disease categories, the age trend was consistently upward among male adults, more erratic among females: benign neoplasms, blood diseases, disorders of the digestive system, urinary tract diseases, allergic-metabolic disorders.

In certain categories the trend was downward—infective diseases, skin disorders, injuries among males, disorders of female sex organs.

The incidence of ear conditions was comparatively steady after age 25.

Except for conditions most frequent in childhood—infective, respiratory, minor digestive and ear disorders—males past 65 showed generally highest rates, whereas among females, highest rates were frequently encountered at ages 35 to 44—e.g. benign neoplasms, urinary tract disorders, injuries, allergic-metabolic disorders.

The relative importance of different disease categories to each adult age-sex subgroup changed gradually with increasing age, except for respiratory diseases.

Among males, skin disorders went from second place, at 20–24, to third, at 25–34, to fourth, at 35–44, after which circulatory disorders assumed third place, at ages 45–54, second at 55–64, and first at 65 and over. Digestive diseases went from fifth to fourth to third to second place by ages 45–54. Injuries went from second place, at 25–44, to fourth at ages 45–64 and fifth thereafter. Diseases of bones and joints, outranked by injuries to age 54, surpassed them in frequency after that point.

Female disorders were a leading type of illness among women at every age from 20 through 54. Skin conditions, a leader at ages 20 to 24, were displaced by allergic-metabolic and intestinal disorders, at ages 25 to 44. Allergic-metabolic conditions (including treatment of obesity) were most important at ages 35 to 44. Disorders of bones and joints were fifth in importance among women aged 45 to 54, moved to fourth at the next interval, 55 to 64, and were third at ages 65 on. At the same time, circulatory disorders moved from fourth, to second, to first place.

# INCIDENCE OF ATTENDED ILLNESS OR PREVENTIVE CARE.
## BY DIAGNOSTIC CATEGORY, BY AGE AND SEX

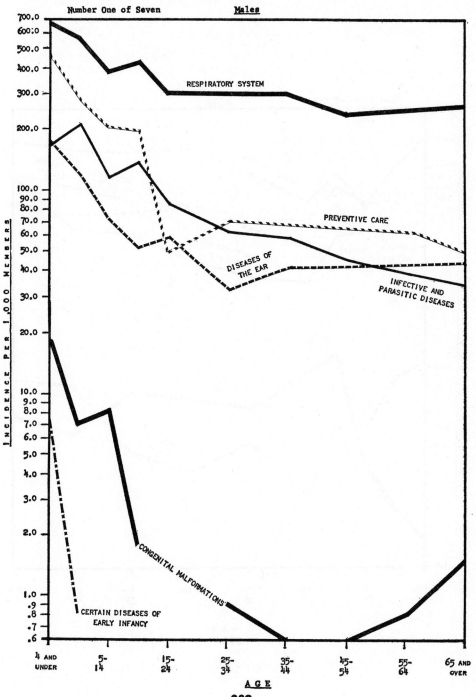

# INCIDENCE OF ATTENDED ILLNESS OR PREVENTIVE CARE
## BY DIAGNOSTIC CATEGORY, BY AGE AND SEX

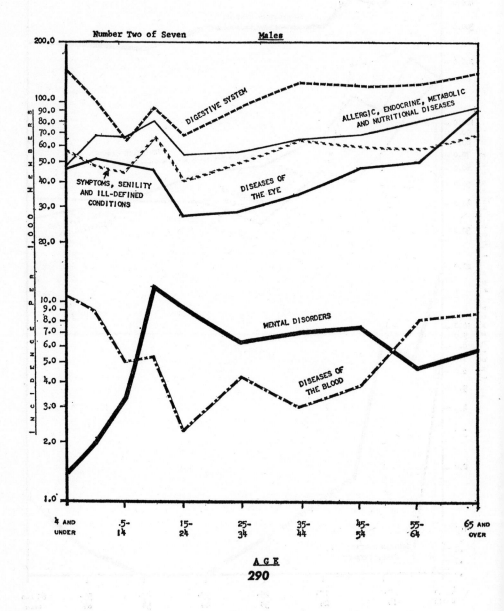

# INCIDENCE OF ATTENDED ILLNESS OR PREVENTIVE CARE
## BY DIAGNOSTIC CATEGORY, BY AGE AND SEX

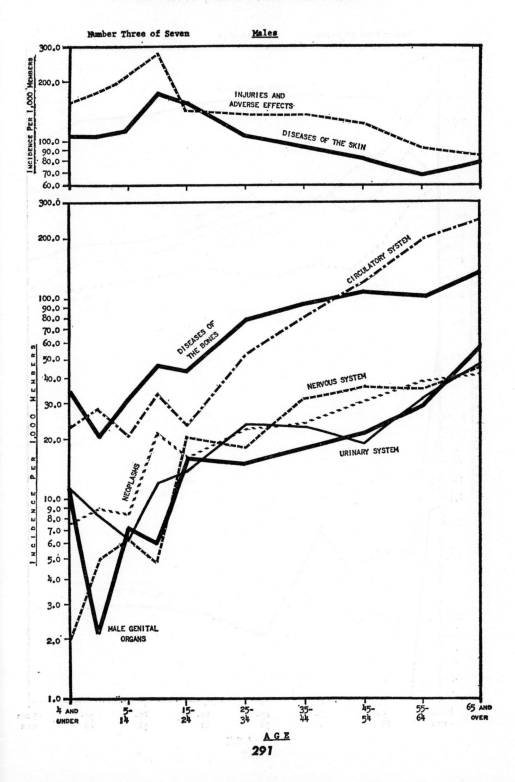

# INCIDENCE OF ATTENDED ILLNESS OR PREVENTIVE CARE
## BY DIAGNOSTIC CATEGORY, BY AGE AND SEX

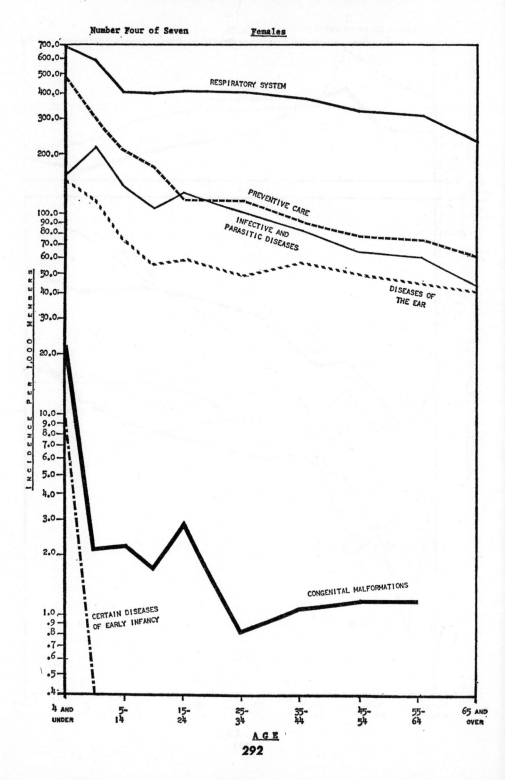

# INCIDENCE OF ATTENDED ILLNESS OR PREVENTIVE CARE
## BY DIAGNOSTIC CATEGORY, BY AGE AND SEX

Females

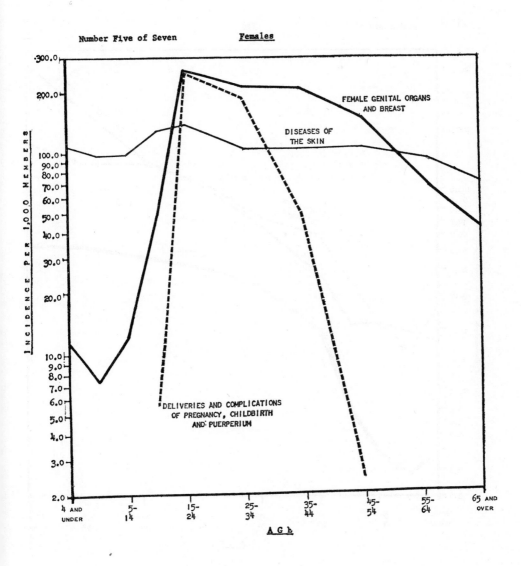

# INCIDENCE OF ATTENDED ILLNESS OR PREVENTIVE CARE
## BY DIAGNOSTIC CATEGORY, BY AGE AND SEX

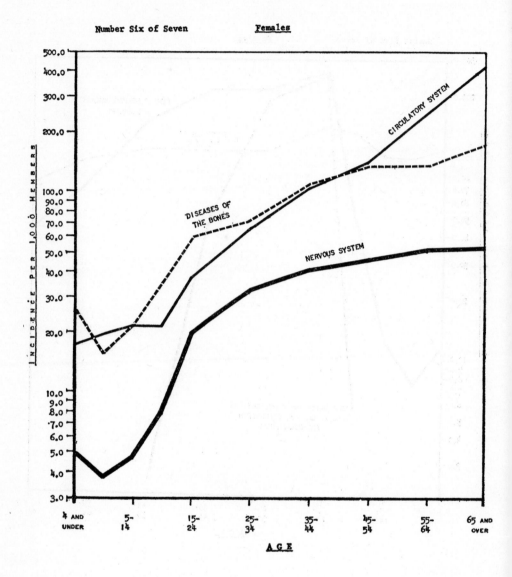

Number Six of Seven          **Females**

# INCIDENCE OF ATTENDED ILLNESS OR PREVENTIVE CARE
## BY DIAGNOSTIC CATEGORY, BY AGE AND SEX

Females

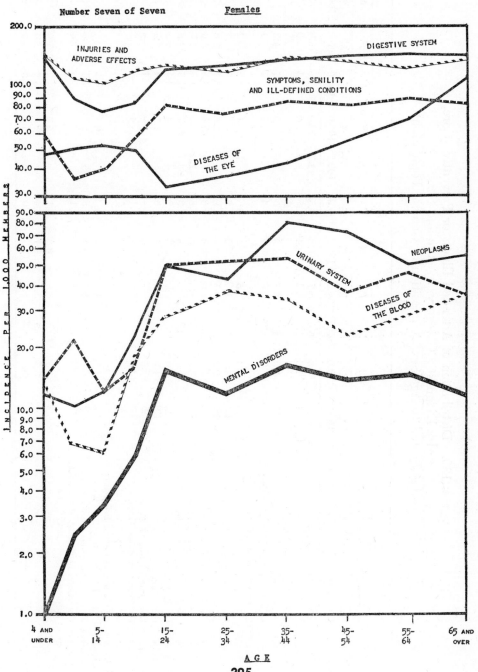

295

## TABLE 130. Distribution of Attended Illness or Preventive Care, by Diagnostic Category, by Age and Sex (and Adjusted to Age-Sex Composition of General Population)

Part I: to Age 19

| DIAGNOSTIC CATEGORY | Adjusted Total* | ALL | | | UNDER 5 | | 5-9 | | 10-14 | | 15-19 | |
|---|---|---|---|---|---|---|---|---|---|---|---|---|
| | | Total | M | F | M | F | M | F | M | F | M | F |
| | % | % | % | % | % | % | % | % | % | % | % | % |
| TOTAL | 100.0 | 100.0 | 100.0 | 100.0 | 100.0 | 100.0 | 100.0 | 100.0 | 100.0 | 100.0 | 100.0 | 100.0 |
| Infective and Parasitic Diseases | 5.2 | 5.8 | 6.0 | 5.7 | 6.6 | 6.5 | 11.3 | 12.0 | 7.6 | 9.6 | 7.6 | 6.8 |
| Neoplasms | 2.1 | 1.9 | 1.4 | 2.3 | .4 | .5 | .5 | .5 | .5 | .9 | 1.1 | 1.4 |
| Allergic, Endocrine System, Metabolic and Nutritional Diseases | 5.1 | 5.0 | 4.3 | 5.6 | 1.9 | 1.6 | 3.6 | 2.5 | 4.7 | 4.3 | 4.6 | 7.1 |
| Diseases of Blood and Blood Forming Organs | .8 | .7 | .3 | 1.0 | .4 | .4 | .4 | .3 | .3 | .4 | .3 | 1.0 |
| Mental, Psychoneurotic and Personality Disorders | .5 | .4 | .3 | .5 | .1 | 0 | .1 | .1 | .2 | .2 | .6 | .4 |
| Diseases of Nervous System | 1.4 | 1.2 | 1.2 | 1.3 | .1 | .2 | .2 | .2 | .5 | .3 | .2 | .5 |
| Diseases of the Eye | 2.9 | 2.6 | 2.8 | 2.5 | 1.9 | 1.9 | 2.4 | 2.5 | 3.1 | 3.6 | 2.5 | 3.2 |
| Diseases of the Ear | 3.5 | 3.8 | 4.1 | 3.6 | 6.5 | 5.6 | 5.6 | 5.8 | 4.5 | 5.0 | 2.8 | 3.5 |
| Diseases of the Circulatory System | 7.2 | 5.2 | 5.6 | 4.9 | .8 | .8 | 1.3 | .9 | 1.3 | 1.5 | 1.8 | 1.5 |
| Diseases of the Respiratory System | 27.4 | 29.4 | 30.6 | 28.3 | 41.8 | 42.6 | 38.7 | 41.7 | 31.5 | 34.8 | 28.7 | 31.5 |
| Diseases of the Digestive System | 7.2 | 7.0 | 7.3 | 6.7 | 5.9 | 5.8 | 4.7 | 4.4 | 4.4 | 5.2 | 5.3 | 5.6 |
| Diseases of the Urinary System | 1.6 | 1.5 | 1.1 | 1.7 | .4 | .6 | .4 | 1.1 | .4 | .9 | .6 | 1.0 |
| Diseases of the Male Genital Organs | .5 | .4 | .9 | — | .4 | — | .1 | — | .4 | — | .3 | — |
| Diseases of the Female Genital Organs and Breast | 3.3 | 3.2 | — | 5.8 | — | .4 | — | .4 | — | .8 | — | 3.0 |
| Deliveries and Complications of Pregnancy, Childbirth and Puerperium | 1.2 | 1.0 | — | 1.9 | — | 0 | — | 0 | — | 0 | — | .4 |
| Diseases of Skin and Subcutaneous Tissues | 5.9 | 6.0 | 6.6 | 5.5 | 4.5 | 4.5 | 5.1 | 5.0 | 7.5 | 7.0 | 10.1 | 8.4 |
| Diseases of Bones and Organs of Movement | 4.9 | 4.3 | 4.5 | 4.1 | 1.3 | 1.1 | .9 | .8 | 1.9 | 1.4 | 2.5 | 2.4 |
| Injuries and Adverse Effects of External Causes | 8.0 | 8.3 | 10.0 | 6.8 | 6.6 | 6.1 | 9.1 | 5.7 | 14.9 | 7.9 | 17.0 | 8.3 |
| Other† | 3.8 | 3.7 | 3.9 | 3.7 | 3.1 | 3.4 | 2.6 | 1.9 | 3.3 | 3.0 | 3.7 | 3.7 |
| Preventive Care | 7.5 | 8.6 | 9.1 | 8.1 | 17.3 | 18.0 | 13.0 | 14.2 | 13.0 | 13.2 | 10.3 | 10.3 |

*Part II: Ages 20 and Over*

| DIAGNOSTIC CATEGORY | 20–24 M % | 20–24 F % | 25–34 M % | 25–34 F % | 35–44 M % | 35–44 F % | 45–54 M % | 45–54 F % | 55–64 M % | 55–64 F % | 65 AND OVER M % | 65 AND OVER F % |
|---|---|---|---|---|---|---|---|---|---|---|---|---|
| TOTAL | 100.0 | 100.0 | 100.0 | 100.0 | 100.0 | 100.0 | 100.0 | 100.0 | 100.0 | 100.0 | 100.0 | 100.0 |
| Infective and Parasitic Diseases | 6.8 | 5.6 | 4.9 | 4.7 | 4.2 | 3.7 | 3.5 | 3.1 | 2.7 | 2.9 | 2.0 | 2.2 |
| Neoplasms | 1.3 | 2.2 | 1.7 | 1.9 | 1.7 | 3.7 | 2.4 | 4.0 | 3.2 | 3.0 | 2.6 | 3.5 |
| Allergic, Endocrine System, Metabolic and Nutritional Diseases | 4.5 | 5.3 | 4.9 | 6.9 | 5.0 | 7.4 | 5.2 | 7.5 | 5.4 | 6.1 | 5.6 | 5.4 |
| Diseases of Blood and Blood Forming Organs | .1 | 1.2 | .3 | 1.6 | .2 | 1.4 | .3 | 1.1 | .5 | 1.3 | .5 | 1.5 |
| Mental, Psychoneurotic and Personality Disorders | .7 | .7 | .5 | .5 | .5 | .7 | .5 | .7 | .3 | .7 | .5 | .7 |
| Diseases of Nervous System | 1.6 | 1.0 | 1.3 | 1.5 | 2.2 | 1.8 | 2.5 | 2.3 | 2.3 | 2.5 | 2.6 | 2.3 |
| Diseases of the Eye | 2.3 | 1.4 | 2.4 | 1.7 | 2.6 | 1.9 | 3.5 | 2.9 | 3.5 | 3.6 | 5.4 | 6.0 |
| Diseases of the Ear | 4.8 | 2.8 | 2.8 | 2.4 | 3.2 | 2.8 | 3.2 | 2.6 | 2.9 | 2.4 | 2.6 | 1.8 |
| Diseases of the Circulatory System | 1.8 | 1.6 | 4.0 | 3.2 | 6.4 | 5.1 | 10.1 | 7.9 | 16.4 | 15.2 | 19.3 | 26.3 |
| Diseases of the Respiratory System | 30.6 | 22.5 | 30.2 | 24.0 | 27.6 | 23.1 | 22.4 | 20.8 | 21.7 | 19.3 | 19.0 | 13.1 |
| Diseases of the Digestive System | 5.9 | 6.0 | 8.1 | 6.7 | 9.8 | 7.4 | 10.2 | 8.4 | 9.8 | 9.2 | 9.1 | 7.6 |
| Diseases of the Urinary System | 1.1 | 2.3 | 1.7 | 2.5 | 1.6 | 2.6 | 1.4 | 1.9 | 2.1 | 2.3 | 2.8 | 1.7 |
| Diseases of the Male Genital Organs | 1.3 | — | 1.1 | — | 1.2 | — | 1.4 | — | 1.8 | — | 2.9 | — |
| Diseases of the Female Genital Organs and Breast | — | 12.2 | — | 10.7 | — | 10.5 | — | 8.2 | — | 3.6 | — | 1.8 |
| Deliveries and Complications of Pregnancy, Childbirth and Puerperium | — | 10.6 | — | 8.2 | — | 2.1 | — | .1 | — | 0 | — | 0 |
| Diseases of Skin and Subcutaneous Tissues | 14.0 | 6.8 | 9.3 | 5.1 | 7.1 | 5.1 | 6.4 | 5.6 | 4.8 | 4.9 | 4.8 | 3.2 |
| Diseases of Bones and Organs of Movement | 3.8 | 2.8 | 6.1 | 3.5 | 7.1 | 5.6 | 8.8 | 7.4 | 7.5 | 7.9 | 7.9 | 9.1 |
| Injuries and Adverse Effects of External Causes | 12.3 | 6.0 | 11.4 | 5.9 | 10.2 | 6.8 | 8.9 | 7.6 | 6.7 | 7.1 | 5.5 | 6.9 |
| Other † | 3.2 | 3.8 | 4.0 | 3.7 | 4.7 | 4.3 | 4.8 | 4.3 | 4.2 | 4.5 | 4.1 | 4.1 |
| Preventive Care | 3.9 | 5.2 | 5.3 | 5.3 | 4.7 | 4.0 | 4.5 | 3.6 | 4.2 | 3.5 | 2.8 | 2.8 |

* Adjusted to age-sex composition of general population of area.
† Other includes: Symptoms, Senility and Ill-Defined Conditions; Congenital Malformations; and Certain Diseases of Early Infancy.

297

TABLE 131. Summary: Incidence of Attended Illness or
Preventive Care, by Diagnostic Category, by Age and Sex
(and Adjusted to Age-Sex Composition of General Population)

*Part I: to Age 19*

| DIAGNOSTIC CATEGORY | | Adjusted Total‡ | GROSS AND NET INCIDENCE PER 1000 EXPOSURE YEARS | | | | | | | | | | | |
|---|---|---|---|---|---|---|---|---|---|---|---|---|---|---|
| | | | Total | 5-9 | | 10-14 | | 15-19 | | ALL | | UNDER 5 | |
| | | | | M | F | M | F | M | F | M | F | M | F |
| Total—Including Undetermined | Gross* | 2077.5 | 2063.8 | 1850.8 | 2285.0 | 2887.0 | 2771.6 | 2310.4 | 2227.2 | 1735.9 | 1610.1 | 2069.9 | 1786.9 |
| | Net† | 802.5 | 801.8 | 754.0 | 851.5 | 988.8 | 1003.5 | 874.5 | 867.2 | 759.3 | 732.5 | 936.6 | 800.7 |
| Infective and Parasitic Diseases | Gross | 101.1 | 113.1 | 104.9 | 121.6 | 184.4 | 173.9 | 249.7 | 258.2 | 125.6 | 147.7 | 147.0 | 113.8 |
| | Net | 93.1 | 103.4 | 95.5 | 111.5 | 167.1 | 158.1 | 213.2 | 218.9 | 114.3 | 133.7 | 137.5 | 108.2 |
| Neoplasms | Gross | 40.2 | 36.4 | 24.8 | 48.4 | 10.3 | 13.4 | 10.7 | 11.6 | 8.8 | 13.1 | 22.1 | 24.3 |
| | Net | 34.5 | 31.9 | 21.3 | 43.9 | 7.5 | 11.9 | 9.0 | 10.3 | 8.3 | 12.2 | 21.5 | 23.2 |
| Malignant Neoplasms | Gross | 8.6 | 6.5 | 5.9 | 7.0 | 1.4 | 2.0 | 2.1 | .4 | .4 | .4 | .6 | 1.7 |
| | Net | 7.3 | 5.5 | 4.8 | 6.2 | 1.4 | 2.0 | 1.2 | .4 | .4 | .4 | .6 | 1.7 |
| Allergic, Endocrine System, Metabolic and Nutritional Diseases | Gross | 100.0 | 97.3 | 75.8 | 119.7 | 54.2 | 42.6 | 80.4 | 53.4 | 78.4 | 66.0 | 90.3 | 119.8 |
| | Net | 89.6 | 86.6 | 67.8 | 106.1 | 48.1 | 40.6 | 69.3 | 50.5 | 66.3 | 56.8 | 81.3 | 103.8 |
| Diseases of Blood and Blood Forming Organs | Gross | 15.4 | 13.9 | 5.9 | 22.2 | 10.7 | 13.4 | 9.0 | 6.6 | 5.0 | 6.1 | 5.4 | 18.2 |
| | Net | 15.4 | 13.9 | 5.9 | 22.2 | 10.7 | 13.4 | 9.0 | 6.6 | 5.0 | 6.1 | 5.4 | 18.2 |
| Mental, Psychoneurotic and Personality Disorders | Gross | 8.8 | 8.0 | 5.9 | 10.1 | 1.4 | 1.0 | 2.1 | 2.5 | 3.7 | 3.5 | 12.6 | 6.1 |
| | Net | 8.3 | 7.7 | 5.7 | 9.8 | 1.4 | 1.0 | 2.1 | 2.5 | 3.3 | 3.5 | 12.0 | 6.1 |
| Diseases of Nervous System | Gross | 27.7 | 24.2 | 21.0 | 27.5 | 1.9 | 5.0 | 4.9 | 3.7 | 7.1 | 4.8 | 4.8 | 8.8 |
| | Net | 26.9 | 23.4 | 20.5 | 26.6 | 1.9 | 5.0 | 4.9 | 3.7 | 6.3 | 4.8 | 4.8 | 8.3 |
| Diseases of the Eye | Gross | 56.1 | 51.2 | 48.6 | 53.9 | 52.3 | 49.6 | 53.7 | 53.8 | 50.5 | 55.9 | 48.4 | 54.1 |
| | Net | 51.6 | 47.9 | 45.6 | 50.4 | 47.6 | 47.1 | 52.5 | 51.3 | 49.2 | 52.0 | 46.6 | 50.2 |

| | | 1 | 2 | 3 | 4 | 5 | 6 | 7 | 8 | 9 | 10 | 11 | 12 |
|---|---|---|---|---|---|---|---|---|---|---|---|---|---|
| Diseases of the Ear | Gross | 68.8 | 73.9 | 71.2 | 76.7 | 179.7 | 150.7 | 123.8 | 125.4 | 74.3 | 77.4 | 53.8 | 58.5 |
| | Net | 64.1 | 68.7 | 66.9 | 70.6 | 172.3 | 147.7 | 116.0 | 117.5 | 70.9 | 72.1 | 53.8 | 55.2 |
| Diseases of the Circulatory System | Gross | 139.0 | 100.4 | 97.0 | 103.8 | 22.9 | 20.3 | 28.3 | 19.9 | 21.7 | 23.2 | 34.7 | 22.6 |
| | Net | 108.9 | 82.4 | 78.5 | 86.4 | 22.4 | 18.3 | 28.3 | 19.9 | 20.9 | 21.9 | 33.5 | 21.9 |
| Diseases of the Respiratory System | Gross | 532.4 | 569.2 | 533.4 | 606.4 | 1159.7 | 1139.7 | 858.5 | 892.0 | 521.9 | 535.8 | 555.9 | 527.9 |
| | Net | 377.1 | 399.0 | 374.3 | 424.6 | 672.7 | 698.2 | 560.9 | 585.4 | 388.0 | 402.1 | 435.7 | 398.7 |
| Diseases of the Digestive System | Gross | 140.9 | 135.7 | 127.8 | 144.0 | 164.3 | 154.6 | 104.1 | 93.9 | 71.8 | 80.4 | 101.6 | 93.9 |
| | Net | 119.9 | 116.4 | 111.2 | 121.7 | 149.4 | 143.7 | 99.6 | 89.8 | 64.7 | 76.5 | 95.0 | 85.6 |
| Diseases of the Urinary System | Gross | 31.1 | 28.2 | 19.3 | 37.4 | 12.6 | 15.4 | 8.2 | 24.4 | 6.3 | 13.5 | 12.5 | 16.0 |
| | Net | 28.5 | 25.9 | 18.1 | 34.0 | 11.6 | 13.9 | 8.2 | 21.9 | 6.3 | 12.2 | 12.0 | 16.0 |
| Diseases of the Male Genital Organs | Gross | 9.8 | 8.1 | 15.9 | — | 11.2 | — | 2.1 | — | 7.1 | 6.0 | 6.0 | — |
| | Net | 9.8 | 8.1 | 15.9 | — | 11.2 | — | 2.1 | — | 7.1 | 6.0 | 6.0 | — |
| Diseases of the Female Genital Organs and Breast | Gross | 63.9 | 61.3 | — | 125.0 | — | 11.9 | — | 7.9 | — | 12.7 | — | 50.8 |
| | Net | 55.5 | 53.0 | — | 108.0 | — | 11.9 | — | 7.4 | — | 12.2 | — | 49.7 |
| Deliveries and Complications of Pregnancy, Childbirth and Puerperium | Gross | 24.0 | 19.9 | — | 40.5 | — | 0 | — | 0 | — | 0 | — | 6.1 |
| | Net | 23.5 | 19.5 | — | 39.8 | — | 0 | — | 0 | — | 0 | — | 5.5 |
| Diseases of Skin and Subcutaneous Tissues | Gross | 114.9 | 116.1 | 114.7 | 117.5 | 125.6 | 120.4 | 112.3 | 107.1 | 125.2 | 107.0 | 196.7 | 140.8 |
| | Net | 101.8 | 103.2 | 102.3 | 104.2 | 109.2 | 109.5 | 105.4 | 96.8 | 114.7 | 98.3 | 175.7 | 128.7 |
| Diseases of Bones and Organs of Movement | Gross | 95.1 | 83.5 | 79.2 | 88.0 | 37.3 | 28.3 | 20.1 | 16.5 | 32.1 | 22.3 | 49.0 | 40.9 |
| | Net | 82.9 | 73.1 | 70.7 | 75.6 | 34.5 | 26.8 | 20.1 | 15.7 | 31.3 | 21.4 | 46.0 | 35.3 |
| Injuries and Adverse Effects of External Causes | Gross | 156.1 | 160.0 | 174.5 | 144.9 | 182.1 | 162.0 | 202.5 | 122.5 | 247.8 | 121.9 | 330.5 | 139.7 |
| | Net | 130.9 | 139.6 | 152.2 | 126.4 | 156.4 | 143.2 | 174.3 | 112.1 | 211.5 | 106.2 | 273.8 | 120.9 |
| Symptoms, Senility and Ill-Defined Conditions | Gross | 70.3 | 67.6 | 60.8 | 74.7 | 59.3 | 61.9 | 50.0 | 38.9 | 47.1 | 43.3 | 69.3 | 60.2 |
| | Net | 65.1 | 62.6 | 56.8 | 68.6 | 56.5 | 59.0 | 48.0 | 36.8 | 44.6 | 41.5 | 66.3 | 58.0 |
| Preventive Care | Gross | 146.5 | 166.3 | 159.2 | 173.8 | 481.8 | 480.7 | 290.3 | 304.9 | 215.3 | 202.8 | 199.0 | 172.8 |
| | Net | 143.1 | 162.4 | 155.1 | 170.0 | 471.1 | 472.7 | 275.9 | 291.3 | 210.3 | 201.0 | 196.7 | 170.1 |
| Other (Congenital Malformations and Certain Diseases of Early Infancy) | Gross | 4.1 | 4.6 | 5.0 | 4.3 | 26.1 | 30.7 | 7.8 | 2.5 | 8.3 | 2.2 | 1.8 | 1.7 |
| | Net | 4.1 | 4.6 | 5.0 | 4.3 | 26.1 | 30.7 | 7.8 | 2.5 | 8.3 | 2.2 | 1.8 | 1.7 |

*†‡ See footnotes at end of table.

TABLE 131. (Cont'd) Summary: Incidence of Attended Illness or Preventive Care, by Diagnostic Category, by Age and Sex (and Adjusted to Age-Sex Composition of General Population)

GROSS AND NET INCIDENCE PER 1000 EXPOSURE YEARS

| DIAGNOSTIC CATEGORY | | 20–24 M | 20–24 F | 25–34 M | 25–34 F | 35–44 M | 35–44 F | 45–54 M | 45–54 F | 55–64 M | 55–64 F | 65 AND OVER M | 65 AND OVER F |
|---|---|---|---|---|---|---|---|---|---|---|---|---|---|
| Total—Including Undetermined | Gross* | 1384.8 | 2613.8 | 1427.7 | 2475.0 | 1582.8 | 2504.3 | 1563.5 | 2300.2 | 1696.0 | 2292.3 | 2022.2 | 2415.7 |
|  | Net† | 668.2 | 972.6 | 672.1 | 896.2 | 673.2 | 865.4 | 650.0 | 802.4 | 664.5 | 808.9 | 745.6 | 898.3 |
| Infective and Parasitic Diseases | Gross | 87.6 | 134.0 | 66.5 | 106.5 | 62.2 | 84.8 | 51.2 | 66.1 | 42.2 | 61.8 | 37.0 | 49.4 |
|  | Net | 85.3 | 126.8 | 63.9 | 99.2 | 60.5 | 82.6 | 47.5 | 64.1 | 39.0 | 61.2 | 35.5 | 43.6 |
| Neoplasms | Gross | 16.1 | 53.3 | 22.9 | 43.0 | 24.5 | 85.7 | 34.8 | 84.5 | 51.0 | 64.1 | 48.8 | 78.5 |
|  | Net | 16.1 | 50.4 | 22.0 | 42.6 | 23.1 | 78.1 | 30.0 | 72.1 | 37.5 | 49.7 | 41.4 | 55.2 |
| Malignant Neoplasms | Gross | 0 | 4.3 | .9 | 3.5 | 3.1 | 7.4 | 9.3 | 13.8 | 22.7 | 23.1 | 23.6 | 29.1 |
|  | Net | 0 | 4.3 | .9 | 3.5 | 2.2 | 7.4 | 7.6 | 12.4 | 18.3 | 17.9 | 20.7 | 23.3 |
| Allergic, Endocrine System, Metabolic and Nutritional Diseases | Gross | 57.6 | 126.8 | 65.7 | 158.8 | 73.3 | 170.0 | 76.0 | 159.4 | 85.7 | 129.3 | 103.5 | 122.1 |
|  | Net | 55.3 | 112.3 | 57.5 | 137.9 | 66.1 | 150.5 | 69.6 | 139.3 | 80.5 | 117.8 | 94.7 | 116.3 |
| Diseases of Blood and Blood Forming Organs | Gross | 2.3 | 28.8 | 4.3 | 37.2 | 3.1 | 33.4 | 3.9 | 22.4 | 8.4 | 28.3 | 8.9 | 34.9 |
|  | Net | 2.3 | 28.8 | 4.3 | 37.2 | 3.1 | 33.4 | 3.9 | 22.4 | 8.4 | 28.3 | 8.9 | 34.9 |
| Mental Psychoneurotic and Personality Disorders | Gross | 9.2 | 15.8 | 6.9 | 12.0 | 7.3 | 17.0 | 7.6 | 14.9 | 4.8 | 14.4 | 8.9 | 14.5 |
|  | Net | 9.2 | 15.8 | 6.5 | 12.0 | 7.3 | 16.4 | 7.6 | 13.8 | 4.8 | 14.4 | 5.9 | 11.6 |
| Diseases of Nervous System | Gross | 20.7 | 23.1 | 18.2 | 33.3 | 32.1 | 42.4 | 36.2 | 48.0 | 35.5 | 52.5 | 47.3 | 52.3 |
|  | Net | 20.7 | 20.2 | 17.7 | 32.9 | 31.5 | 40.2 | 35.3 | 46.8 | 34.7 | 50.8 | 44.4 | 52.3 |
| Diseases of the Eye | Gross | 30.0 | 34.6 | 32.4 | 38.0 | 37.6 | 43.3 | 51.2 | 62.3 | 55.0 | 76.2 | 99.1 | 136.6 |
|  | Net | 27.6 | 33.1 | 28.9 | 37.2 | 35.7 | 42.7 | 47.8 | 55.7 | 50.2 | 70.4 | 91.7 | 110.5 |

| Category | Rate | | | | | | | | | | | | |
|---|---|---|---|---|---|---|---|---|---|---|---|---|---|
| Diseases of the Ear | Gross | 62.2 | 67.7 | 37.2 | 53.9 | 46.8 | 64.8 | 46.4 | 56.3 | 45.0 | 51.4 | 48.8 | 40.7 |
| | Net | 59.9 | 59.1 | 33.7 | 48.8 | 42.7 | 56.6 | 43.0 | 49.1 | 42.6 | 44.5 | 45.9 | 40.7 |
| Diseases of the Circulatory System | Gross | 23.1 | 38.9 | 54.0 | 72.8 | 94.0 | 118.2 | 145.9 | 168.9 | 258.6 | 323.9 | 356.5 | 595.9 |
| | Net | 23.1 | 38.9 | 51.4 | 67.4 | 80.0 | 105.5 | 117.0 | 140.8 | 192.4 | 245.4 | 248.5 | 418.6 |
| Diseases of the Respiratory System | Gross | 394.0 | 541.8 | 408.2 | 549.8 | 408.2 | 532.8 | 324.3 | 444.1 | 341.0 | 409.3 | 350.6 | 296.5 |
| | Net | 308.8 | 407.8 | 308.9 | 400.6 | 308.1 | 378.1 | 248.5 | 326.1 | 257.0 | 312.9 | 267.8 | 229.7 |
| Diseases of the Digestive System | Gross | 76.0 | 144.1 | 109.7 | 154.2 | 144.5 | 170.0 | 147.9 | 178.4 | 153.8 | 194.6 | 167.2 | 171.5 |
| | Net | 69.1 | 126.8 | 95.9 | 127.5 | 124.7 | 138.0 | 121.9 | 142.8 | 124.3 | 147.2 | 140.5 | 145.3 |
| Diseases of the Urinary System | Gross | 13.8 | 54.8 | 23.3 | 56.6 | 24.0 | 58.8 | 19.8 | 40.5 | 34.2 | 49.7 | 51.8 | 37.8 |
| | Net | 13.8 | 49.0 | 22.5 | 51.1 | 22.3 | 53.5 | 18.9 | 36.2 | 30.7 | 45.6 | 45.9 | 34.9 |
| Diseases of the Male Genital Organs | Gross | 16.1 | — | 14.7 | — | 17.8 | — | 20.9 | — | 29.1 | — | 54.7 | — |
| | Net | 16.1 | — | 14.7 | — | 17.8 | — | 20.9 | — | 29.1 | — | 54.7 | — |
| Diseases of the Female Genital Organs and Breast | Gross | — | 295.3 | 245.7 | — | 242.7 | — | 173.8 | — | 76.8 | — | — | 40.7 |
| | Net | — | 253.6 | 211.2 | — | 206.2 | — | 147.1 | — | 70.4 | — | — | 40.7 |
| Deliveries and Complications of Pregnancy, Childbirth and Puerperium | Gross | — | 256.5 | 186.7 | — | 47.5 | — | 2.3 | — | 0 | — | — | 0 |
| | Net | — | 250.7 | 182.9 | — | 47.5 | — | 2.3 | — | 0 | — | — | 0 |
| Diseases of Skin and Subcutaneous Tissues | Gross | 179.7 | 164.3 | 125.3 | 117.8 | 104.3 | 117.9 | 92.4 | 118.6 | 75.7 | 105.1 | 88.7 | 72.7 |
| | Net | 156.7 | 138.3 | 108.4 | 102.3 | 93.4 | 101.8 | 80.6 | 103.7 | 67.7 | 92.4 | 76.9 | 69.8 |
| Diseases of Bones and Organs of Movement | Gross | 48.4 | 67.7 | 82.1 | 80.6 | 104.6 | 128.4 | 127.8 | 156.9 | 117.5 | 168.0 | 145.0 | 206.4 |
| | Net | 43.8 | 59.1 | 77.8 | 71.7 | 92.3 | 110.0 | 108.8 | 133.9 | 101.2 | 136.3 | 133.1 | 171.5 |
| Injuries and Adverse Effects of External Causes | Gross | 159.0 | 144.1 | 154.2 | 134.4 | 150.9 | 156.4 | 129.5 | 160.9 | 104.8 | 150.1 | 133.1 | 157.0 |
| | Net | 140.6 | 129.7 | 135.6 | 119.7 | 135.2 | 139.1 | 121.6 | 134.2 | 92.0 | 125.3 | 102.1 | 133.7 |
| Symptoms, Senility and Ill-Defined Conditions | Gross | 41.5 | 89.3 | 53.1 | 84.1 | 69.4 | 96.4 | 67.6 | 91.6 | 64.9 | 94.7 | 74.0 | 93.0 |
| | Net | 41.5 | 83.6 | 50.5 | 74.4 | 65.0 | 86.8 | 60.5 | 81.9 | 59.0 | 89.5 | 69.5 | 84.3 |
| Preventive Care | Gross | 50.7 | 125.4 | 70.8 | 120.5 | 69.4 | 93.0 | 65.6 | 77.3 | 65.3 | 75.1 | 51.8 | 64.0 |
| | Net | 50.7 | 118.2 | 70.8 | 118.6 | 68.3 | 91.3 | 64.5 | 76.7 | 63.3 | 73.9 | 50.3 | 61.0 |
| Other (Congenital Malformations and Certain Diseases of Early Infancy) | Gross | 0 | 2.9 | .9 | .8 | .6 | 1.1 | .6 | 1.2 | .8 | 1.2 | 1.5 | 0 |
| | Net | 0 | 2.9 | .9 | .8 | .6 | 1.1 | .6 | 1.2 | .8 | 1.2 | 1.5 | 0 |

* Gross rate is based on sum of patients reported for each component of a category; this represents duplicate count of persons treated for more than one condition in that category.

† Net rate is based on number of patients with any condition listed for a specified category.

‡ Adjusted to age-sex composition of general population of area.

*Part I: to Age 19*

## TABLE 132. Incidence of Attended Illness or Preventive Care, by Diagnosis, by Age and Sex (and Adjusted to Age-Sex Composition of General Population)

| DIAGNOSIS | | Adjusted Total § | NUMBER OF MEMBERS WITH INDICATED DIAGNOSIS PER 1,000 EXPOSURE YEARS | | | | | | | | | | |
|---|---|---|---|---|---|---|---|---|---|---|---|---|---|
| | | | ALL | | | UNDER 5 | | 5–9 | | 10–14 | | 15–19 | |
| | | | Total | M | F | M | F | M | F | M | F | M | F |
| TOTAL | Gross † | 2077.5 | 2063.8 | 1850.8 | 2285.0 | 2887.0 | 2771.6 | 2310.4 | 2227.2 | 1735.9 | 1610.1 | 2069.9 | 1786.9 |
| | Net ‡ | 802.5 | 801.8 | 754.0 | 851.5 | 988.8 | 1003.5 | 874.5 | 867.2 | 759.3 | 732.5 | 936.6 | 800.7 |
| **I** | | | | | | | | | | | | | |
| Infective and Parasitic Diseases | Gross | 101.1 | 113.1 | 104.9 | 121.6 | 184.4 | 173.9 | 249.7 | 258.2 | 125.6 | 147.7 | 147.0 | 113.8 |
| | Net | 93.1 | 103.4 | 95.5 | 111.5 | 167.1 | 158.1 | 213.2 | 218.9 | 114.3 | 133.7 | 137.5 | 108.2 |
| Streptococcal Sore Throat | | 15.2 | 17.2 | 15.4 | 19.0 | 24.7 | 25.3 | 28.7 | 30.6 | 17.5 | 23.2 | 21.5 | 20.4 |
| Measles | | 5.1 | 6.7 | 7.0 | 6.5 | 17.3 | 14.4 | 34.4 | 28.1 | 8.3 | 8.3 | 4.8 | 3.9 |
| Rubella (German Measles) | | 19.1 | 24.3 | 21.8 | 27.0 | 50.0 | 42.6 | 75.4 | 83.2 | 40.0 | 55.1 | 39.4 | 34.2 |
| Chicken Pox | | 3.6 | 4.8 | 5.0 | 4.5 | 14.9 | 11.9 | 25.4 | 21.1 | 4.2 | 6.5 | 2.4 | 1.1 |
| Mumps | | 2.5 | 3.4 | 3.2 | 3.6 | 4.7 | 4.9 | 16.4 | 20.7 | 2.5 | 3.1 | 1.8 | 0 |
| Infectious Hepatitis | | .3 | .3 | .4 | .2 | 0 | .5 | .4 | 0 | .8 | .4 | 1.8 | .6 |
| Glandular Fever (Infectious Mononucleosis) | | 1.4 | 1.5 | 1.4 | 1.6 | .5 | .5 | 3.3 | 2.1 | 1.7 | .9 | 7.2 | 6.1 |
| Intestinal Virus | | 40.4 | 42.3 | 38.7 | 45.9 | 56.5 | 60.4 | 52.9 | 52.1 | 40.1 | 37.5 | 50.2 | 35.9 |
| Dermatophytoses | | 6.0 | 5.8 | 6.4 | 5.3 | 6.5 | 4.0 | 6.6 | 5.0 | 6.3 | 6.1 | 13.7 | 5.5 |
| Other | | 7.5 | 6.8 | 5.6 | 8.0 | 9.3 | 9.4 | 6.2 | 15.3 | 4.2 | 6.6 | 4.2 | 6.1 |

| Cause | Basis | | | | | | | | | | | | |
|---|---|---|---|---|---|---|---|---|---|---|---|---|---|
| Neoplasms | Gross | 40.2 | 36.4 | 24.8 | 48.4 | 10.3 | 13.4 | 10.7 | 11.6 | 8.8 | 13.1 | 22.1 | 24.3 |
| | Net | 34.5 | 31.9 | 21.3 | 43.9 | 7.5 | 11.9 | 9.0 | 10.3 | 8.3 | 12.2 | 21.5 | 23.2 |
| Malignant Neoplasms | Gross | 8.6 | 6.5 | 5.9 | 7.0 | 1.4 | 2.0 | 2.1 | .4 | .4 | .4 | .6 | 1.7 |
| | Net | 7.3 | 5.5 | 4.8 | 6.2 | 1.4 | 2.0 | 1.2 | .4 | .4 | .4 | .6 | 1.7 |
| Digestive System—Including Mouth | | 1.5 | .9 | 1.2 | .6 | 0 | 0 | .4 | 0 | 0 | 0 | 0 | 0 |
| Respiratory System | | 1.1 | .7 | 1.0 | .4 | 0 | 0 | 0 | 0 | 0 | 0 | 0 | 0 |
| Breast | | 1.4 | 1.1 | — | 2.2 | — | 0 | — | — | — | 0 | — | .6 |
| Female Genital Organs | | .5 | .5 | .5 | 1.0 | — | — | — | — | — | 0 | — | 0 |
| Male Genital Organs | | .4 | .3 | .4 | — | 0 | 0 | 0 | 0 | 0 | 0 | 0 | 0 |
| Urinary System | | .3 | .3 | .9 | .1 | 0 | 0 | 0 | 0 | 0 | 0 | 0 | 0 |
| Skin | | 1.2 | .8 | 0 | .6 | 0 | .5 | 0 | 0 | 0 | 0 | 0 | .6 |
| Eye | | .1 | 0* | 0 | .1 | 0 | 0 | 0 | 0 | 0 | 0 | 0 | 0 |
| Nervous System—Including Brain | | .2 | .2 | .3 | .1 | 0 | 0 | 0 | 0 | 0 | 0 | 0 | 0 |
| Endocrine Glands | | .2 | .2 | .1 | .3 | 0 | .5 | .5 | 0 | 0 | 0 | 0 | 0 |
| Bone | | .2 | .1 | .1 | .1 | 0 | 0 | 0 | 0 | 0 | 0 | 0 | 0 |
| Connective Tissue | | 0 | 0 | 0* | 0 | 0 | 0 | 0 | 0 | 0 | 0 | 0 | 0 |
| Lymphosarcoma | | .1 | .1 | 0* | .1 | 0 | 0 | 0 | 0 | 0 | 0 | 0 | 0 |
| Hodgkin's Disease | | .1 | .1 | 0* | .1 | 0 | .5 | 0 | 0 | 0 | 0 | 0 | 0 |
| Other Lymphoma | | .1 | .1 | .2 | .1 | .5 | .5 | .4 | 0 | 0 | .4 | 0 | 0 |
| Multiple Myeloma | | .1 | 0* | 0* | .1 | .5 | 0 | 0 | 0 | 0 | 0 | 0 | 0 |
| Leukemia | | .2 | .2 | .2 | .3 | 0 | 0 | .4 | 0 | 0 | 0 | 0 | 0 |
| Not Elsewhere Classified | | 1.1 | .9 | 1.0 | .8 | .4 | 0 | .4 | .4 | .4 | 0 | .6 | .5 |
| Benign Neoplasms | Gross | 29.5 | 28.0 | 17.6 | 38.8 | 6.6 | 10.9 | 7.8 | 8.7 | 7.5 | 11.8 | 20.9 | 22.1 |
| | Net | 27.3 | 26.6 | 17.0 | 36.5 | 5.6 | 9.9 | 7.8 | 7.9 | 7.1 | 11.4 | 20.3 | 21.0 |
| Mouth | | 1.1 | .9 | .6 | 1.3 | 0 | 0 | .8 | 1.6 | 0 | .9 | .6 | .5 |
| Rectum | | .9 | .8 | .8 | .6 | 0 | 0 | .4 | 0 | — | 0 | 0 | 0 |
| Breast | | 1.7 | 1.6 | — | 3.3 | — | .5 | — | 0 | 0 | 0 | — | 2.8 |
| Female Genital Organs | | 7.3 | 7.4 | 10.5 | 15.2 | 3.8 | 2.5 | 5.4 | 5.0 | 5.4 | .9 | 17.3 | 2.8 |
| Skin | | 11.6 | 11.0 | 5.7 | 11.5 | 2.8 | 7.9 | 1.2 | 2.1 | 2.1 | 7.8 | 3.0 | 9.4 |
| Other | | 6.9 | 6.3 | 1.3 | 6.9 | 2.3 | .5 | .8 | 2.5 | .9 | 2.5 | .6 | 6.6 |
| Unspecified Neoplasms | Gross | 2.1 | 1.9 | 1.3 | 2.6 | 2.3 | .5 | .8 | 2.5 | .9 | .9 | .6 | .5 |
| | Net | 2.1 | 1.9 | 1.3 | 2.6 | 2.3 | .5 | .8 | 2.5 | .9 | .9 | .6 | .5 |
| Rectum | | .1 | .1 | 0 | .2 | 0 | 0 | 0 | .4 | 0 | .4 | 0 | 0 |
| Breast | | .3 | .3 | — | .6 | — | 0 | — | 0 | — | 0 | — | 0 |
| Female Genital Organs | | .1 | .1 | — | .3 | — | 0 | — | 2.1 | — | 0 | — | 0 |
| Other | | 1.6 | 1.4 | 1.3 | 1.5 | 2.3 | .5 | .8 | 0 | .9 | .5 | .6 | .5 |

303

TABLE 132. (*Cont'd*) Incidence of Attended Illness or Preventive Care, by Diagnosis, by Age and Sex (and Adjusted to Age-Sex Composition of General Population)

*Part I: to Age 19 (Cont'd)*

NUMBER OF MEMBERS WITH INDICATED DIAGNOSIS PER 1,000 EXPOSURE YEARS

| DIAGNOSIS | | Adjusted Total § | ALL | | | UNDER 5 | | 5–9 | | 10–14 | | 15–19 | |
|---|---|---|---|---|---|---|---|---|---|---|---|---|---|
| | | | *Total* | *M* | *F* | *M* | *F* | *M* | *F* | *M* | *F* | *M* | *F* |
| **III** | | | | | | | | | | | | | |
| Allergic, Endocrine System, Metabolic and Nutritional Diseases | Gross | 100.0 | 97.3 | 75.8 | 119.7 | 54.2 | 42.6 | 80.4 | 53.4 | 78.4 | 66.0 | 90.3 | 119.8 |
| | Net | 89.6 | 86.6 | 67.8 | 106.1 | 48.1 | 40.6 | 69.3 | 50.5 | 66.3 | 56.8 | 81.3 | 103.8 |
| Hay Fever | | 16.7 | 17.8 | 17.6 | 18.1 | 11.7 | 8.4 | 28.3 | 17.8 | 28.4 | 18.4 | 32.3 | 23.2 |
| Asthma | | 14.1 | 14.5 | 15.0 | 14.0 | 21.5 | 13.8 | 27.5 | 16.1 | 19.2 | 13.5 | 20.3 | 12.2 |
| Other Allergic Diseases | | 13.3 | 13.9 | 12.8 | 15.0 | 15.9 | 14.9 | 19.3 | 13.3 | 21.3 | 13.1 | 14.3 | 23.7 |
| Diseases of Thyroid Gland | | 11.0 | 10.4 | 2.9 | 18.2 | 0 | .5 | 1.2 | 0 | 1.2 | 4.4 | 3.0 | 18.8 |
| Diabetes Mellitus | | 12.9 | 9.3 | 10.6 | 8.0 | .5 | .5 | .8 | .4 | 1.2 | 1.3 | 3.6 | 4.4 |
| Obesity (Not Otherwise Specified) | | 25.2 | 24.6 | 10.7 | 39.0 | 1.4 | 2.0 | 2.1 | 3.7 | 3.8 | 12.7 | 10.8 | 30.9 |
| Other | | 6.8 | 6.8 | 6.2 | 7.4 | 3.2 | 2.5 | 1.2 | 2.1 | 3.3 | 2.6 | 6.0 | 6.6 |
| **IV** | | | | | | | | | | | | | |
| Diseases of Blood and Blood Forming Organs | Gross | 15.4 | 13.9 | 5.9 | 22.2 | 10.7 | 13.4 | 9.0 | 6.6 | 5.0 | 6.1 | 5.4 | 18.2 |
| | Net | 15.4 | 13.9 | 5.9 | 22.2 | 10.7 | 13.4 | 9.0 | 6.6 | 5.0 | 6.1 | 5.4 | 18.2 |
| Anemias | | 13.8 | 12.6 | 4.7 | 20.8 | 9.8 | 12.4 | 7.8 | 5.4 | 4.6 | 5.2 | 3.6 | 18.2 |
| Other | | 1.6 | 1.3 | 1.2 | 1.4 | .9 | 1.0 | 1.2 | 1.2 | .4 | .9 | 1.8 | 0 |

| | | 1 | 2 | 3 | 4 | 5 | 6 | 7 | 8 | 9 | 10 | 11 | 12 |
|---|---|---|---|---|---|---|---|---|---|---|---|---|---|
| **v** | | | | | | | | | | | | | |
| Mental, Psychoneurotic and Personality Disorders | Gross | 8.8 | 8.0 | 5.9 | 10.1 | 1.4 | 1.0 | 2.1 | 2.5 | 3.7 | 3.5 | 12.6 | 6.1 |
| | Net | 8.3 | 7.7 | 5.7 | 9.8 | 1.4 | 1.0 | 2.1 | 2.5 | 3.3 | 3.5 | 12.0 | 6.1 |
| Chronic Brain Disorders | | .4 | .3 | .4 | .2 | .9 | 1.0 | 0 | 0 | .8 | 0 | 0 | .5 |
| Psychoses | | 1.2 | 1.0 | .6 | 1.4 | 0 | 0 | .4 | .9 | 0 | .9 | 1.8 | 1.1 |
| Psychophysiologic, Autonomic and Visceral Disorders | | .2 | .2 | .1 | .3 | 0 | 0 | 0 | 0 | 0 | 0 | 0 | 0 |
| Psychoneuroses | | 6.1 | 5.7 | 4.2 | 7.2 | 0 | 0 | .4 | .8 | 1.7 | 2.2 | 9.0 | 3.9 |
| Personality Disorders | | .8 | .6 | .4 | .9 | .5 | 0 | .9 | .8 | 0 | .4 | 1.8 | .6 |
| Mental Deficiency | | .1 | .2 | .2 | .1 | 0 | 0 | .4 | 0 | 1.2 | 0 | 0 | 0 |
| **vi** | | | | | | | | | | | | | |
| Diseases of Nervous System | Gross | 27.7 | 24.2 | 21.0 | 27.5 | 1.9 | 5.0 | 4.9 | 3.7 | 7.1 | 4.8 | 4.8 | 8.8 |
| | Net | 26.9 | 23.4 | 20.5 | 26.6 | 1.9 | 5.0 | 4.9 | 3.7 | 6.3 | 4.8 | 4.8 | 8.3 |
| Stroke | | .2 | .1 | .1 | 0 | 0 | 0 | 0 | 0 | 0 | 0 | 0 | 0 |
| Multiple Sclerosis | | .3 | .3 | .1 | .5 | 0 | 0 | 0 | 0 | 0 | 0 | 0 | 0 |
| Migraine | | 3.3 | 3.3 | 2.0 | 4.8 | 0 | .5 | .8 | .8 | 1.7 | .4 | 1.2 | 1.7 |
| Epilepsy | | .5 | .6 | .7 | .5 | 0 | 0 | 1.6 | 0 | 1.7 | 1.3 | 0 | .5 |
| Sciatica | | 4.5 | 3.9 | 3.6 | 4.2 | 0 | 0 | 0 | 0 | 0 | 0 | 0 | .5 |
| Other | | 18.9 | 16.0 | 14.5 | 17.5 | 1.9 | 4.5 | 2.5 | 2.9 | 3.7 | 3.1 | 3.6 | 6.1 |
| **vii** | | | | | | | | | | | | | |
| Diseases of Eye | Gross | 56.1 | 51.2 | 48.6 | 53.9 | 52.3 | 49.6 | 53.7 | 53.8 | 50.5 | 55.9 | 48.4 | 54.1 |
| | Net | 51.6 | 47.9 | 45.6 | 50.4 | 47.6 | 47.1 | 52.5 | 51.3 | 49.2 | 52.0 | 46.6 | 50.2 |
| Conjunctivitis and Ophthalmia | | 22.4 | 22.4 | 21.9 | 23.0 | 32.2 | 26.8 | 28.7 | 21.1 | 27.5 | 28.4 | 20.3 | 27.6 |
| Strabismus | | 4.2 | 5.1 | 4.4 | 5.9 | 9.3 | 9.4 | 11.9 | 18.2 | 9.2 | 11.3 | 6.6 | 5.0 |
| Cataract | | 3.7 | 1.9 | 1.9 | 1.8 | 0 | .5 | 0 | 0 | .9 | 0 | .6 | .5 |
| Glaucoma | | 4.0 | 2.1 | 2.1 | 2.0 | 0 | 0 | 0 | 0 | 0 | 0 | .6 | .5 |
| Detachment of Retina | | .3 | .1 | .1 | .2 | 0 | 0 | 0 | 0 | 0 | 0 | 0 | .6 |
| Other | | 21.5 | 19.6 | 18.2 | 21.0 | 10.8 | 12.9 | 13.1 | 14.5 | 12.9 | 16.2 | 20.3 | 19.9 |
| **viii** | | | | | | | | | | | | | |
| Diseases of Ear | Gross | 68.8 | 73.9 | 71.2 | 76.7 | 179.7 | 150.7 | 123.8 | 125.4 | 74.3 | 77.4 | 53.8 | 58.5 |
| | Net | 64.1 | 68.7 | 66.9 | 70.6 | 172.3 | 147.7 | 116.0 | 117.5 | 70.9 | 72.1 | 53.8 | 55.2 |
| Otitis Externa | | 8.7 | 9.0 | 8.6 | 9.4 | 11.7 | 7.9 | 11.9 | 9.9 | 11.3 | 11.8 | 11.3 | 9.4 |
| Otitis Media | | 42.8 | 48.5 | 45.8 | 51.4 | 159.6 | 138.8 | 102.9 | 101.8 | 54.2 | 56.0 | 30.5 | 38.1 |
| Deafness | | 1.2 | 1.1 | 1.0 | 1.1 | 1.4 | 0 | .4 | 2.5 | 1.3 | .4 | 1.2 | 0 |
| Other | | 16.1 | 15.3 | 15.8 | 14.8 | 7.0 | 4.0 | 8.6 | 11.2 | 7.5 | 9.2 | 10.8 | 11.0 |

**TABLE 132.** *(Cont'd)* Incidence of Attended Illness or Preventive Care, by Diagnosis, by Age and Sex (and Adjusted to Age-Sex Composition of General Population)

*Part I: to Age 19 (Cont'd)*

| DIAGNOSIS | | Adjusted Total § | ALL | | | UNDER 5 | | 5–9 | | 10–14 | | 15–19 | |
|---|---|---|---|---|---|---|---|---|---|---|---|---|---|
| | | | Total | M | F | M | F | M | F | M | F | M | F |
| IX Diseases of Circulatory System | Gross | 139.0 | 100.4 | 97.0 | 103.8 | 22.9 | 20.3 | 28.3 | 19.9 | 21.7 | 23.2 | 34.7 | 22.6 |
| | Net | 108.9 | 82.4 | 78.5 | 86.4 | 22.4 | 18.3 | 28.3 | 19.9 | 20.9 | 21.9 | 33.5 | 21.9 |
| Rheumatic Fever without Mention of Heart | | .4 | .5 | .4 | .6 | 0 | .5 | 0 | .4 | 1.2 | 2.6 | 1.2 | 1.1 |
| Diseases of Heart | Gross | 55.0 | 35.7 | 41.4 | 29.7 | 4.2 | 4.0 | 4.5 | 3.3 | 3.8 | 5.7 | 5.4 | 3.3 |
| | Net | 42.2 | 27.6 | 31.0 | 24.2 | 4.2 | 3.0 | 4.5 | 3.3 | 3.3 | 5.2 | 5.3 | 3.3 |
| Rheumatic Heart Disease | | 3.0 | 2.8 | 2.0 | 3.6 | .4 | .5 | .8 | .8 | 1.3 | 3.1 | 3.0 | 1.7 |
| Arteriosclerotic Heart Disease | | 13.2 | 7.0 | 9.1 | 4.9 | 0 | 1.0 | 0 | 0 | 0 | 0 | 0 | 0 |
| Acute Coronary Occlusion | | 4.5 | 3.0 | 4.7 | 1.3 | 0 | 0 | 0 | 0 | 0 | 0 | 0 | 0 |
| Coronary Insufficiency | | 9.5 | 6.2 | 7.9 | 4.5 | .5 | 0 | 0 | 0 | .4 | 0 | 0 | .5 |
| Angina Pectoris | | 7.1 | 5.2 | 6.2 | 4.0 | 0 | 0 | .4 | .8 | 0 | 0 | .6 | 0 |
| Hypertensive Heart Disease | | 7.8 | 4.0 | 3.2 | 4.9 | .5 | .5 | .4 | 0 | 0 | 0 | 0 | 0 |
| Other | | 9.9 | 7.5 | 8.3 | 6.5 | 2.8 | 2.0 | 2.9 | 1.7 | 2.1 | 2.6 | 1.8 | 1.1 |
| Diseases of Veins and Arteries Other than Heart | Gross | 83.6 | 64.2 | 55.2 | 73.5 | 18.7 | 15.8 | 23.8 | 16.2 | 16.7 | 14.9 | 28.1 | 18.2 |
| | Net | 79.0 | 60.9 | 53.2 | 68.9 | 18.6 | 15.4 | 23.8 | 16.2 | 16.7 | 14.9 | 27.5 | 17.1 |
| Hypertensive Diseases | | 46.1 | 30.9 | 25.1 | 36.9 | 1.9 | 2.4 | 0 | 1.7 | 2.1 | 1.3 | 6.0 | 3.3 |
| Hypotension | | 3.0 | 2.6 | 1.7 | 3.7 | 0 | 0 | 0 | 0 | .4 | 0 | .6 | 2.2 |
| Hemorrhoids | | 11.9 | 10.8 | 11.0 | 10.5 | .9 | .5 | .4 | 0 | .4 | 0 | 1.8 | 3.3 |
| General Arteriosclerosis | | 2.3 | 1.0 | 1.0 | 1.0 | 0 | 0 | 0 | 0 | 0 | 0 | 0 | 0 |
| Varicose Veins of Lower Extremities | | 3.1 | 2.6 | 1.5 | 3.8 | .5 | .5 | 0 | 0 | 0 | 0 | 1.2 | 0 |
| Pulmonary Embolism and Infarction | | .2 | .3 | .2 | .3 | 0 | 0 | 0 | 0 | 0 | 0 | 0 | 0 |
| Lymphadenitis | | 6.5 | 7.9 | 7.9 | 7.9 | 13.5 | 10.9 | 21.3 | 14.5 | 12.5 | 12.7 | 14.9 | 6.6 |
| Other | | 10.5 | 8.1 | 6.8 | 9.4 | 1.9 | 1.5 | 2.1 | 0 | 1.3 | .9 | 3.6 | 2.8 |

| x | | 1 | 2 | 3 | 4 | 5 | 6 | 7 | 8 | 9 | 10 | 11 | 12 |
|---|---|---|---|---|---|---|---|---|---|---|---|---|---|
| Diseases of Respiratory System | Gross | 532.4 | 569.2 | 533.4 | 606.4 | 1159.7 | 1139.7 | 858.5 | 892.0 | 521.9 | 535.8 | 555.9 | 527.9 |
| | Net | 377.1 | 399.0 | 374.3 | 424.6 | 672.7 | 698.2 | 560.9 | 585.4 | 388.0 | 402.1 | 435.7 | 398.7 |
| Acute Nasopharyngitis | | 30.9 | 33.7 | 30.9 | 36.7 | 74.7 | 73.8 | 39.8 | 40.1 | 31.7 | 35.4 | 32.3 | 42.0 |
| Pharyngitis | | 82.9 | 91.8 | 83.1 | 100.8 | 176.5 | 191.3 | 149.6 | 165.9 | 98.0 | 114.5 | 101.0 | 106.6 |
| Tonsillitis | | 52.9 | 63.1 | 62.5 | 63.6 | 225.0 | 205.7 | 158.7 | 176.7 | 73.8 | 70.8 | 58.0 | 50.8 |
| Hypertrophy of Tonsils | | 9.7 | 12.3 | 12.8 | 11.8 | 37.4 | 34.7 | 58.6 | 48.0 | 12.1 | 11.4 | 6.6 | 6.6 |
| Laryngitis and Tracheitis | | 17.7 | 18.6 | 17.1 | 20.1 | 50.9 | 36.2 | 25.4 | 23.2 | 15.8 | 9.6 | 11.9 | 17.1 |
| Sinusitis | | 22.5 | 22.9 | 20.2 | 25.6 | 6.5 | 9.4 | 16.8 | 11.6 | 13.8 | 11.8 | 26.3 | 24.3 |
| Influenza | | 29.8 | 30.0 | 28.1 | 32.0 | 29.0 | 24.8 | 21.3 | 23.6 | 24.2 | 24.9 | 28.1 | 27.0 |
| Pneumonia | | 11.6 | 11.1 | 10.5 | 11.8 | 17.7 | 12.3 | 12.3 | 12.0 | 7.1 | 7.0 | 7.8 | 3.9 |
| Bronchitis | | 87.7 | 89.7 | 85.7 | 93.9 | 162.0 | 151.1 | 118.1 | 104.2 | 67.2 | 62.9 | 78.9 | 69.6 |
| Other Diseases of Respiratory Tract | | 178.9 | 189.4 | 175.4 | 204.1 | 375.8 | 397.4 | 255.8 | 285.0 | 176.1 | 186.2 | 202.0 | 178.9 |
| Diseases of Lungs | | 7.8 | 6.6 | 7.1 | 6.0 | 4.2 | 3.0 | 2.1 | 1.7 | 2.1 | 1.3 | 3.0 | 1.1 |
| **xi** | | | | | | | | | | | | | |
| Diseases of the Digestive System | Gross | 140.9 | 135.7 | 127.8 | 144.0 | 164.3 | 154.6 | 104.1 | 93.9 | 71.8 | 80.4 | 101.6 | 93.9 |
| | Net | 119.9 | 116.4 | 111.2 | 121.7 | 149.4 | 143.7 | 99.6 | 89.8 | 64.7 | 76.5 | 95.0 | 85.6 |
| Stomatitis | | 2.8 | 3.3 | 2.8 | 3.8 | 5.1 | 9.4 | 6.1 | 3.7 | 4.6 | 5.2 | 3.6 | 3.3 |
| Other Diseases of the Buccal Cavity and Esophagus | | 4.8 | 4.7 | 4.2 | 5.2 | 8.9 | 7.9 | 2.5 | 2.5 | 2.1 | 2.6 | 6.0 | 5.0 |
| Ulcers | | 11.1 | 10.0 | 12.1 | 7.8 | .5 | 0 | .8 | 0 | 1.3 | .4 | 2.4 | 2.2 |
| Gastritis and Duodenitis | | 21.9 | 20.8 | 19.5 | 22.2 | 11.2 | 9.9 | 9.0 | 9.5 | 8.8 | 10.1 | 13.7 | 14.9 |
| Other Diseases of Stomach and Duodenum | | 5.2 | 4.9 | 4.6 | 5.2 | 3.3 | 4.0 | 2.0 | 2.5 | 2.5 | 4.4 | 3.0 | 2.2 |
| Appendicitis | | 2.1 | 2.5 | 2.5 | 2.5 | 1.4 | 1.0 | 2.5 | 3.7 | 5.8 | 4.8 | 9.5 | 6.1 |
| Hernia of Abdominal Cavity | | 7.6 | 6.5 | 8.2 | 4.7 | 13.5 | 4.5 | 7.4 | 1.3 | 2.9 | .9 | 4.8 | .6 |
| Gastroenteritis and Colitis (Except Ulcerative) | | 54.7 | 55.8 | 49.7 | 62.3 | 105.5 | 110.0 | 64.4 | 62.9 | 38.4 | 47.2 | 48.4 | 48.6 |
| Other Diseases of Intestines and Peritoneum | | 18.1 | 16.4 | 16.8 | 16.1 | 13.5 | 7.4 | 7.4 | 6.6 | 4.6 | 3.9 | 7.2 | 7.7 |
| Diseases of Liver, Gall Bladder and Pancreas | Gross | 12.6 | 10.8 | 7.4 | 14.2 | 1.4 | .5 | 2.0 | 1.2 | .8 | .9 | 3.0 | 3.3 |
| | Net | 12.2 | 10.4 | 7.0 | 13.9 | 1.4 | .5 | 2.0 | 1.2 | .8 | .9 | 3.0 | 3.3 |
| Diseases of Liver | | 1.9 | 1.9 | 2.4 | 1.3 | 0 | 0 | .8 | .8 | .4 | .9 | 2.4 | .5 |
| Diseases of Gall Bladder | | 9.7 | 8.1 | 4.2 | 12.1 | .5 | .5 | 1.2 | .4 | .4 | 0 | .6 | 2.8 |
| Diseases of Pancreas | | 1.0 | .8 | .8 | .8 | .9 | 0 | 0 | 0 | 0 | 0 | 0 | 0 |

**TABLE 132. (Cont'd)** Incidence of Attended Illness or Preventive Care, by Diagnosis, by Age and Sex (and Adjusted to Age-Sex Composition of General Population)

*Part I: to Age 19 (Cont'd)*

| DIAGNOSIS | | Adjusted Total § | Total | ALL | | UNDER 5 | | 5–9 | | 10–14 | | 15–19 | |
|---|---|---|---|---|---|---|---|---|---|---|---|---|---|
| | | | | M | F | M | F | M | F | M | F | M | F |
| **XII** | | | | | | | | | | | | | |
| Diseases of Urinary System | Gross | 31.1 | 28.2 | 19.3 | 37.4 | 12.6 | 15.4 | 8.2 | 24.4 | 6.3 | 13.5 | 12.5 | 16.0 |
| | Net | 28.5 | 25.9 | 18.1 | 34.0 | 11.6 | 13.9 | 8.2 | 21.9 | 6.3 | 12.2 | 12.0 | 16.0 |
| Nephritis and Nephrosis | | .9 | .9 | .7 | 1.2 | 1.9 | .5 | 0 | .8 | 2.1 | .9 | .6 | 1.6 |
| Cystitis | | 16.3 | 14.6 | 7.3 | 22.2 | 4.2 | 7.0 | 3.7 | 11.6 | 2.1 | 4.3 | 5.4 | 9.4 |
| Other | | 13.9 | 12.7 | 11.3 | 14.0 | 6.5 | 7.9 | 4.5 | 12.0 | 2.1 | 8.3 | 6.5 | 5.0 |
| **XIII** | | | | | | | | | | | | | |
| Diseases of Male Genital Organs (Excluding Neoplasms) | Gross | 9.8 | 8.1 | 15.9 | — | 11.2 | — | 2.1 | — | 7.1 | — | 6.0 | — |
| | Net | 9.8 | 8.1 | 15.9 | — | 11.2 | — | 2.1 | — | 7.1 | — | 6.0 | — |
| **XIV** | | | | | | | | | | | | | |
| Diseases of Female Genital Organs and Breast (Excluding Neoplasms) | Gross | 63.9 | 61.3 | — | 125.0 | — | 11.9 | — | 7.9 | — | 12.7 | — | 50.8 |
| | Net | 55.5 | 53.0 | — | 108.0 | — | 11.9 | — | 7.4 | — | 12.2 | — | 49.7 |
| Diseases of Breast | | 4.3 | 4.2 | — | 8.6 | — | 1.0 | — | 1.2 | — | 2.2 | — | 4.4 |
| Diseases of Ovaries, Fallopian Tubes and Parametrium | | 3.0 | 2.7 | — | 5.5 | — | 0 | — | .8 | — | 0 | — | 2.8 |
| Cervicitis | | 15.2 | 14.2 | — | 28.9 | — | 2.0 | — | .8 | — | 1.3 | — | 2.2 |
| Vaginitis and Vulvitis | | 11.3 | 10.4 | — | 21.1 | — | 3.5 | — | 4.2 | — | 3.1 | — | 8.8 |
| Menstrual Disorders | | 14.0 | 14.1 | — | 28.8 | — | 0 | — | .4 | — | 5.2 | — | 30.9 |
| Menopausal Symptoms | | 6.6 | 7.1 | — | 14.5 | — | 0 | — | 0 | — | 0 | — | 0 |
| Other | | 9.5 | 8.6 | — | 17.6 | — | 5.4 | — | .4 | — | .9 | — | 1.7 |

NUMBER OF MEMBERS WITH INDICATED DIAGNOSIS PER 1,000 EXPOSURE YEARS

The following data table is printed rotated on the page. Values are organized into 12 data columns (unlabeled on this page), with "Gross" and "Net" rows for each major category.

| | 1 | 2 | 3 | 4 | 5 | 6 | 7 | 8 | 9 | 10 | 11 | 12 |
|---|---|---|---|---|---|---|---|---|---|---|---|---|
| **XV** | | | | | | | | | | | | |
| Deliveries and Complications of Pregnancy, Childbirth and Puerperium — Gross | 24.0 | 19.9 | — | 40.5 | — | 0 | — | 0 | — | 0 | — | 6.1 |
| Net | 23.5 | 19.5 | — | 39.8 | — | 0 | — | 0 | — | 0 | — | 5.5 |
| Normal Deliveries | 20.6 | 16.9 | — | 34.3 | — | 0 | — | 0 | — | 0 | — | 5.0 |
| Complicated Deliveries | .4 | .3 | — | .6 | — | 0 | — | 0 | — | 0 | — | 0 |
| Abortion | 2.6 | 2.3 | — | 4.8 | — | 0 | — | 0 | — | 0 | — | .6 |
| Ectopic Pregnancy | .1 | .1 | — | .2 | — | 0 | — | 0 | — | 0 | — | .5 |
| Other | .3 | .3 | — | .6 | — | 0 | — | 0 | — | 0 | — | 0 |
| **XVI** | | | | | | | | | | | | |
| Diseases of Skin and Subcutaneous Tissues — Gross | 114.9 | 116.1 | 114.7 | 117.5 | 125.6 | 120.4 | 112.3 | 107.1 | 125.2 | 107.0 | 196.7 | 140.8 |
| Net | 101.8 | 103.2 | 102.3 | 104.2 | 109.2 | 109.5 | 105.4 | 96.8 | 114.7 | 98.3 | 175.7 | 128.7 |
| Boil and Carbuncle | 9.5 | 9.1 | 10.5 | 7.7 | 7.0 | 6.4 | 5.8 | 5.8 | 9.6 | 6.6 | 12.0 | 7.2 |
| Cellulitis | 20.3 | 20.6 | 22.2 | 18.9 | 17.3 | 14.4 | 18.0 | 18.6 | 25.0 | 17.0 | 24.5 | 13.8 |
| Impetigo | 4.7 | 5.8 | 6.7 | 4.8 | 19.1 | 15.3 | 20.9 | 16.1 | 12.9 | 3.9 | 4.8 | 3.3 |
| Infectious Wart | 10.0 | 10.7 | 10.1 | 11.4 | 1.4 | 2.5 | 9.8 | 5.8 | 18.0 | 19.2 | 27.5 | 22.1 |
| Dermatitis | 29.8 | 30.7 | 27.4 | 34.0 | 50.4 | 59.0 | 31.6 | 36.4 | 31.7 | 31.9 | 40.0 | 33.1 |
| Acne | 4.8 | 5.0 | 4.7 | 5.3 | .5 | 0 | .8 | .4 | 2.9 | 6.6 | 45.4 | 31.5 |
| Sebaceous Cyst | 6.4 | 5.7 | 6.7 | 4.7 | .9 | 0 | 1.6 | .4 | 1.7 | .4 | 6.0 | 1.6 |
| Other | 29.4 | 28.5 | 26.4 | 30.7 | 29.0 | 22.8 | 23.8 | 23.6 | 23.4 | 21.4 | 36.5 | 28.2 |
| **XVII** | | | | | | | | | | | | |
| Diseases of Bones and Organs of Movement — Gross | 95.1 | 83.5 | 79.2 | 88.0 | 37.3 | 28.3 | 20.1 | 16.5 | 32.1 | 22.3 | 49.0 | 40.9 |
| Net | 82.9 | 73.1 | 70.7 | 75.6 | 34.5 | 26.8 | 20.1 | 15.7 | 31.3 | 21.4 | 46.0 | 35.3 |
| Arthritis and Rheumatism | 30.3 | 24.3 | 21.4 | 27.3 | 2.8 | 3.5 | 5.3 | 2.1 | 4.2 | 3.5 | 7.8 | 7.7 |
| Osteomyelitis and Other Diseases of Bones and Joints | 10.0 | 8.5 | 8.4 | 8.6 | 4.7 | 3.0 | 4.1 | 3.3 | 9.6 | 4.8 | 9.6 | 3.3 |
| Synovitis, Bursitis and Tenosynovitis | 28.2 | 25.3 | 24.4 | 26.2 | 2.3 | 1.5 | 2.1 | 3.3 | 6.2 | 4.8 | 13.7 | 11.6 |
| Infective Myositis | 17.8 | 16.5 | 16.7 | 16.3 | 0 | .5 | 2.1 | 2.9 | 5.8 | 3.9 | 10.7 | 8.3 |
| Muscular Dystrophy | .1 | .1 | .1 | .1 | .9 | 0 | 0 | 0 | 0 | 0 | 0 | 0 |
| Scoliosis | 1.1 | 1.1 | .9 | 1.4 | .5 | 0 | .8 | .4 | 1.7 | 2.2 | .6 | 3.9 |
| Other Deformities | 3.9 | 4.2 | 4.3 | 4.2 | 23.8 | 17.8 | 4.9 | 4.1 | 2.9 | 2.2 | 3.0 | 3.3 |
| Other Diseases of Musculoskeletal System | 3.7 | 3.5 | 3.0 | 3.9 | 2.3 | 2.0 | .8 | .4 | 1.7 | .9 | 3.6 | 2.8 |

**TABLE 132.** *(Cont'd)* Incidence of Attended Illness or Preventive Care, by Diagnosis, by Age and Sex (and Adjusted to Age-Sex Composition of General Population)

Part I: to Age 19 (Cont'd)

| DIAGNOSIS | | Adjusted Total § | Total | ALL | | UNDER 5 | | 5–9 | | 10–14 | | 15–19 | |
|---|---|---|---|---|---|---|---|---|---|---|---|---|---|
| | | | | M | F | M | F | M | F | M | F | M | F |
| **XVIII** Injuries and Adverse Effects of External Causes | Gross | 156.1 | 160.0 | 174.5 | 144.9 | 182.1 | 162.0 | 202.5 | 122.5 | 247.8 | 121.9 | 330.5 | 139.7 |
| | Net | 130.9 | 139.6 | 152.2 | 126.4 | 156.4 | 143.2 | 174.3 | 112.1 | 211.5 | 106.2 | 273.8 | 120.9 |
| Fractures | Gross | 14.3 | 15.0 | 17.4 | 12.4 | 10.7 | 7.9 | 18.9 | 9.9 | 33.8 | 14.9 | 47.8 | 9.4 |
| | Net | 13.3 | 13.8 | 16.1 | 11.5 | 9.3 | 7.9 | 16.8 | 8.7 | 32.5 | 13.1 | 43.0 | 8.8 |
| Skull and Face | | 1.2 | 1.3 | 2.1 | .5 | .9 | 2.0 | 1.2 | .4 | 3.3 | .9 | 8.4 | 0 |
| Torso | Gross | 1.5 | 1.5 | 1.4 | 1.5 | 0 | .5 | 0 | 0 | 0 | .4 | 1.2 | 0 |
| Spine (Vertical Column) | | .4 | .4 | .2 | .7 | 0 | 0 | 0 | 0 | 0 | 0 | 0 | 0 |
| Ribs, Sternum and Larynx | | 1.1 | 1.1 | 1.2 | .8 | 0 | .5 | 0 | 0 | 0 | .4 | 1.2 | 0 |
| UPPER EXTREMITIES | Gross | 6.5 | 7.4 | 9.6 | 5.2 | 7.9 | 5.5 | 14.0 | 6.6 | 21.7 | 9.2 | 26.9 | 5.5 |
| Clavicle | | .7 | .8 | 1.1 | .5 | 2.4 | 1.5 | 2.9 | .4 | .4 | 1.3 | 2.4 | 0 |
| Scapula | | .1 | .1 | .1 | .1 | 0 | 0 | 0 | 0 | .4 | 0 | 0 | 0 |
| Humerus | | .6 | .6 | .7 | .5 | .9 | 1.0 | 2.1 | .8 | .8 | .9 | .6 | .5 |
| Radius and Ulna | | 1.8 | 2.2 | 2.9 | 1.6 | 2.8 | 1.5 | 4.5 | 4.2 | 9.2 | 3.1 | 6.6 | 1.7 |
| Wrist | | .8 | .8 | .8 | .8 | .9 | 1.0 | .8 | .4 | 2.5 | 1.7 | 1.8 | .5 |
| Hand-Finger | | 2.5 | 2.9 | 4.0 | 1.7 | .9 | .5 | 3.7 | .8 | 8.4 | 2.2 | 15.5 | 2.8 |
| LOWER EXTREMITIES | Gross | 5.0 | 4.7 | 4.3 | 5.1 | 1.9 | 0 | 3.7 | 2.9 | 8.8 | 4.4 | 11.3 | 3.9 |
| Pelvis | | .1 | .1 | 0* | .1 | 0 | 0 | 0 | 0 | .4 | .5 | 0 | 0 |
| Femur | | .7 | .3 | .2 | .4 | 0 | 0 | .4 | 0 | .4 | .5 | .6 | 0 |
| Patella | | .1 | .2 | .4 | 0 | 0 | 0 | 0 | 0 | .8 | 0 | 1.8 | 0 |
| Tibia and Fibula | | 1.1 | 1.2 | 1.2 | 1.2 | 1.9 | 0 | 1.3 | .8 | 2.1 | 2.2 | 3.0 | 1.1 |
| Ankle | | .7 | .7 | .6 | .9 | 0 | 0 | .8 | 1.3 | .9 | .4 | 1.2 | 0 |
| Foot and Toe | | 2.3 | 2.2 | 1.9 | 2.5 | 0 | 0 | .4 | .8 | 4.2 | .8 | 4.7 | 2.8 |
| Late Effects of Fractures | | .1 | .1 | 0 | .1 | 0 | 0 | 0 | 0 | 0 | 0 | 0 | 0 |

NUMBER OF MEMBERS WITH INDICATED DIAGNOSIS PER 1,000 EXPOSURE YEARS

| | 1 | 2 | 3 | 4 | 5 | 6 | 7 | 8 | 9 | 10 | 11 | 12 |
|---|---|---|---|---|---|---|---|---|---|---|---|---|
| *Injuries (Cont'd)* | | | | | | | | | | | | |
| Dislocations | 1.8 | 1.9 | 2.2 | 1.6 | 2.3 | 4.5 | .4 | 1.2 | 4.6 | 1.7 | 7.2 | .5 |
| Sprains and Strains | 47.9 | 47.7 | 50.8 | 44.5 | 7.0 | 8.9 | 16.8 | 9.1 | 48.8 | 25.8 | 93.8 | 56.3 |
| Head Injuries (Other than Fractures) | 10.1 | 11.0 | 14.5 | 7.3 | 41.6 | 28.2 | 29.9 | 12.4 | 22.9 | 6.1 | 19.1 | 5.0 |
| Internal Injuries | .3 | .3 | .3 | .3 | 1.9 | .5 | 0 | 0 | .4 | .4 | 0 | 0 |
| Lacerations and Open Wounds | 29.7 | 32.3 | 37.1 | 27.3 | 57.0 | 41.6 | 69.7 | 45.5 | 63.4 | 28.4 | 68.1 | 24.3 |
| Superficial Injuries | 10.3 | 11.1 | 11.3 | 11.1 | 21.9 | 25.8 | 22.5 | 14.1 | 16.3 | 15.7 | 20.3 | 9.4 |
| Foreign Body | 3.9 | 4.0 | 4.2 | 3.8 | 5.1 | 6.9 | 4.5 | 6.2 | 1.7 | 2.2 | 5.4 | 2.8 |
| Contusions | 24.3 | 24.5 | 25.4 | 23.6 | 21.0 | 19.3 | 30.3 | 19.9 | 46.3 | 23.2 | 58.0 | 23.7 |
| Complications of Surgical or Medical Procedures | 7.6 | 6.6 | 5.2 | 8.0 | 3.3 | 4.0 | 2.5 | 2.5 | 4.2 | .4 | 2.4 | 2.8 |
| Other | 5.9 | 5.6 | 6.1 | 5.0 | 10.3 | 14.4 | 7.0 | 1.7 | 5.4 | 3.1 | 8.4 | 5.5 |
| **xix** Congenital Malformations — Gross | 3.3 | 3.7 | 4.1 | 3.3 | 18.2 | 21.3 | 7.0 | 2.1 | 8.3 | 2.2 | 1.8 | 1.7 |
| Congenital Malformations — Net | 3.3 | 3.7 | 4.1 | 3.3 | 18.2 | 21.3 | 7.0 | 2.1 | 8.3 | 2.2 | 1.8 | 1.7 |
| **xx** Certain Diseases of Early Infancy — Gross | .8 | .9 | .9 | 1.0 | 7.9 | 9.4 | .8 | .4 | — | — | — | — |
| Certain Diseases of Early Infancy — Net | .8 | .9 | .9 | 1.0 | 7.9 | 9.4 | .8 | .4 | — | — | — | — |
| **xxi** Symptoms, Senility and Ill-Defined Conditions — Gross | 70.3 | 67.6 | 60.8 | 74.7 | 59.3 | 61.9 | 50.0 | 38.9 | 47.1 | 43.3 | 69.3 | 60.2 |
| Symptoms, Senility and Ill-Defined Conditions — Net | 65.1 | 62.6 | 56.8 | 68.6 | 56.5 | 59.0 | 48.0 | 36.8 | 44.6 | 41.5 | 66.3 | 58.0 |
| Symptoms Referrable to Nervous System | 7.5 | 7.1 | 6.8 | 7.5 | 3.7 | 4.0 | 2.9 | .8 | 2.9 | 2.6 | 6.0 | 8.3 |
| Symptoms Referrable to Cardiovascular System | 6.7 | 6.3 | 4.7 | 7.9 | .9 | 2.0 | 1.6 | 2.5 | 6.3 | 3.9 | 4.8 | 3.9 |
| Symptoms Referrable to Respiratory System | 12.3 | 12.1 | 14.2 | 10.0 | 13.1 | 6.9 | 13.5 | 10.4 | 12.5 | 7.9 | 20.3 | 4.4 |
| Symptoms Referrable to Upper and Lower Gastrointestinal System | 11.2 | 10.9 | 9.2 | 12.7 | 15.4 | 15.3 | 10.2 | 9.9 | 7.5 | 7.0 | 8.3 | 10.5 |

TABLE 132. (Cont'd)  Incidence of Attended Illness or Preventive Care, by Diagnosis, by Age and Sex (and Adjusted to Age-Sex Composition of General Population)

Part I: to Age 19 (Concluded)

NUMBER OF MEMBERS WITH INDICATED DIAGNOSIS PER 1,000 EXPOSURE YEARS

| DIAGNOSIS | Adjusted Total§ | Total | ALL M | ALL F | UNDER 5 M | UNDER 5 F | 5–9 M | 5–9 F | 10–14 M | 10–14 F | 15–19 M | 15–19 F |
|---|---|---|---|---|---|---|---|---|---|---|---|---|
| *Symptoms (Cont'd)* | | | | | | | | | | | | |
| Symptoms Referrable to Urinary System | 3.0 | 2.8 | 2.9 | 2.7 | .9 | 1.5 | 2.5 | .4 | 2.5 | .9 | 0 | 1.1 |
| Pain in Back | 5.6 | 5.0 | 4.1 | 5.8 | 1.4 | 2.5 | 1.2 | 1.7 | 3.8 | 4.4 | 7.2 | 3.8 |
| Other Referrable Symptoms (Not Elsewhere Classified) | 8.8 | 8.7 | 8.3 | 9.2 | 22.0 | 26.7 | 10.7 | 8.3 | 5.8 | 6.5 | 9.0 | 5.0 |
| Headache | 7.7 | 7.7 | 6.0 | 9.5 | 1.4 | 2.0 | 5.3 | 4.1 | 5.4 | 5.7 | 9.5 | 12.7 |
| Other Ill-Defined Diseases | 7.5 | 7.0 | 4.6 | 9.4 | .5 | 1.0 | 2.1 | .8 | .4 | 4.4 | 4.2 | 10.5 |
| **XXII** Supplementary Classifications  Gross | 146.5 | 166.3 | 159.2 | 173.8 | 481.8 | 480.7 | 290.3 | 304.9 | 215.3 | 202.8 | 199.0 | 172.8 |
|  Net | 143.1 | 162.4 | 155.1 | 170.0 | 471.1 | 472.7 | 275.9 | 291.3 | 210.3 | 201.0 | 196.7 | 170.1 |
| General Medical Examinations (Including Immunizations) | 69.6 | 80.8 | 73.9 | 88.0 | — | — | 125.5 | 133.2 | 205.7 | 191.0 | 183.5 | 162.3 |
| Well Baby and Child Care (Including Immunizations) | 54.8 | 65.1 | 65.2 | 65.2 | 481.8 | 479.7 | 156.6 | 163.0 | — | — | — | — |
| Diagnostic Screening | 19.7 | 18.3 | 20.1 | 16.3 | 0 | 1.0 | 8.2 | 8.7 | 9.6 | 11.8 | 15.5 | 9.9 |
| Other | 2.4 | 2.1 | — | 4.3 | — | 0 | — | 0 | — | 0 | — | .6 |
| **XXIII** Undetermined Classifications  Gross | 131.3 | 124.9 | 105.9 | 144.6 | 109.2 | 96.1 | 91.9 | 81.5 | 78.0 | 70.4 | 128.5 | 109.9 |
|  Net | 131.3 | 124.9 | 105.9 | 144.6 | 109.2 | 96.1 | 91.9 | 81.5 | 78.0 | 70.4 | 128.5 | 109.9 |

TABLE 132. (Cont'd) Incidence of Attended Illness or Preventive Care, by Diagnosis, by Age and Sex (and Adjusted to Age-Sex Composition of General Population)

*Part II: Ages 20 and Over*

| DIAGNOSIS | | NUMBER OF MEMBERS WITH INDICATED DIAGNOSIS PER 1,000 EXPOSURE YEARS | | | | | | | | | | | |
|---|---|---|---|---|---|---|---|---|---|---|---|---|---|
| | | 20–24 | | 25–34 | | 35–44 | | 45–54 | | 55–64 | | 65 AND OVER | |
| | | M | F | M | F | M | F | M | F | M | F | M | F |
| TOTAL | Gross † | 1384.8 | 2613.8 | 1427.7 | 2475.0 | 1582.8 | 2504.3 | 1563.5 | 2300.2 | 1696.0 | 2292.2 | 2022.2 | 2415.7 |
| | Net ‡ | 668.2 | 972.6 | 672.1 | 896.2 | 673.2 | 865.4 | 650.0 | 802.4 | 664.5 | 808.9 | 745.6 | 898.3 |
| Infective and Parasitic Diseases | Gross | 87.6 | 134.0 | 66.5 | 106.5 | 62.2 | 84.8 | 51.2 | 66.1 | 42.2 | 61.8 | 37.0 | 49.4 |
| | Net | 85.3 | 126.8 | 63.9 | 99.2 | 60.5 | 82.6 | 47.5 | 64.1 | 39.0 | 61.2 | 35.5 | 43.6 |
| Streptococcal Sore Throat | | 13.8 | 18.7 | 13.4 | 22.9 | 11.1 | 16.1 | 9.9 | 12.1 | 7.5 | 5.8 | 3.0 | 2.9 |
| Measles | | 0 | 4.3 | 1.3 | 2.7 | 0 | .6 | 0 | 0 | 0 | 0 | 0 | 0 |
| Rubella (German Measles) | | 9.2 | 27.4 | 2.2 | 16.6 | 2.0 | 5.9 | .8 | 1.4 | 0 | .6 | 0 | 0 |
| Chicken Pox | | 0 | 0 | 0 | .4 | .3 | .3 | 0 | 0 | 0 | 0 | 0 | 0 |
| Mumps | | 0 | 0 | 0 | 1.2 | 1.4 | 1.1 | .9 | .3 | 1.2 | .6 | 0 | 0 |
| Infectious Hepatitis | | 0 | 0 | 0 | .4 | .3 | 0 | .6 | 0 | 0 | .6 | 0 | 0 |
| Glandular Fever (Infectious Mononucleosis) | | 4.6 | 4.3 | .4 | 2.7 | .6 | .9 | 0 | 0 | 0 | 1.2 | 0 | 0 |
| Intestinal Virus | | 34.6 | 60.5 | 35.0 | 46.9 | 37.9 | 49.2 | 29.4 | 41.4 | 24.7 | 41.5 | 19.2 | 23.3 |
| Dermatophytoses | | 16.2 | 5.8 | 7.3 | 4.6 | 5.3 | 5.9 | 5.1 | 5.5 | 3.6 | 4.0 | 1.5 | 8.7 |
| Other | | 9.2 | 13.0 | 6.9 | 8.1 | 3.3 | 4.8 | 4.5 | 5.4 | 5.2 | 7.5 | 13.3 | 14.5 |

**TABLE 132.** (*Cont'd*)  Incidence of Attended Illness or Preventive Care, by Diagnosis, by Age and Sex (and Adjusted to Age-Sex Composition of General Population)

*Part II: Ages 20 and Over (Cont'd)*

NUMBER OF MEMBERS WITH INDICATED DIAGNOSIS PER 1,000 EXPOSURE YEARS

| DIAGNOSIS | 20–24 M | 20–24 F | 25–34 M | 25–34 F | 35–44 M | 35–44 F | 45–54 M | 45–54 F | 55–64 M | 55–64 F | 65 AND OVER M | 65 AND OVER F |
|---|---|---|---|---|---|---|---|---|---|---|---|---|
| II Neoplasms — Gross | 16.1 | 53.3 | 22.9 | 43.0 | 24.5 | 85.7 | 34.8 | 84.5 | 51.0 | 64.1 | 48.8 | 78.5 |
| Neoplasms — Net | 16.1 | 50.4 | 22.0 | 42.6 | 23.1 | 78.1 | 30.0 | 72.1 | 37.5 | 49.7 | 41.4 | 55.2 |
| Malignant Neoplasms — Gross | 0 | 4.3 | .9 | 3.5 | 3.1 | 7.9 | 9.3 | 13.8 | 22.7 | 23.1 | 23.6 | 29.1 |
| Malignant Neoplasms — Net | 0 | 4.3 | .9 | 3.5 | 2.2 | 7.4 | 7.6 | 12.4 | 18.3 | 17.9 | 20.7 | 23.3 |
| Digestive System— Including Mouth | 0 | 0 | 0 | 0 | .3 | .3 | 2.3 | .9 | 4.4 | 3.5 | 8.9 | 5.8 |
| Respiratory System | 0 | 1.5 | .4 | 0 | 0 | .8 | 1.4 | .6 | 4.8 | 1.2 | 5.9 | 2.9 |
| Breast | — | 1.4 | — | 1.5 | — | 2.8 | — | 5.2 | — | 5.8 | — | 5.8 |
| Female Genital Organs | — | 0 | — | .4 | — | 2.3 | — | 1.4 | — | 3.5 | — | 0 |
| Male Genital Organs | 0 | — | 0 | — | .3 | — | .6 | — | 2.4 | — | 2.9 | — |
| Urinary System | 0 | 0 | 0 | 0 | .3 | 0 | .6 | 0 | 2.4 | 0 | 0 | 0 |
| Skin | 0 | 0 | .5 | .8 | .8 | 0 | 1.4 | 1.4 | 3.2 | 1.7 | 2.9 | 8.8 |
| Eye | 0 | 0 | 0 | 0 | 0 | 0 | 0 | .3 | 0 | .6 | 0 | 0 |
| Nervous System— Including Brain | 0 | 0 | 0 | 0 | 0 | .3 | .6 | .3 | 1.6 | 0 | 0 | 0 |
| Endocrine Glands | 0 | 1.4 | 0 | 0 | 0 | .3 | .3 | .6 | 0 | .6 | 0 | 0 |
| Bone | 0 | 0 | 0 | 0 | 0 | 0 | 0 | .6 | .4 | 0 | 0 | 2.9 |
| Connective Tissue | 0 | 0 | 0 | 0 | 0 | 0 | .3 | 0 | 0 | .6 | 0 | 0 |
| Lymphosarcoma | 0 | 0 | 0 | 0 | .3 | 0 | 0 | 0 | 0 | .6 | 0 | 0 |
| Hodgkin's Disease | 0 | 0 | 0 | 0 | .3 | .6 | .2 | 0 | 0 | .5 | 0 | 0 |
| Other Lymphoma | 0 | 0 | 0 | 0 | 0 | 0 | 0 | 0 | 0 | .5 | 0 | 0 |
| Multiple Myeloma | 0 | 0 | 0 | 0 | 0 | 0 | 0 | 0 | 0 | 0 | 0 | 0 |
| Leukemia | 0 | 0 | 0 | 0 | 0 | .3 | .2 | 1.4 | .8 | 0 | 0 | 0 |
| Not Elsewhere Classified | 0 | 0 | 0 | .8 | .8 | .2 | 1.4 | 1.1 | 2.7 | 4.0 | 3.0 | 2.9 |

*Neoplasms (Cont'd)*

| | | | | | | | | | | | | | |
|---|---|---|---|---|---|---|---|---|---|---|---|---|---|
| **Benign Neoplasms** | Gross | 16.1 | 47.6 | 22.0 | 38.0 | 20.3 | 74.1 | 24.6 | 66.1 | 24.3 | 35.8 | 23.7 | 43.6 |
| | Net | 16.1 | 47.6 | 21.6 | 37.6 | 20.1 | 70.4 | 23.5 | 60.6 | 23.9 | 32.3 | 23.7 | 37.8 |
| Mouth | | 0 | 1.4 | .4 | .8 | .3 | 2.0 | 1.2 | 1.2 | 1.2 | 1.7 | 0 | 5.8 |
| Rectum | | 0 | 0 | .4 | .4 | .3 | .8 | 1.4 | 1.2 | 2.4 | 2.9 | 5.9 | 0 |
| Breast | | — | 8.7 | — | 2.7 | — | 7.1 | — | 6.0 | — | 1.7 | — | 2.9 |
| Female Genital Organs | | — | 15.9 | — | 19.4 | — | 39.3 | — | 27.9 | — | 5.8 | — | 5.8 |
| Skin | | 11.5 | 13.0 | 17.3 | 12.0 | 12.5 | 17.0 | 12.7 | 16.9 | 9.6 | 13.9 | 7.4 | 17.5 |
| Other | | 4.6 | 8.6 | 3.9 | 2.7 | 7.2 | 7.9 | 9.3 | 12.9 | 11.1 | 9.8 | 10.4 | 11.6 |
| | | | | | | | | | | | | | |
| **Unspecified Neoplasms** | Gross | 0 | 1.4 | 0 | 1.5 | 1.1 | 3.7 | .9 | 4.6 | 4.0 | 5.2 | 1.5 | 5.8 |
| | Net | 0 | 1.4 | 0 | 1.5 | 1.1 | 3.7 | .9 | 4.6 | 4.0 | 5.2 | 1.5 | 5.8 |
| Rectum | | — | 0 | 0 | 0 | 0 | .3 | 0 | .6 | 0 | .6 | 0 | 0 |
| Breast | | — | — | — | 0 | — | 1.7 | — | .6 | — | 1.7 | — | 0 |
| Female Genital Organs | | — | 1.4 | — | 1.1 | — | .3 | — | .3 | — | 0 | — | 0 |
| Other | | 0 | 0 | 0 | .4 | 1.1 | 1.4 | .9 | 2.8 | 4.0 | 2.9 | 1.4 | 5.8 |
| | | | | | | | | | | | | | |
| **III** | | | | | | | | | | | | | |
| **Allergic, Endocrine System, Metabolic and Nutritional Diseases** | Gross | 57.6 | 126.8 | 65.7 | 158.8 | 73.3 | 170.0 | 76.0 | 159.4 | 85.7 | 129.3 | 103.5 | 122.1 |
| | Net | 55.3 | 112.3 | 57.5 | 137.9 | 66.1 | 150.5 | 69.6 | 139.3 | 80.5 | 117.8 | 94.7 | 116.3 |
| Hay Fever | | 16.1 | 18.7 | 16.9 | 23.6 | 15.9 | 18.1 | 9.9 | 19.8 | 8.0 | 14.4 | 13.3 | 5.8 |
| Asthma | | 6.9 | 8.7 | 10.8 | 12.4 | 8.4 | 13.6 | 8.8 | 16.9 | 13.5 | 13.9 | 14.8 | 14.6 |
| Other Allergic Diseases | | 18.5 | 17.3 | 12.1 | 15.9 | 9.8 | 15.6 | 7.6 | 15.5 | 6.0 | 8.7 | 11.8 | 5.8 |
| Diseases of Thyroid Gland | | 0 | 23.1 | 5.2 | 26.3 | 3.6 | 32.5 | 4.2 | 29.9 | 4.0 | 15.0 | 3.0 | 20.3 |
| Diabetes Mellitus | | 4.6 | 1.4 | 1.7 | 5.4 | 8.6 | 7.6 | 16.1 | 12.9 | 36.2 | 30.0 | 47.3 | 43.6 |
| Obesity (Not Otherwise Specified) | | 11.5 | 53.3 | 13.8 | 64.7 | 20.6 | 71.8 | 16.7 | 52.0 | 10.0 | 39.8 | 4.4 | 26.2 |
| Other | | 0 | 4.3 | 5.2 | 10.5 | 6.4 | 10.8 | 12.7 | 12.4 | 8.0 | 7.5 | 8.9 | 5.8 |
| | | | | | | | | | | | | | |
| **IV** | | | | | | | | | | | | | |
| **Diseases of Blood and Blood Forming Organs** | Gross | 2.3 | 28.8 | 4.3 | 37.2 | 3.1 | 33.4 | 3.9 | 22.4 | 8.4 | 28.3 | 8.9 | 34.9 |
| | Net | 2.3 | 28.8 | 4.3 | 37.2 | 3.1 | 33.4 | 3.9 | 22.4 | 8.4 | 28.3 | 8.9 | 34.9 |
| Anemias | | 2.3 | 28.8 | 3.4 | 36.0 | 2.0 | 31.1 | 3.1 | 21.5 | 6.8 | 24.3 | 3.0 | 32.0 |
| Other | | 0 | 0 | .9 | 1.2 | 1.1 | 2.3 | .8 | .9 | 1.6 | 4.0 | 5.9 | 2.9 |

315

TABLE 132. (Cont'd)  Incidence of Attended Illness or Preventive Care, by Diagnosis, by Age and Sex (and Adjusted to Age-Sex Composition of General Population)

*Part II: Ages 20 and Over (Cont'd)*

NUMBER OF MEMBERS WITH INDICATED DIAGNOSIS PER 1,000 EXPOSURE YEARS

| DIAGNOSIS | | 20–24 | | 25–34 | | 35–44 | | 45–54 | | 55–64 | | 65 AND OVER | |
|---|---|---|---|---|---|---|---|---|---|---|---|---|---|
| | | M | F | M | F | M | F | M | F | M | F | M | F |
| **V** | | | | | | | | | | | | | |
| Mental, Psychoneurotic and Personality Disorders | Gross | 9.2 | 15.8 | 6.9 | 12.0 | 7.3 | 17.0 | 7.6 | 14.9 | 4.8 | 14.4 | 8.9 | 14.5 |
| | Net | 9.2 | 15.8 | 6.5 | 12.0 | 7.3 | 16.4 | 7.6 | 13.8 | 4.8 | 14.4 | 5.9 | 11.6 |
| Chronic Brain Disorders | | 0 | 0 | 0 | 0 | .3 | 0 | .3 | .3 | .4 | 0 | 3.0 | 0 |
| Psychoses | | 0 | 2.9 | 2.2 | 1.1 | .6 | 2.3 | 0 | 1.7 | 0 | 1.7 | 3.0 | 2.9 |
| Psychophysiologic, Autonomic and Visceral Disorders | | 0 | 0 | 0 | .4 | .3 | .8 | .3 | .3 | 0 | .6 | 0 | 0 |
| Psychoneuroses | | 9.2 | 10.1 | 4.3 | 8.5 | 5.8 | 13.3 | 6.8 | 10.6 | 4.4 | 11.5 | 2.9 | 8.7 |
| Personality Disorders | | 0 | 2.8 | .4 | 1.2 | .3 | .3 | .2 | 2.0 | 0 | .6 | 0 | 2.9 |
| Mental Deficiency | | 0 | 0 | 0 | .8 | 0 | .3 | 0 | 0 | 0 | 0 | 0 | 0 |
| **VI** | | | | | | | | | | | | | |
| Diseases of Nervous System | Gross | 20.7 | 23.1 | 18.2 | 33.3 | 32.1 | 42.4 | 36.2 | 48.0 | 35.5 | 52.5 | 47.3 | 52.3 |
| | Net | 20.7 | 20.2 | 17.7 | 32.9 | 31.5 | 40.2 | 35.3 | 46.8 | 34.7 | 50.8 | 44.4 | 52.3 |
| Stroke | | 0 | 0 | 0 | 0 | .3 | 0 | 0 | 0 | .4 | 1.1 | 2.9 | 0 |
| Multiple Sclerosis | | 0 | 0 | 0 | .4 | .3 | 1.7 | 0 | .6 | 0 | 0 | 0 | 0 |
| Migraine | | 6.9 | 2.9 | 1.3 | 10.1 | 5.6 | 8.7 | 1.4 | 6.9 | 1.6 | 5.8 | 1.5 | 0 |
| Epilepsy | | 0 | 0 | .4 | .4 | .5 | .6 | .6 | .3 | 0 | 1.2 | 0 | 0 |
| Sciatica | | 2.3 | 4.3 | 3.5 | 4.2 | 5.0 | 5.4 | 8.2 | 9.8 | 7.6 | 9.8 | 5.9 | 8.7 |
| Other | | 11.5 | 15.9 | 13.0 | 18.2 | 20.4 | 26.0 | 26.0 | 30.4 | 25.9 | 34.6 | 37.0 | 43.6 |

| | | | | | | | | | | | | | |
|---|---|---|---|---|---|---|---|---|---|---|---|---|---|
| **VII Diseases of Eye** | Gross | 30.0 | 34.6 | 32.4 | 38.0 | 37.6 | 43.3 | 51.2 | 62.3 | 55.0 | 76.2 | 99.1 | 136.6 |
| | Net | 27.6 | 33.1 | 28.9 | 37.2 | 35.7 | 42.7 | 47.8 | 55.7 | 50.2 | 70.4 | 91.7 | 110.5 |
| Conjunctivitis and Ophthalmia | | 18.5 | 20.2 | 17.7 | 17.5 | 17.3 | 19.3 | 18.7 | 24.1 | 16.7 | 23.1 | 25.1 | 29.1 |
| Strabismus | | 2.3 | 5.8 | .9 | 2.3 | 1.1 | 1.4 | 1.7 | 2.0 | .4 | .6 | 0 | 2.9 |
| Cataract | | 0 | 0 | .4 | .4 | 0 | 1.4 | 2.5 | 2.3 | 5.6 | 8.1 | 22.2 | 23.2 |
| Glaucoma | | 0 | 0 | 0 | 0 | 1.1 | 2.0 | 4.0 | 3.2 | 6.8 | 6.9 | 13.3 | 32.0 |
| Detachment of Retina | | 0 | 0 | 0 | .4 | 0 | 0 | 0 | 0 | .4 | 1.1 | 0 | 2.9 |
| Other | | 9.2 | 8.6 | 13.4 | 17.4 | 18.1 | 19.2 | 24.3 | 30.7 | 25.1 | 36.4 | 38.5 | 46.5 |
| **VIII Diseases of Ear** | Gross | 62.2 | 67.7 | 37.2 | 53.9 | 46.8 | 64.8 | 46.4 | 56.3 | 45.0 | 51.4 | 48.8 | 40.7 |
| | Net | 59.9 | 59.1 | 33.7 | 48.8 | 42.7 | 56.6 | 43.0 | 49.1 | 42.6 | 44.5 | 45.9 | 40.7 |
| Otitis Externa | | 11.5 | 11.5 | 6.5 | 7.8 | 8.4 | 11.1 | 6.2 | 9.2 | 4.0 | 6.9 | 5.9 | 8.7 |
| Otitis Media | | 34.6 | 44.7 | 16.9 | 33.3 | 18.1 | 32.0 | 14.7 | 24.4 | 15.1 | 19.1 | 17.8 | 8.7 |
| Deafness | | 2.3 | 1.4 | 0 | .4 | .8 | .6 | 0 | .9 | 2.4 | 5.2 | 4.4 | 0 |
| Other | | 13.8 | 10.1 | 13.8 | 12.4 | 19.5 | 21.1 | 25.5 | 21.8 | 23.5 | 20.2 | 20.7 | 23.3 |
| **IX Diseases of Circulatory System** | Gross | 23.1 | 38.9 | 54.0 | 72.8 | 94.0 | 118.2 | 145.9 | 168.9 | 258.6 | 323.9 | 356.5 | 595.9 |
| | Net | 23.1 | 38.9 | 51.4 | 67.4 | 80.0 | 105.5 | 117.0 | 140.8 | 192.4 | 245.4 | 248.5 | 418.6 |
| Rheumatic Fever without Mention of Heart | | 0 | 0 | 0 | .4 | .3 | .3 | .6 | .3 | .4 | 0 | 0 | 0 |
| **Diseases of Heart** | Gross | 2.3 | 5.8 | 11.7 | 13.1 | 35.1 | 21.5 | 65.9 | 44.5 | 129.1 | 132.8 | 221.9 | 250.0 |
| | Net | 2.3 | 5.8 | 9.9 | 11.2 | 27.6 | 20.1 | 47.5 | 36.2 | 94.0 | 101.6 | 159.8 | 194.8 |
| Rheumatic Heart Disease | | 0 | 0 | .9 | 6.6 | 2.5 | 3.1 | 2.8 | 4.3 | 4.0 | 9.8 | 1.5 | 5.8 |
| Arteriosclerotic Heart Disease | | 0 | 0 | 1.3 | .4 | 4.2 | 2.0 | 10.5 | 6.9 | 34.7 | 25.4 | 81.4 | 69.8 |
| Acute Coronary Occlusion | | 0 | 0 | .9 | .8 | 3.9 | .3 | 11.3 | .9 | 13.9 | 8.1 | 16.3 | 20.3 |
| Coronary Insufficiency | | 0 | 1.5 | 3.5 | 1.5 | 7.8 | 3.4 | 13.6 | 7.2 | 24.7 | 20.8 | 34.0 | 46.5 |
| Angina Pectoris | | 0 | 0 | 1.7 | 1.1 | 7.0 | 4.2 | 12.7 | 7.7 | 16.7 | 15.6 | 25.1 | 26.2 |
| Hypertensive Heart Disease | | 0 | 0 | 0 | 1.2 | 1.9 | 2.3 | 4.0 | 6.6 | 9.6 | 28.9 | 34.0 | 49.4 |
| Other | | 2.3 | 4.3 | 3.4 | 1.5 | 7.8 | 6.2 | 11.0 | 10.9 | 25.5 | 24.2 | 29.6 | 32.0 |

TABLE 132. (Cont'd)  Incidence of Attended Illness or Preventive Care, by Diagnosis, by Age and Sex (and Adjusted to Age-Sex Composition of General Population)

Part II: Ages 20 and Over (Cont'd)

| DIAGNOSIS | | NUMBER OF MEMBERS WITH INDICATED DIAGNOSIS PER 1,000 EXPOSURE YEARS | | | | | | | | | | | |
| | | 20–24 | | 25–34 | | 35–44 | | 45–54 | | 55–64 | | 65 AND OVER | |
| | | M | F | M | F | M | F | M | F | M | F | M | F |
| Diseases of Veins and Arteries | Gross | 20.8 | 33.1 | 42.3 | 59.3 | 58.6 | 96.4 | 79.4 | 124.1 | 129.1 | 191.1 | 134.6 | 345.9 |
| Other than Heart | Net | 20.8 | 33.1 | 42.3 | 56.6 | 55.5 | 89.4 | 76.1 | 124.1 | 123.5 | 179.0 | 127.2 | 308.1 |
| Hypertensive Diseases | | 4.6 | 1.4 | 13.4 | 18.6 | 22.9 | 35.3 | 41.0 | 75.8 | 82.4 | 131.1 | 87.3 | 255.8 |
| Hypotension | | 0 | 8.6 | 2.6 | 6.2 | 3.6 | 7.6 | 2.3 | 4.3 | 2.4 | 4.0 | 1.5 | 5.8 |
| Hemorrhoids | | 13.9 | 8.7 | 19.4 | 13.6 | 19.8 | 22.1 | 21.5 | 17.0 | 12.4 | 16.2 | 5.9 | 20.4 |
| General Arteriosclerosis | | 0 | 0 | 0 | 0 | 0 | .3 | .3 | 1.1 | 6.0 | 5.8 | 7.4 | 20.3 |
| Varicose Veins of Lower Extremities | | 0 | 2.9 | .9 | 6.2 | 2.5 | 6.8 | 2.2 | 6.3 | 2.8 | 6.3 | 4.4 | 8.7 |
| Pulmonary Embolism and Infarction | | 0 | 0 | 0 | .4 | 0 | .8 | 1.1 | 0 | .4 | 1.2 | 0 | 0 |
| Lymphadenitis | | 2.3 | 10.1 | 2.6 | 5.4 | 3.6 | 6.8 | 2.2 | 5.2 | 2.8 | 2.3 | 0 | 0 |
| Other | | 0 | 1.4 | 3.4 | 8.9 | 6.2 | 16.7 | 8.8 | 14.4 | 19.9 | 24.2 | 28.1 | 34.9 |
| x | Gross | 394.0 | 541.8 | 408.2 | 549.8 | 408.2 | 532.8 | 324.3 | 444.1 | 341.0 | 409.3 | 350.6 | 296.5 |
| Diseases of Respiratory System | Net | 308.8 | 407.8 | 308.9 | 400.6 | 308.1 | 378.1 | 248.5 | 326.1 | 257.0 | 312.9 | 267.8 | 229.7 |
| Acute Nasopharyngitis | | 20.7 | 31.7 | 23.8 | 32.9 | 24.8 | 31.7 | 19.2 | 27.3 | 20.7 | 27.1 | 14.8 | 5.8 |
| Pharyngitis | | 59.9 | 96.5 | 67.8 | 92.6 | 60.2 | 78.6 | 44.1 | 56.3 | 29.5 | 42.7 | 41.4 | 32.0 |
| Tonsillitis | | 39.2 | 36.0 | 31.5 | 32.9 | 18.1 | 22.6 | 11.3 | 8.6 | 5.6 | 7.5 | 7.4 | 2.9 |
| Hypertrophy of Tonsils | | 9.2 | 1.4 | .9 | 2.7 | 1.1 | 2.6 | .3 | 1.2 | 1.2 | 1.2 | 1.5 | 0 |
| Laryngitis and Tracheitis | | 2.3 | 17.3 | 12.5 | 18.2 | 14.2 | 21.5 | 9.9 | 19.0 | 7.6 | 18.5 | 11.8 | 14.5 |
| Sinusitis | | 18.4 | 33.2 | 25.1 | 40.7 | 29.6 | 34.2 | 22.1 | 35.0 | 19.5 | 24.8 | 11.8 | 8.7 |
| Influenza | | 20.8 | 37.5 | 31.5 | 40.3 | 34.0 | 41.6 | 29.7 | 32.8 | 27.1 | 32.9 | 20.7 | 23.3 |
| Pneumonia | | 6.9 | 7.2 | 8.6 | 10.9 | 7.8 | 13.3 | 7.4 | 14.9 | 17.9 | 18.5 | 10.4 | 17.5 |
| Bronchitis | | 69.1 | 87.9 | 61.8 | 89.9 | 71.4 | 96.7 | 66.4 | 95.9 | 80.5 | 86.0 | 99.1 | 52.3 |
| Other Diseases of Respiratory Tract | | 142.9 | 183.0 | 139.1 | 180.9 | 140.0 | 180.7 | 106.3 | 144.8 | 112.3 | 140.3 | 109.5 | 127.9 |
| Diseases of Lungs | | 4.6 | 10.1 | 5.6 | 7.8 | 7.0 | 9.3 | 7.6 | 8.3 | 19.1 | 9.8 | 22.2 | 11.6 |

| | | 1 | 2 | 3 | 4 | 5 | 6 | 7 | 8 | 9 | 10 | 11 | 12 |
|---|---|---|---|---|---|---|---|---|---|---|---|---|---|
| **XI** | | | | | | | | | | | | | |
| Diseases of the Digestive System | Gross | 76.0 | 144.1 | 109.7 | 154.2 | 144.5 | 170.0 | 147.9 | 178.4 | 153.8 | 194.6 | 167.2 | 171.5 |
| | Net | 69.1 | 126.8 | 95.9 | 127.5 | 124.7 | 138.0 | 121.9 | 142.8 | 124.3 | 147.2 | 140.5 | 145.3 |
| Stomatitis | | 2.3 | 0 | 1.7 | 3.5 | 1.7 | 3.1 | 2.0 | 3.2 | 0 | 1.7 | 0 | 0 |
| Other Diseases of the Buccal Cavity and Esophagus | | 6.9 | 7.2 | 3.9 | 4.3 | 5.3 | 5.4 | 3.7 | 6.0 | 2.4 | 8.7 | 1.5 | 2.9 |
| Ulcers | | 9.2 | 7.2 | 9.9 | 10.1 | 18.4 | 13.9 | 24.6 | 14.9 | 20.7 | 12.7 | 31.0 | 8.7 |
| Gastritis and Duodenitis | | 13.8 | 20.2 | 26.3 | 31.8 | 26.5 | 30.3 | 28.3 | 29.6 | 20.7 | 32.9 | 26.6 | 23.3 |
| Other Diseases of Stomach and Duodenum | | 4.6 | 2.9 | 3.4 | 5.0 | 5.9 | 5.6 | 6.2 | 6.3 | 6.8 | 13.3 | 10.4 | 2.9 |
| Appendicitis | | 0 | 2.9 | .9 | 2.7 | 1.1 | 1.4 | 2.0 | .9 | 1.2 | 1.7 | 0 | 0 |
| Hernia of Abdominal Cavity | | 0 | 0 | 3.5 | 2.3 | 6.1 | 4.8 | 9.9 | 8.9 | 14.8 | 12.7 | 20.7 | 17.4 |
| Gastroenteritis and Colitis (Except Ulcerative) | | 27.7 | 69.1 | 36.3 | 61.2 | 47.4 | 60.8 | 34.2 | 57.2 | 45.8 | 52.5 | 31.1 | 61.0 |
| Other Diseases of Intestines and Peritoneum | | 9.2 | 21.6 | 19.0 | 14.3 | 21.8 | 24.9 | 23.7 | 26.1 | 25.5 | 24.3 | 31.1 | 26.2 |
| Diseases of Liver, Gall Bladder and Pancreas | Gross | 2.3 | 13.0 | 4.8 | 19.0 | 10.3 | 19.8 | 13.3 | 25.3 | 15.9 | 34.1 | 14.8 | 29.1 |
| | Net | 2.3 | 13.0 | 4.8 | 19.0 | 9.8 | 19.5 | 12.2 | 24.4 | 15.5 | 32.9 | 13.3 | 29.1 |
| Diseases of Liver | | 0 | 1.5 | .5 | 1.9 | 3.3 | 2.3 | 5.4 | 1.7 | 4.4 | 1.7 | 4.4 | 0 |
| Diseases of Gall Bladder | | 2.3 | 11.5 | 3.0 | 16.7 | 5.9 | 16.4 | 5.9 | 22.1 | 11.1 | 29.5 | 8.9 | 26.2 |
| Diseases of Pancreas | | 0 | 0 | 1.3 | .4 | 1.1 | 1.1 | 2.0 | 1.5 | .4 | 2.9 | 1.5 | 2.9 |
| **XII** | | | | | | | | | | | | | |
| Diseases of Urinary System | Gross | 13.8 | 54.8 | 23.3 | 56.6 | 24.0 | 58.8 | 19.8 | 40.5 | 34.2 | 49.7 | 51.8 | 37.8 |
| | Net | 13.8 | 49.0 | 22.5 | 51.1 | 22.3 | 53.5 | 18.9 | 36.2 | 30.7 | 45.6 | 45.9 | 34.9 |
| Nephritis and Nephrosis | | 0 | 0 | .9 | 1.2 | .3 | 1.7 | .6 | .8 | .4 | 2.3 | 0 | 0 |
| Cystitis | | 2.3 | 40.4 | 8.2 | 35.6 | 9.2 | 33.6 | 6.2 | 25.9 | 15.9 | 33.5 | 16.3 | 26.2 |
| Other | | 11.5 | 14.4 | 14.2 | 19.8 | 14.5 | 23.5 | 13.0 | 13.8 | 17.9 | 13.9 | 35.5 | 11.6 |
| **XIII** | | | | | | | | | | | | | |
| Diseases of Male Genital Organs (Excluding Neoplasms) | Gross | 16.1 | — | 14.7 | — | 17.8 | — | 20.9 | — | 29.1 | — | 54.7 | — |
| | Net | 16.1 | — | 14.7 | — | 17.8 | — | 20.9 | — | 29.1 | — | 54.7 | — |

TABLE 132. (*Cont'd*) Incidence of Attended Illness or Preventive Care, by Diagnosis, by Age and Sex (and Adjusted to Age-Sex Composition of General Population)

*Part II: Ages 20 and Over (Cont'd)*

| DIAGNOSIS | | NUMBER OF MEMBERS WITH INDICATED DIAGNOSIS PER 1,000 EXPOSURE YEARS | | | | | | | | | | | |
|---|---|---|---|---|---|---|---|---|---|---|---|---|---|
| | | 20–24 | | 25–34 | | 35–44 | | 45–54 | | 55–64 | | 65 AND OVER | |
| | | M | F | M | F | M | F | M | F | M | F | M | F |
| **xiv** | | | | | | | | | | | | | |
| Diseases of Female Genital Organs and Breast (Excluding Neoplasms) | Gross | — | 295.3 | — | 245.7 | — | 242.7 | — | 173.8 | — | 76.8 | — | 40.7 |
| | Net | — | 253.6 | — | 211.2 | — | 206.2 | — | 147.1 | — | 70.4 | — | 40.7 |
| Diseases of Breast | | — | 17.3 | — | 12.8 | — | 14.4 | — | 15.2 | — | 6.4 | — | 2.9 |
| Diseases of Ovaries, Fallopian Tubes and Parametrium | | — | 28.8 | — | 17.4 | — | 9.3 | — | 2.6 | — | .6 | — | 0 |
| Cervicitis | | — | 90.8 | — | 67.4 | — | 63.6 | — | 30.5 | — | 12.1 | — | 8.8 |
| Vaginitis and Vulvitis | | — | 53.3 | — | 42.6 | — | 42.7 | — | 19.5 | — | 17.3 | — | 14.5 |
| Menstrual Disorders | | — | 72.0 | — | 63.2 | — | 58.6 | — | 30.7 | — | 3.5 | — | 0 |
| Menopausal Symptoms | | — | 1.4 | — | 1.2 | — | 20.1 | — | 54.9 | — | 21.9 | — | 0 |
| Other | | — | 31.7 | — | 41.1 | — | 34.0 | — | 20.4 | — | 15.0 | — | 14.5 |
| **xv** | | | | | | | | | | | | | |
| Deliveries and Complications of Pregnancy, Childbirth and Puerperium | Gross | — | 256.5 | — | 186.7 | — | 47.5 | — | 2.3 | — | 0 | — | 0 |
| | Net | — | 250.7 | — | 182.9 | — | 47.5 | — | 2.3 | — | 0 | — | 0 |
| Normal Deliveries | | — | 230.6 | — | 160.0 | — | 37.6 | — | .9 | — | 0 | — | 0 |
| Complicated Deliveries | | — | 4.3 | — | 3.1 | — | .5 | — | 0 | — | 0 | — | 0 |
| Abortion | | — | 17.3 | — | 20.1 | — | 8.5 | — | 1.4 | — | 0 | — | 0 |
| Ectopic Pregnancy | | — | 0 | — | .8 | — | .3 | — | 0 | — | 0 | — | 0 |
| Other | | — | 4.3 | — | 2.7 | — | .6 | — | 0 | — | 0 | — | 0 |

320

**XVI**

| | | | | | | | | | | | | | |
|---|---|---|---|---|---|---|---|---|---|---|---|---|---|
| Diseases of Skin and Subcutaneous Tissues | Gross | 179.7 | 164.3 | 125.3 | 117.8 | 104.3 | 117.9 | 92.4 | 118.6 | 75.7 | 105.1 | 88.7 | 72.7 |
| | Net | 156.7 | 138.3 | 108.4 | 102.3 | 93.4 | 101.8 | 80.6 | 103.7 | 67.7 | 92.4 | 76.9 | 69.8 |
| Boil and Carbuncle | | 20.7 | 8.6 | 16.0 | 8.5 | 11.2 | 9.6 | 11.0 | 8.0 | 9.6 | 8.1 | 10.3 | 5.8 |
| Cellulitis | | 36.9 | 17.3 | 31.5 | 21.3 | 25.9 | 21.8 | 19.5 | 22.4 | 15.1 | 19.1 | 17.7 | 5.8 |
| Impetigo | | 6.9 | 4.3 | .9 | 1.9 | 2.0 | .8 | .3 | .6 | .4 | 1.2 | 0 | 0 |
| Infectious Wart | | 13.8 | 15.9 | 9.1 | 10.9 | 7.2 | 11.0 | 9.0 | 12.6 | 6.3 | 6.4 | 3.0 | 5.8 |
| Dermatitis | | 39.2 | 37.5 | 20.3 | 32.2 | 20.6 | 32.3 | 19.2 | 28.4 | 17.1 | 24.8 | 25.1 | 20.3 |
| Acne | | 18.4 | 20.2 | 2.1 | 5.8 | .6 | 1.7 | .6 | .9 | 0 | 0 | 0 | 0 |
| Sebaceous Cyst | | 11.5 | 11.5 | 12.1 | 7.4 | 10.6 | 6.8 | 9.0 | 9.5 | 6.4 | 4.6 | 8.9 | 5.8 |
| Other | | 32.3 | 49.0 | 33.3 | 29.8 | 26.2 | 33.9 | 23.8 | 36.2 | 20.7 | 41.0 | 23.7 | 29.2 |

**XVII**

| | | | | | | | | | | | | | |
|---|---|---|---|---|---|---|---|---|---|---|---|---|---|
| Diseases of Bones and Organs of Movement | Gross | 48.4 | 67.7 | 82.1 | 80.6 | 104.6 | 128.4 | 127.8 | 156.9 | 117.5 | 168.0 | 145.0 | 206.4 |
| | Net | 43.8 | 59.1 | 77.8 | 71.7 | 92.3 | 110.0 | 108.8 | 133.9 | 101.2 | 136.3 | 133.1 | 171.5 |
| Arthritis and Rheumatism | | 6.9 | 10.1 | 16.4 | 17.8 | 25.9 | 38.2 | 37.3 | 55.4 | 44.2 | 71.0 | 66.6 | 93.0 |
| Osteomyelitis and Other Diseases of Bones and Joints | | 4.6 | 8.7 | 6.5 | 5.8 | 8.4 | 10.2 | 11.9 | 15.2 | 9.2 | 17.3 | 16.3 | 29.1 |
| Synovitis, Bursitis and Tenosynovitis | | 11.5 | 18.7 | 25.9 | 22.5 | 38.2 | 43.0 | 42.4 | 55.2 | 40.2 | 41.0 | 42.9 | 55.2 |
| Infective Myositis | | 25.4 | 21.6 | 28.5 | 29.1 | 26.0 | 26.0 | 29.1 | 23.6 | 17.9 | 21.9 | 11.8 | 20.3 |
| Muscular Dystrophy | | 0 | 0 | 0 | 0 | 0 | 0 | .3 | .3 | 0 | .6 | 0 | 0 |
| Scoliosis | | 0 | 1.4 | .9 | 1.5 | 1.4 | 2.0 | .6 | .3 | .8 | 1.2 | 0 | 2.9 |
| Other Deformities | | 0 | 4.3 | 1.3 | .4 | 1.1 | 2.2 | 1.7 | 2.3 | 1.6 | 5.8 | 1.5 | 0 |
| Other Diseases of Musculoskeletal System | | 0 | 2.9 | 2.6 | 3.5 | 3.6 | 6.8 | 4.5 | 4.6 | 3.6 | 9.2 | 5.9 | 5.8 |

TABLE 132. (Cont'd)  Incidence of Attended Illness or Preventive Care, by Diagnosis, by Age and Sex (and Adjusted to Age-Sex Composition of General Population)

*Part II: Ages 20 and Over (Cont'd)*

| DIAGNOSIS | | NUMBER OF MEMBERS WITH INDICATED DIAGNOSIS PER 1,000 EXPOSURE YEARS | | | | | | | | | | | |
|---|---|---|---|---|---|---|---|---|---|---|---|---|---|
| | | 20–24 | | 25–34 | | 35–44 | | 45–54 | | 55–64 | | 65 AND OVER | |
| | | M | F | M | F | M | F | M | F | M | F | M | F |
| XVIII Injuries and Adverse Effects of External Causes | Gross | 159.0 | 144.1 | 154.2 | 134.4 | 150.9 | 156.4 | 129.5 | 160.9 | 104.8 | 150.1 | 102.1 | 157.0 |
| | Net | 140.6 | 129.7 | 135.6 | 119.7 | 135.2 | 139.1 | 121.6 | 134.2 | 92.0 | 125.3 | 85.8 | 133.7 |
| Fractures | Gross | 16.1 | 10.1 | 11.2 | 7.7 | 15.1 | 12.4 | 10.2 | 14.9 | 9.6 | 23.7 | 3.0 | 14.5 |
| | Net | 13.8 | 10.1 | 10.4 | 6.6 | 13.9 | 11.9 | 9.9 | 14.1 | 8.4 | 21.9 | 3.0 | 14.5 |
| Skull and Face | Gross | 2.3 | 0 | 1.7 | .4 | 2.2 | .8 | .8 | 0 | 1.2 | 0 | 1.5 | 0 |
| Torso | Gross | 2.3 | 1.5 | .9 | .7 | 1.7 | 1.4 | 3.7 | 3.1 | 2.4 | 4.6 | 0 | 0 |
| Spine (Vertical Column) | | 0 | 0 | 0 | 0 | .6 | .3 | .3 | .5 | .4 | 1.7 | 0 | 0 |
| Ribs, Sternum and Larynx | | 2.3 | 1.5 | .9 | .7 | 1.1 | 1.1 | 3.4 | 2.6 | 2.0 | 2.9 | 0 | 0 |
| UPPER EXTREMITIES | Gross | 6.9 | 1.4 | 3.4 | 2.7 | 7.6 | 3.4 | 3.4 | 4.3 | 4.0 | 9.3 | 1.5 | 2.9 |
| Clavicle | | 2.3 | 1.4 | .8 | .4 | .3 | .3 | .3 | .3 | .4 | .6 | 0 | 0 |
| Scapula | | 0 | 0 | 0 | 0 | .3 | .3 | 0 | .3 | 0 | 0 | 0 | 0 |
| Humerus | | 0 | 0 | .4 | 0 | .6 | 0 | .3 | .3 | .4 | 0 | 1.5 | 2.9 |
| Radius and Ulna | | 2.3 | 0 | 0 | .4 | 1.1 | .6 | 1.1 | 1.1 | .8 | 2.9 | 0 | 0 |
| Wrist | | 2.3 | 0 | .4 | .7 | .3 | 0 | 0 | 1.1 | 1.2 | .6 | 0 | 0 |
| Hand-Finger | | 0 | 0 | 1.8 | 1.2 | 5.0 | 2.3 | 1.7 | 1.2 | 1.2 | 5.2 | 0 | 0 |
| LOWER EXTREMITIES | Gross | 4.6 | 7.2 | 5.2 | 3.9 | 3.6 | 6.2 | 2.3 | 7.5 | 2.0 | 9.2 | 0 | 11.6 |
| Pelvis | | 0 | 0 | 0 | .4 | 0 | 0 | 0 | 0 | 0 | .6 | 0 | 0 |
| Femur | | 0 | 0 | 0 | 0 | 0 | 0 | 0 | .3 | .4 | 1.7 | 0 | 8.7 |
| Patella | | 0 | 0 | 0 | 0 | 0 | 0 | .3 | 0 | 0 | 0 | 0 | 0 |
| Tibia and Fibula | | 0 | 0 | 1.7 | .8 | .8 | 1.4 | .3 | 1.8 | .8 | 1.2 | 0 | 0 |
| Ankle | | 0 | 1.4 | 1.3 | .8 | .6 | 1.7 | 0 | 1.4 | .4 | .6 | 0 | 2.9 |
| Foot and Toe | | 4.6 | 5.8 | 2.2 | 1.9 | 2.2 | 3.1 | 1.7 | 4.0 | .4 | 5.1 | 0 | 0 |
| Late Effects of Fractures | | 0 | 0 | 0 | 0 | 0 | .3 | 0 | 0 | 0 | .6 | 0 | 0 |

322

## Injuries (Cont'd)

| Category | | | | | | | | | | | | | |
|---|---|---|---|---|---|---|---|---|---|---|---|---|---|
| Dislocations | 4.6 | 1.4 | 1.7 | 1.1 | .8 | 1.7 | 2.0 | 1.2 | .8 | 1.7 | 0 | 0 | |
| Sprains and Strains | 43.8 | 54.8 | 65.2 | 56.6 | 71.4 | 64.8 | 61.6 | 63.8 | 42.6 | 46.8 | 32.5 | 40.7 | |
| Head Injuries (Other than Fractures) | 6.9 | 2.9 | 5.2 | 3.9 | 4.7 | 2.0 | 5.7 | 2.9 | 4.4 | 5.2 | 4.4 | 11.6 | |
| Internal Injuries | 0 | 1.4 | 0 | 1.1 | 0 | 0 | 0 | 0 | .4 | 0 | 0 | 0 | |
| Lacerations and Open Wounds | 32.3 | 37.5 | 26.4 | 21.7 | 22.9 | 22.3 | 14.4 | 21.6 | 12.8 | 13.8 | 10.3 | 23.3 | |
| Superficial Injuries | 6.9 | 5.8 | 7.3 | 7.0 | 5.3 | 5.7 | 4.8 | 8.9 | 2.8 | 9.2 | 8.9 | 8.7 | |
| Foreign Body | 2.3 | 0 | 6.5 | 3.1 | 5.0 | 4.0 | 4.8 | 3.4 | 2.4 | 2.9 | 0 | 5.8 | |
| Contusions | 27.7 | 23.0 | 22.0 | 21.7 | 15.6 | 29.7 | 16.1 | 23.8 | 13.1 | 23.7 | 23.7 | 29.1 | |
| Complications of Surgical or Medical Procedures | 2.3 | 7.2 | 2.6 | 7.4 | 4.5 | 9.3 | 6.8 | 16.1 | 11.1 | 16.2 | 16.3 | 14.6 | |
| Other | 16.1 | 0 | 6.1 | 3.1 | 5.6 | 4.8 | 3.1 | 4.3 | 4.8 | 6.9 | 3.0 | 8.7 | |

## XIX Congenital Malformations

| | Gross/Net | | | | | | | | | | | | |
|---|---|---|---|---|---|---|---|---|---|---|---|---|---|
| Congenital Malformations — Gross | 0 | 2.9 | .9 | .8 | .6 | 1.1 | .6 | 1.2 | .8 | 1.2 | 1.5 | 0 | |
| Congenital Malformations — Net | 0 | 2.9 | .9 | .8 | .6 | 1.1 | .6 | 1.2 | .8 | 1.2 | 1.5 | 0 | |

## XX Certain Diseases of Early Infancy

| | Gross/Net | | | | | | | | | | | | |
|---|---|---|---|---|---|---|---|---|---|---|---|---|---|
| Certain Diseases of Early Infancy — Gross | — | — | — | — | — | — | — | — | — | — | — | — | |
| Certain Diseases of Early Infancy — Net | — | — | — | — | — | — | — | — | — | — | — | — | |

## XXI Symptoms, Senility and Ill-Defined Conditions

| | Gross/Net | | | | | | | | | | | | |
|---|---|---|---|---|---|---|---|---|---|---|---|---|---|
| Symptoms, Senility and Ill-Defined Conditions — Gross | 41.5 | 89.3 | 53.1 | 84.1 | 69.4 | 96.4 | 67.6 | 91.6 | 64.9 | 94.7 | 74.0 | 93.0 | |
| Symptoms, Senility and Ill-Defined Conditions — Net | 41.5 | 83.6 | 50.5 | 74.4 | 65.0 | 86.8 | 60.5 | 81.9 | 59.0 | 89.5 | 69.5 | 84.3 | |
| Symptoms Referrable to Nervous System | 2.3 | 5.8 | 6.0 | 8.2 | 9.8 | 12.5 | 8.5 | 10.9 | 11.5 | 8.6 | 8.9 | 11.6 | |
| Symptoms Referrable to Cardiovascular System | 2.3 | 10.1 | 2.2 | 5.8 | 5.8 | 12.5 | 6.5 | 14.7 | 6.4 | 11.0 | 11.8 | 8.7 | |
| Symptoms Referrable to Respiratory System | 6.9 | 10.1 | 12.5 | 10.1 | 13.1 | 10.7 | 15.6 | 12.6 | 15.1 | 13.3 | 16.3 | 14.5 | |
| Symptoms Referrable to Upper and Lower Gastro-intestinal System | 4.6 | 21.6 | 7.8 | 11.6 | 9.2 | 13.0 | 7.9 | 12.3 | 9.9 | 20.8 | 5.9 | 14.6 | |
| Symptoms Referrable to Urinary System | 0 | 1.4 | 1.3 | 5.8 | 3.1 | 4.2 | 6.0 | 2.0 | 2.8 | 6.3 | 8.9 | 0 | |
| Pain in Back | 2.3 | 11.5 | 3.9 | 6.2 | 5.0 | 8.2 | 6.2 | 8.0 | 3.6 | 5.8 | 5.9 | 14.6 | |
| Other Referrable Symptoms (Not Elsewhere Classified) | 4.6 | 5.8 | 4.7 | 8.5 | 6.7 | 6.5 | 5.9 | 7.5 | 6.0 | 8.1 | 7.4 | 14.5 | |
| Headache | 9.3 | 11.5 | 6.5 | 12.8 | 8.1 | 13.0 | 6.5 | 12.4 | 4.8 | 9.8 | 3.0 | 5.8 | |
| Other Ill-Defined Diseases | 9.2 | 11.5 | 8.2 | 15.1 | 8.6 | 15.8 | 4.5 | 11.2 | 4.8 | 11.0 | 5.9 | 8.7 | |

TABLE 132. (*Concluded*)  Incidence of Attended Illness or Preventive Care, by Diagnosis, by Age and Sex (and Adjusted to Age-Sex Composition of General Population)

*Part II: Ages 20 and Over (Concluded)*

| DIAGNOSIS | | NUMBER OF MEMBERS WITH INDICATED DIAGNOSIS PER 1,000 EXPOSURE YEARS | | | | | | | | | | | |
|---|---|---|---|---|---|---|---|---|---|---|---|---|---|
| | | 20–24 | | 25–34 | | 35–44 | | 45–54 | | 55–64 | | 65 AND OVER | |
| | | M | F | M | F | M | F | M | F | M | F | M | F |
| XXII Supplementary Classifications | Gross | 50.7 | 125.4 | 70.8 | 120.5 | 69.4 | 93.0 | 65.6 | 77.3 | 65.3 | 75.1 | 51.8 | 64.0 |
| | Net | 50.7 | 118.2 | 70.8 | 118.6 | 68.3 | 91.3 | 64.5 | 76.7 | 63.3 | 73.9 | 50.3 | 61.0 |
| General Medical Examinations (Including Immunizations) | | 48.4 | 90.8 | 48.4 | 87.2 | 44.6 | 68.7 | 35.3 | 48.6 | 25.5 | 43.9 | 23.7 | 32.0 |
| Well Baby and Child Care (Including Immunizations) | | — | — | — | — | — | — | — | — | — | — | — | — |
| Diagnostic Screening | | 2.3 | 13.0 | 22.4 | 12.4 | 24.8 | 18.9 | 30.3 | 28.7 | 39.8 | 31.2 | 28.1 | 32.0 |
| Other | | — | 21.6 | — | 20.9 | — | 5.4 | — | 0 | — | 0 | — | 0 |
| XXIII Undetermined Classifications | Gross | 96.8 | 204.6 | 77.3 | 188.3 | 18.2 | 199.7 | 113.9 | 171.8 | 122.7 | 165.7 | 176.0 | 151.2 |
| | Net | 96.8 | 204.6 | 77.3 | 188.3 | 18.2 | 199.7 | 113.9 | 171.8 | 122.7 | 165.7 | 176.0 | 151.2 |

* Less than .05.
† Gross rate is based on sum of patients reported for each component of a category; this represents duplicate count of persons treated for more than one condition in that category.
‡ Net rate is based on number of patients with *any* condition listed for a specified category.
§ Adjusted to age-sex composition of general population of area.

## Occupation Class Variations

In the absence of data permitting more specific measurement, subscriber occupation has been used in the present studies as a crude index of social class. It is introduced briefly below, in the analysis of incidence rates, to probe for possible indications of class-related treated illness patterns.

The analysis emphasizes the combined experience of the professional-executive-sales classes vs. that of the blue-collar groups; if there were divergent class patterns, they would presumably emerge most clearly in a comparison of these two categories. It can only be conjectured in each instance, however, whether such differences as have been found resulted from differences in actual illness rates (need for medical care), variations in patient attitudes toward seeking care (demand) or, as is also conceivable, variations in physician attitudes toward defining illness in patients from different classes.

Differences in attitudes toward seeking care appear to be implicit in some of the findings, especially where blue-collar rates were lower. In other instances, a class pattern favoring higher blue-collar rates is seen, but with no ready explanation. In a third group of diagnoses showing occupation class differences, the significance of class as a factor is nullified by sex variations. Finally, there are a number of conditions for which incidence was the same irrespective of occupation class. Each of these classifications is illustrated below. The observations derive from Table 133.

### Category 1. Higher Professional-Executive-Sales Class Rates

The diagnoses for which rates in the professional-executive-sales class were definitely higher than in blue-collar groups generally contain some connotation of class differences in attitudes toward seeking preventive, early, or minor care, rather than in disease rates.

The neoplasm treatment rate was considerably higher in the professional-executive-sales group, particularly for males, among whom the treated malignancy rate more than doubled that of males in the blue-collar class. Since there is no reason to credit blue-collar class males with greater immunity to cancer, their lower rate of treatment may be attributed to a lower discovery rate.

Similar findings occurred for eye conditions; the professional-executive-sales incidence was nearly 50 per cent higher. In the case of glaucoma, the male rate was more than double that found for blue-collar males, while the comparable female ratio was over three to one. Treatment of strabismus (cross-eyes) was also substantially lower among blue-collar families.

Skin conditions, over 20 per cent higher in the professional-executive-sales group, constitute another category where class-generated definitions of what is necessary medical care may have exerted some influence.

Further evidence tending to substantiate the same hypothesis comes from the category of general medical examinations (no positive diagnosis reported), for which the professional-executive-sales class showed rates about 50 per cent higher.

Finally, a diagnosis of sprain or strain occurred much more frequently among the professional-executive-sales group, perhaps indicating a tendency to seek attention for minor conditions which the blue-collar groups were likelier to ignore or self-treat; supporting this view is the finding that in the case of lacerations, where care was obviously required, there was not much class difference in treatment rates.

## Category 2. Higher Blue-Collar Class Rates

In contrast to most diagnoses in the previous category, theories as to varying degrees of medical motivation do not generally emerge to explain instances where higher blue-collar class incidence rates occurred.

Members of blue-collar families were treated more frequently for infective diseases, tonsillitis, pneumonia, influenza, bronchitis, other respiratory conditions, gall bladder disorders, duodenal ulcers. It is probably reasonable to surmise that these conditions occurred more frequently, during the study year, among the blue-collar classes; but whether this is a regular occurrence and if so why must be left to further investigation. It is certainly difficult to reconcile the higher ulcer rates found for blue-collar members, particularly the 60 per cent higher rate of the males, with common assumptions as to greater ulcer susceptibility among those in positions of greatest responsibility.

Maternity care was used about 40 per cent more frequently in the blue-collar families. But it may be noteworthy that the reported abortion rate, in proportion to number of deliveries, was identical in the two groups discussed—one abortion to 7.53 deliveries.

*Category 3. Class Differences Varying for Males and Females*

The incidence of treated arthritis was a third higher among males of the blue-collar group than in the professional-executive-sales class.

Females of the latter class, however, experienced the highest rates—over 10 per cent higher than blue-collar class females.

A somewhat similar pattern was found for synovitis, and in fact for the total category of diseases of bones, joints and muscles.

The reverse pattern occurred for heart diseases. Here, the rate for males of the professional-executive-sales category was 25 per cent higher than among males of the blue-collar group, whereas treated incidence among females of the blue-collar group was 50 per cent higher than among females of the professional-executive-sales group.

Still another pattern was found for a miscellaneous group of diagnoses in which males of different classes experienced similar rates, while females of the blue-collar group showed higher rates than those in the professional-executive-sales category. Examples include diabetes (blue-collar female rate nearly a third higher than professional-executive-sales females), hernia (blue-collar female rate over 80 per cent higher), liver

TABLE 133. Incidence of Attended Illness or Preventive
Care, by Diagnosis, by Sex and Class: Comparison of
Professional-Executive-Sales and
Blue-Collar Class Rates

| DIAGNOSIS | | NUMBER OF MEMBERS WITH INDICATED DIAGNOSIS PER 1,000 EXPOSURE YEARS, INCLUDING DEPENDENTS | | | |
|---|---|---|---|---|---|
| | | MALE | | FEMALE | |
| | | Professional, Executive and Sales | Blue Collar | Professional, Executive and Sales | Blue Collar |
| TOTAL | Gross * | 1923.5 | 1787.2 | 2301.8 | 2259.1 |
| | Net † | 771.4 | 733.1 | 841.3 | 847.5 |
| I | Gross | 74.5 | 108.3 | 121.9 | 126.0 |
| Infective and Parasitic Diseases | Net | 68.8 | 98.2 | 112.5 | 115.0 |
| Streptococcal Sore Throat | | 9.8 | 15.5 | 17.8 | 19.5 |
| Measles | | 3.6 | 6.8 | 6.7 | 6.1 |
| Rubella (German Measles) | | 15.9 | 23.5 | 34.5 | 27.9 |
| Chicken Pox | | 2.6 | 5.5 | 2.2 | 5.2 |
| Mumps | | 1.6 | 3.4 | 3.9 | 3.8 |
| Infectious Hepatitis | | .5 | .2 | 0 | .2 |
| Glandular Fever (Infectious Mononucleosis) | | 1.5 | 1.2 | .6 | 1.8 |
| Intestinal Virus | | 30.8 | 39.2 | 36.2 | 49.4 |
| Dermatophytoses | | 3.1 | 7.0 | 8.3 | 5.0 |
| Other | | 5.1 | 6.0 | 11.7 | 7.1 |
| II | Gross | 36.0 | 22.0 | 54.0 | 46.1 |
| Neoplasms | Net | 29.8 | 18.5 | 46.2 | 40.7 |
| Malignant Neoplasms | Gross | 11.3 | 5.4 | 7.8 | 6.2 |
| | Net | 9.2 | 4.1 | 6.7 | 5.3 |
| Digestive System—Including Mouth | | 2.6 | .7 | 0 | .4 |
| Respiratory System | | 1.5 | 1.0 | 1.1 | .2 |
| Breast | | — | — | 1.7 | 1.9 |
| Female Genital Organs | | — | — | 1.1 | .8 |
| Male Genital Organs | | 0 | .7 | — | — |
| Urinary System | | 0 | .6 | 0 | 0 |
| Skin | | 2.6 | .6 | 1.7 | .3 |
| Eye | | 0 | 0 | .5 | .1 |
| Nervous System—Including Brain | | 1.0 | .3 | .5 | .1 |
| Endocrine Glands | | 0 | .1 | 0 | .5 |
| Bone | | 0 | .1 | .6 | .2 |
| Connective Tissue | | 0 | 0 | 0 | 0 |
| Lymphosarcoma | | 0 | 0 | 0 | .1 |
| Hodgkin's Disease | | 0 | .1 | 0 | .1 |
| Other Lymphoma | | .5 | .2 | 0 | 0 |
| Multiple Myeloma | | 0 | .1 | 0 | .1 |
| Leukemia | | .5 | .1 | 0 | .4 |
| Not Elsewhere Classified | | 2.6 | .8 | .6 | 1.0 |
| Benign Neoplasms | Gross | 23.7 | 15.4 | 44.5 | 37.7 |
| | Net | 22.1 | 15.1 | 41.2 | 35.3 |
| Mouth | | 1.6 | .4 | 1.1 | 1.4 |
| Rectum | | 1.5 | .9 | .5 | .5 |
| Breast | | — | — | 1.7 | 3.7 |
| Female Genital Organs | | — | — | 15.6 | 15.3 |
| Skin | | 13.4 | 8.7 | 18.4 | 10.3 |
| Other | | 7.2 | 5.4 | 7.2 | 6.5 |

TABLE 133. (Cont'd)

| DIAGNOSIS | | NUMBER OF MEMBERS WITH INDICATED DIAGNOSIS PER 1,000 EXPOSURE YEARS, INCLUDING DEPENDENTS | | | |
|---|---|---|---|---|---|
| | | MALE | | FEMALE | |
| | | Professional, Executive and Sales | Blue Collar | Professional, Executive and Sales | Blue Collar |
| *Neoplasms (Cont'd)* | | | | | |
| | Gross | 1.0 | 1.2 | 1.7 | 2.2 |
| Unspecified Neoplasms | Net | 1.0 | 1.2 | 1.7 | 2.2 |
| Rectum | | 0 | 0 | 0 | .2 |
| Breast | | — | — | 0 | .6 |
| Female Genital Organs | | — | — | 0 | .3 |
| Other | | 1.0 | 1.2 | 1.7 | 1.1 |
| **III** | | | | | |
| Allergic, Endocrine System, Meta- | Gross | 90.4 | 70.8 | 126.4 | 116.7 |
| bolic and Nutritional Diseases | Net | 81.7 | 63.9 | 110.8 | 104.5 |
| Hay Fever | | 23.1 | 15.7 | 25.0 | 16.9 |
| Asthma | | 13.9 | 14.0 | 13.4 | 13.2 |
| Other Allergic Diseases | | 18.0 | 11.2 | 14.5 | 15.3 |
| Diseases of Thyroid Gland | | 2.0 | 3.0 | 25.6 | 16.2 |
| Diabetes Mellitus | | 11.3 | 10.9 | 5.6 | 9.1 |
| Obesity (Not Otherwise Specified) | | 13.9 | 10.3 | 30.1 | 40.0 |
| Other | | 8.2 | 5.7 | 12.2 | 6.0 |
| **IV** | | | | | |
| Diseases of Blood and Blood Form- | Gross | 4.6 | 6.2 | 12.8 | 22.4 |
| ing Organs | Net | 4.6 | 6.2 | 12.8 | 22.4 |
| Anemias | | 4.1 | 4.6 | 12.2 | 20.9 |
| Other | | .5 | 1.6 | .6 | 1.5 |
| **V** | | | | | |
| Mental, Psychoneurotic and Person- | Gross | 6.2 | 5.4 | 11.1 | 9.9 |
| ality Disorders | Net | 6.2 | 5.1 | 10.6 | 9.5 |
| Chronic Brain Disorders | | 0 | .6 | .6 | .1 |
| Psychoses | | .5 | .7 | 1.1 | 1.5 |
| Psychophysiologic, Autonomic and | | | | | |
| Visceral Disorders | | 0 | .1 | 0 | .2 |
| Psychoneuroses | | 5.2 | 3.4 | 6.7 | 7.1 |
| Personality Disorders | | 0 | .4 | 2.2 | .9 |
| Mental Deficiency | | .5 | .2 | .5 | .1 |
| **VI** | Gross | 26.2 | 20.8 | 28.4 | 27.2 |
| Diseases of Nervous System | Net | 25.2 | 20.3 | 26.7 | 26.2 |
| Stroke | | 0 | .1 | 0 | 0 |
| Multiple Sclerosis | | .5 | .1 | 0 | .4 |
| Migraine | | 3.1 | 2.0 | 5.0 | 4.8 |
| Epilepsy | | .5 | .7 | 0 | .7 |
| Sciatica | | 4.1 | 3.9 | 1.7 | 4.7 |
| Other | | 18.0 | 14.0 | 21.7 | 16.6 |
| **VII** | Gross | 67.8 | 44.8 | 69.1 | 50.5 |
| Diseases of Eye | Net | 65.7 | 41.6 | 65.1 | 47.2 |
| Conjunctivitis and Ophthalmia | | 28.8 | 21.8 | 29.0 | 21.6 |
| Strabismus | | 6.7 | 3.7 | 8.9 | 5.2 |
| Cataract | | 1.5 | 1.9 | 0 | 2.2 |
| Glaucoma | | 3.6 | 1.6 | 4.5 | 1.4 |
| Detachment of Retina | | 0 | .1 | 0 | .2 |
| Other | | 27.2 | 15.7 | 26.7 | 19.9 |

TABLE 133. (Cont'd) Incidence of Attended Illness or Preventive
Care, by Diagnosis, by Sex and Class: Comparison of
Professional-Executive-Sales and
Blue-Collar Class Rates

| DIAGNOSIS | | NUMBER OF MEMBERS WITH INDICATED DIAGNOSIS PER 1,000 EXPOSURE YEARS, INCLUDING DEPENDENTS | | | |
|---|---|---|---|---|---|
| | | MALE | | FEMALE | |
| | | Professional, Executive and Sales | Blue Collar | Professional, Executive and Sales | Blue Collar |
| VIII | Gross | 63.7 | 67.8 | 74.6 | 73.0 |
| Diseases of Ear | Net | 59.6 | 63.6 | 68.5 | 67.0 |
| Otitis Externa | | 7.7 | 8.1 | 7.2 | 9.4 |
| Otitis Media | | 37.5 | 42.4 | 50.1 | 48.1 |
| Deafness | | 1.0 | .9 | .6 | 1.1 |
| Other | | 17.5 | 16.4 | 16.7 | 14.4 |
| IX | Gross | 104.8 | 94.5 | 90.2 | 106.6 |
| Diseases of Circulatory System | Net | 86.3 | 75.6 | 77.4 | 87.5 |
| Rheumatic Fever without Mention of Heart | | .5 | .5 | .6 | .9 |
| | Gross | 50.9 | 40.4 | 21.7 | 32.3 |
| Diseases of Heart | Net | 38.5 | 29.4 | 18.4 | 25.8 |
| Rheumatic Heart Disease | | 2.1 | 1.9 | 1.1 | 4.4 |
| Arteriosclerotic Heart Disease | | 12.3 | 8.7 | 4.4 | 4.7 |
| Acute Coronary Occlusion | | 4.1 | 4.8 | 1.7 | 1.3 |
| Coronary Insufficiency | | 11.8 | 8.2 | 2.2 | 5.0 |
| Angina Pectoris | | 5.1 | 6.6 | 2.8 | 4.5 |
| Hypertensive Heart Disease | | 2.1 | 2.9 | 2.8 | 5.1 |
| Other | | 13.4 | 7.3 | 6.7 | 7.3 |
| Diseases of Veins and Arteries | Gross | 53.4 | 53.6 | 67.9 | 73.4 |
| (Other than Heart) | Net | 51.4 | 51.9 | 62.9 | 68.5 |
| Hypertensive Diseases | | 24.1 | 25.3 | 28.4 | 38.2 |
| Hypotension | | 0 | 1.3 | 5.0 | 3.4 |
| Hemorrhoids | | 14.9 | 10.3 | 10.0 | 10.1 |
| General Arteriosclerosis | | 0 | 1.1 | 1.7 | 1.0 |
| Varicose Veins of Lower Extremities | | 2.1 | 1.4 | 5.6 | 3.9 |
| Pulmonary Embolism and Infarction | | 1.0 | .2 | 0 | .3 |
| Lymphadenitis | | 3.6 | 7.6 | 6.1 | 6.9 |
| Other | | 7.7 | 6.4 | 11.1 | 9.6 |
| X | Gross | 483.8 | 528.6 | 546.8 | 615.3 |
| Diseases of Respiratory System | Net | 351.8 | 370.4 | 378.6 | 430.6 |
| Acute Nasopharyngitis | | 24.6 | 31.9 | 29.5 | 38.8 |
| Pharyngitis | | 86.3 | 82.6 | 107.4 | 104.0 |
| Tonsillitis | | 47.8 | 61.9 | 58.5 | 65.4 |
| Hypertrophy of Tonsils | | 12.3 | 10.5 | 12.2 | 11.7 |
| Laryngitis and Tracheitis | | 22.1 | 16.6 | 27.3 | 19.5 |
| Sinusitis | | 23.6 | 19.1 | 31.2 | 23.9 |
| Influenza | | 25.2 | 29.7 | 25.1 | 33.6 |
| Pneumonia | | 7.7 | 11.3 | 8.3 | 12.6 |
| Bronchitis | | 68.3 | 88.6 | 71.3 | 97.7 |
| Other Diseases of Respiratory Tract | | 161.3 | 168.0 | 169.3 | 202.6 |
| Diseases of Lungs | | 4.6 | 8.4 | 6.7 | 5.5 |

TABLE 133. *(Cont'd)*

| DIAGNOSIS | | NUMBER OF MEMBERS WITH INDICATED DIAGNOSIS PER 1,000 EXPOSURE YEARS, INCLUDING DEPENDENTS | | | |
|---|---|---|---|---|---|
| | | MALE | | FEMALE | |
| | | *Professional, Executive and Sales* | *Blue Collar* | *Professional, Executive and Sales* | *Blue Collar* |
| XI | Gross | 127.4 | 125.5 | 121.9 | 151.7 |
| Diseases of the Digestive System | Net | 113.0 | 108.9 | 105.8 | 126.8 |
| Stomatitis | | 3.6 | 2.4 | 2.2 | 4.1 |
| Other Diseases of Buccal Cavity and Esophagus | | 4.1 | 4.0 | 5.0 | 5.8 |
| Ulcers | | 8.2 | 13.1 | 6.7 | 7.9 |
| Gastritis and Duodenitis | | 17.0 | 20.2 | 18.9 | 23.6 |
| Other Diseases of Stomach and Duodenum | | 6.2 | 4.2 | 7.8 | 4.7 |
| Appendicitis | | 3.6 | 2.1 | 1.1 | 3.2 |
| Hernia of Abdominal Cavity | | 8.7 | 7.8 | 2.8 | 5.1 |
| Gastroenteritis and Colitis (Except Ulcerative) | | 48.8 | 47.5 | 51.2 | 65.4 |
| Other Diseases of Intestines and Peritoneum | | 20.0 | 16.0 | 14.5 | 17.0 |
| Diseases of Liver, Gall Bladder and Pancreas | Gross | 7.2 | 8.2 | 11.7 | 14.9 |
| | Net | 7.2 | 7.8 | 11.7 | 14.5 |
| Diseases of Liver | | 2.6 | 2.6 | 1.1 | 1.5 |
| Diseases of Gall Bladder | | 3.6 | 4.8 | 10.0 | 12.3 |
| Diseases of Pancreas | | 1.0 | .8 | .6 | 1.1 |
| XII | Gross | 18.5 | 19.6 | 36.8 | 36.3 |
| Diseases of the Urinary System | Net | 18.0 | 18.0 | 34.0 | 32.8 |
| Nephritis and Nephrosis | | 0 | .7 | .6 | 1.4 |
| Cystitis | | 6.2 | 7.5 | 24.5 | 21.1 |
| Other | | 12.3 | 11.4 | 11.7 | 13.8 |
| XIII | Gross | 22.6 | 15.2 | — | — |
| Diseases of the Male Genital Organs (Excluding Neoplasms) | Net | 22.6 | 15.2 | — | — |
| XIV | | | | | |
| Diseases of the Female Genital Organs and Breast (Excluding Neoplasms) | Gross | — | — | 132.0 | 124.9 |
| | Net | — | — | 117.5 | 106.5 |
| Diseases of Breast | | — | — | 10.0 | 8.6 |
| Diseases of Ovaries, Fallopian Tubes and Parametrium | | — | — | 3.9 | 6.2 |
| Cervicitis | | — | — | 32.3 | 29.5 |
| Vaginitis and Vulvitis | | — | — | 19.5 | 20.1 |
| Menstrual Disorders | | — | — | 34.0 | 27.2 |
| Menopausal Symptoms | | — | — | 17.3 | 15.5 |
| Other | | — | — | 15.0 | 17.8 |
| XV | | | | | |
| Deliveries and Complications of Pregnancy, Childbirth and Puerperium | Gross | — | — | 29.0 | 41.3 |
| | Net | — | — | 29.0 | 40.5 |
| Normal Deliveries | | — | — | 24.5 | 35.3 |
| Complicated Deliveries | | — | — | 0 | .5 |
| Abortion | | — | — | 3.4 | 4.9 |
| Ectopic Pregnancy | | — | — | 0 | .2 |
| Other | | — | — | 1.1 | .4 |

| DIAGNOSIS | | NUMBER OF MEMBERS WITH INDICATED DIAGNOSIS PER 1,000 EXPOSURE YEARS, INCLUDING DEPENDENTS | | | |
|---|---|---|---|---|---|
| | | MALE | | FEMALE | |
| | | Professional, Executive and Sales | Blue Collar | Professional, Executive and Sales | Blue Collar |
| **XVI** | | | | | |
| Diseases of Skin and Subcutaneous | Gross | 135.1 | 107.2 | 138.6 | 111.4 |
| Tissues | Net | 117.6 | 96.1 | 125.8 | 98.2 |
| Boil and Carbuncle | | 10.3 | 11.0 | 11.7 | 7.8 |
| Cellulitis | | 24.7 | 21.4 | 20.0 | 19.5 |
| Impetigo | | 5.6 | 5.7 | 5.6 | 4.7 |
| Infectious Wart | | 12.8 | 8.9 | 17.8 | 9.3 |
| Dermatitis | | 32.4 | 24.7 | 31.2 | 33.6 |
| Acne | | 10.8 | 4.1 | 11.7 | 4.2 |
| Sebaceous Cyst | | 8.7 | 6.1 | 7.8 | 4.2 |
| Other | | 29.8 | 25.3 | 32.8 | 28.1 |
| **XVII** | | | | | |
| Diseases of Bones and Organs of | Gross | 77.0 | 82.4 | 105.8 | 86.3 |
| Movement | Net | 69.9 | 72.9 | 91.9 | 74.6 |
| Arthritis and Rheumatism | | 16.9 | 22.4 | 31.2 | 27.9 |
| Osteomyelitis and Other Diseases of Bones and Joints | | 9.8 | 8.4 | 7.8 | 8.1 |
| Synovitis, Bursitis and Tenosynovitis | | 23.1 | 26.2 | 31.7 | 25.4 |
| Infective Myositis | | 13.9 | 18.2 | 16.7 | 17.3 |
| Muscular Dystrophy | | 0 | .2 | 0 | .1 |
| Scoliosis | | 1.0 | .6 | 3.4 | 1.0 |
| Other Deformities | | 8.7 | 3.8 | 7.8 | 3.6 |
| Other Diseases of Musculoskeletal System | | 3.6 | 2.6 | 7.2 | 2.9 |
| **XVIII** | | | | | |
| Injuries and Adverse Effects of | Gross | 203.4 | 159.5 | 162.0 | 134.5 |
| External Causes | Net | 174.1 | 139.8 | 143.1 | 117.4 |
| | Gross | 20.5 | 14.4 | 15.6 | 11.8 |
| Fractures | Net | 18.0 | 13.3 | 15.0 | 10.8 |
| Skull and Face | | 2.5 | 1.9 | 1.1 | .4 |
| Torso | Gross | .5 | 1.5 | 1.7 | 1.5 |
| Spine | | 0 | .2 | 1.1 | .5 |
| Ribs, Sternum and Larynx | | .5 | 1.3 | .6 | 1.0 |
| UPPER EXTREMITIES | Gross | 11.3 | 7.5 | 8.4 | 4.6 |
| Clavicle | | 0 | .7 | 1.7 | .5 |
| Scapula | | 0 | .1 | 0 | 0 |
| Humerus | | 1.0 | .7 | .6 | .2 |
| Radius and Ulna | | 4.1 | 2.2 | 2.8 | 1.3 |
| Wrist | | 1.6 | .7 | 2.2 | .6 |
| Hand—Finger | | 4.6 | 3.1 | 1.1 | 2.0 |
| LOWER EXTREMITIES | Gross | 6.2 | 3.5 | 3.9 | 5.2 |
| Pelvis | | 0 | .1 | .6 | .1 |
| Femur | | .5 | .1 | .6 | .2 |
| Patella | | .5 | .3 | 0 | 0 |
| Tibia and Fibula | | 1.0 | 1.1 | 1.1 | 1.4 |
| Ankle | | 1.6 | .3 | .5 | .9 |
| Foot—Toe | | 2.6 | 1.6 | 1.1 | 2.6 |
| Late Effects of Fractures | | 0 | 0 | .5 | .1 |

TABLE 133. *(Concluded)*

| DIAGNOSIS | | NUMBER OF MEMBERS WITH INDICATED DIAGNOSIS PER 1,000 EXPOSURE YEARS, INCLUDING DEPENDENTS | | | |
|---|---|---|---|---|---|
| | | MALE | | FEMALE | |
| | | *Professional, Executive and Sales* | *Blue Collar* | *Professional, Executive and Sales* | *Blue Collar* |
| *Injuries (Cont'd)* | | | | | |
| Dislocations | | 2.6 | 2.1 | 2.2 | 1.6 |
| Sprains and Strains | | 69.3 | 47.4 | 56.8 | 40.2 |
| Head Injuries (Other than Fractures) | | 9.2 | 13.5 | 7.8 | 7.4 |
| Internal Injuries | | 0 | .3 | 0 | .2 |
| Lacerations and Open Wounds | | 37.0 | 34.4 | 29.5 | 25.7 |
| Superficial Injuries | | 12.8 | 9.9 | 12.2 | 9.3 |
| Foreign Body | | 5.7 | 3.8 | 6.1 | 3.8 |
| Contusions | | 32.9 | 22.8 | 20.1 | 22.6 |
| Complications of Surgical and Medical Procedures | | 6.7 | 5.0 | 7.8 | 7.4 |
| Other | | 6.7 | 6.0 | 3.9 | 4.5 |
| XIX | Gross | 6.1 | 4.1 | 3.3 | 3.3 |
| Congenital Malformations | Net | 6.1 | 4.1 | 3.3 | 3.3 |
| XX | Gross | 0 | 1.0 | 1.1 | 1.0 |
| Certain Diseases of Early Infancy | Net | 0 | 1.0 | 1.1 | 1.0 |
| XXI | Gross | 64.7 | 57.7 | 72.4 | 76.0 |
| Symptoms, Senility and Ill-Defined Conditions | Net | 61.6 | 53.7 | 67.9 | 69.5 |
| Symptoms Referrable to Nervous System | | 2.6 | 7.5 | 8.9 | 8.2 |
| Symptoms Referrable to Cardiovascular System | | 6.7 | 4.2 | 5.6 | 8.6 |
| Symptoms Referrable to Respiratory System | | 14.4 | 13.7 | 8.9 | 10.3 |
| Symptoms Referrable to Upper and Lower Gastrointestinal System | | 10.3 | 8.2 | 11.7 | 12.3 |
| Symptoms Referrable to Urinary System | | 3.6 | 3.1 | 1.7 | 3.4 |
| Pain in Back | | 4.1 | 4.0 | 7.2 | 5.6 |
| Other Referrable Symptoms (Not Elsewhere Classified) | | 8.2 | 7.5 | 12.8 | 8.6 |
| Headache | | 9.2 | 5.2 | 5.6 | 9.8 |
| Other Ill-Defined Diseases | | 5.6 | 4.3 | 10.0 | 9.2 |
| XXII | Gross | 170.5 | 148.0 | 186.5 | 165.7 |
| Supplementary Classifications | Net | 169.5 | 143.9 | 183.2 | 161.6 |
| General Medical Examinations (Including Immunizations) | | 99.1 | 61.4 | 118.0 | 76.6 |
| Well Baby and Child Care (Including Immunizations) | | 59.1 | 57.6 | 54.6 | 61.7 |
| Other | | 12.3 | 29.0 | 13.9 | 27.4 |
| XXIII | Gross | 140.2 | 97.8 | 177.1 | 133.0 |
| Undetermined Classifications | | | | | |

* Gross rate is based on sum of patients reported for each component of a category; this represents duplicate count of persons treated for more than one condition in that category.
† Net rate is based on number of patients with *any* condition listed for a specified category.

conditions (blue-collar female rate about a fourth higher), anemias (blue-collar female rate about 70 per cent higher), sciatica (blue-collar female rate nearly triple), gastroenteritis and colitis (blue-collar female rate nearly 30 per cent higher).

No hypotheses as to the reasons for these findings are offered or even attempted. The usual cautionary reservation as to conclusions based on one year's multivariate analysis may be particularly applicable here.

### Category 4. No Class Differences

Although the incidence of treated hay fever was nearly 50 per cent higher for both males and females of the professional-executive-sales class, as compared with the blue-collar group, the incidence of asthma was practically identical in the two occupation categories.

Examples of other conditions showing little or no evidence of class differences include ear disorders, acute coronary occlusion, urinary tract conditions, disorders of veins and arteries.

# Chapter 17

# DIAGNOSIS AND TREATMENT:
# STUDIES OF PATIENT CARE

The title of this chapter is not intended to imply that the care of patients can be electronically or otherwise evaluated from insurance records. The limitations of records are quickly evident when the challenge involves determinations of medical care adequacy. This is particularly true in the absence of quantitative standards or norms; but if and when such standards are developed for measurable aspects of medical care, the limitless number of unmeasurable variables affecting the care of individual cases will always circumscribe the range of value judgments entrustable to record readers.

Thus, given minimum standards of adequacy for specified services in relation to specified diagnoses, computers could "kick out" cases falling below the minima; they would be able to report, for example, that of a thousand diabetics, such and such per cent apparently received inadequate amounts of such and such services. But they could not assume the absence of circumstances satisfactorily explaining the apparent inadequacies; nor could they infer that the care received by other cases was good merely on the basis that it met selected criteria.

What records and computers can do is to describe experience with respect to quantifiable components of medical care. When such descriptions relate treatment to diagnosis, they may be of value to qualitative studies, if only as an informed point of departure for further investigation. This observation applies particularly to ambulatory care, where the characteristic confusion and frustration besetting evaluative efforts may in some degree be attributable to lack of data. Since the bulk of ambulatory care is still provided by physicians practicing from private offices, insurance plans covering office and home services should be able to fill part of this information vacuum.

GHI's initial explorations have involved two different approaches to data retrieval programs relating patient care and diagnosis. The first deals with aggregates and averages of measured services associated with each diagnosis; the resulting tabulations contrast average services for one diagnosis with averages for another. In the second approach, individual case listings for selected diagnoses permit comparisons of treatment, by type of physician if desired, for different individuals with the same diagnosis. This approach also integrates diseases and physicians on a patient basis.

## Average Utilization of Principal Types of Service, by Diagnosis

Average services are stated per hundred cases of each diagnosis, rather than per case, to minimize the number of fractional entries. Service rates presented in Table 134 are arithmetic averages derived by dividing the aggregate number of services of each type recorded per diagnosis by the number of cases of that diagnosis, and multiplying by 100.

Although some of the entries appear questionable, much of the data falls within the limits of credibility at least in the sense that volume listed for each type of service is proportionately greater where expected—e.g. more home calls for infective diseases, more laboratory tests for hepatitis, diabetes. Nevertheless, the table is included here primarily to illustrate the possibilities and boundaries of this electronic approach to ambulatory treatment analysis, rather than for content. Cross checking and amplification of source data would be desirable next steps, if this first step were deemed promising enough to warrant expenditures for non-electronic data collection and appraisal.

Theoretically, the analytic process used could be developed in greater detail and depth with respect to type and source of service, and in combination with disease expectancy rates could eventually be applied to the derivation of annual service expectancy rates.

## TABLE 134. Utilization of Principal Types of Service, by Diagnosis

| DIAGNOSIS | NUMBER OF SPECIFIED OUT-OF-HOSPITAL SERVICES PER 100 CASES | | | | | | | HOSPITAL ADMISSIONS PER 100 CASES | | |
| --- | --- | --- | --- | --- | --- | --- | --- | --- | --- | --- |
| | OFFICE VISITS* | | Home Visits | Surgical Procedures | Consultations | Diagnostic x-rays | Laboratory Tests† | TOTAL‡ | Surgical | Medical |
| | G.P. | Spec. | | | | | | | | |
| *Infective and Parasitic Diseases* | 77.7 | 19.7 | 94.0 | .5 | .9 | 1.2 | 8.8 | .8 | — | .8 |
| Streptococcal Sore Throat | 91.4 | 13.7 | 110.5 | .1 | .1 | .1 | 9.5 | .5 | — | .5 |
| Measles | 35.2 | 5.6 | 130.6 | 0 | 0 | 0 | .7 | 0 | 0 | 0 |
| Rubella (German Measles) | 44.3 | 7.8 | 94.6 | .1 | 0 | 0 | 1.9 | .1 | — | .1 |
| Chicken Pox | 32.0 | 12.3 | 90.2 | 0 | 0 | 0 | 0 | 0 | — | 0 |
| Mumps | 62.3 | 11.6 | 85.6 | .7 | .7 | 1.4 | .7 | 0 | — | 0 |
| Infectious Hepatitis | 257.1 | 28.6 | 78.6 | 7.2 | 7.1 | 21.4 | 300.0 | 35.7 | — | 35.7 |
| Glandular Fever (Infectious Mononucleosis) | 112.5 | 76.6 | 82.8 | 0 | 3.1 | 4.7 | 159.4 | 9.4 | — | 9.4 |
| Intestinal Virus | 88.9 | 19.7 | 101.7 | .3 | .5 | .6 | 5.4 | .8 | — | .8 |
| Dermatophytoses | 109.7 | 55.8 | 12.1 | 4.4 | 5.2 | .8 | 11.6 | 0 | — | 0 |
| Other | 131.6 | 56.6 | 46.2 | 2.1 | 5.5 | 12.2 | 20.8 | 2.4 | — | 2.4 |
| *Neoplasms* | 42.1 | 42.0 | 9.5 | 36.8 | 8.2 | 7.7 | 21.3 | 29.1 | 24.5 | 4.6 |
| Malignant Neoplasms | 62.0 | 89.1 | 31.5 | 18.1 | 6.9 | 19.2 | 34.1 | 50.7 | 38.4 | 12.3 |
| Digestive System (Including Mouth) | 59.0 | 84.6 | 82.0 | 12.8 | 2.6 | 10.3 | 5.1 | 66.7 | 53.9 | 12.8 |
| Respiratory System | 46.7 | 130.0 | 36.7 | 10.0 | 20.0 | 33.3 | 10.0 | 83.3 | 53.3 | 30.0 |
| Breast | 67.4 | 86.9 | 37.0 | 4.3 | 6.5 | 28.3 | 43.5 | 50.0 | 41.3 | 8.7 |
| Female Genital Organs | 38.1 | 66.7 | 0 | 14.3 | 9.5 | 4.7 | 47.6 | 76.2 | 71.4 | 4.8 |
| Male Genital Organs | 145.4 | 218.2 | 54.5 | 0 | 0 | 27.3 | 18.2 | 100.0 | 72.7 | 27.3 |
| Urinary System | 0 | 154.6 | 0 | 54.5 | 0 | 45.5 | 72.7 | 72.7 | 72.7 | 0 |
| Skin | 15.6 | 78.1 | 0 | 62.5 | 0 | 3.1 | 12.5 | 28.1 | 28.1 | 0 |
| Eye | 0 | 50.0 | 50.0 | 0 | 0 | 0 | 0 | 50.0 | 50.0 | 0 |
| Nervous System (Including Brain) | 50.0 | 137.5 | 0 | 0 | 0 | 50.0 | 0 | 25.0 | 12.5 | 12.5 |
| Endocrine Glands | 33.3 | 77.8 | 0 | 0 | 11.1 | 0 | 11.1 | 0 | 0 | 0 |
| Bone | 0 | 0 | 0 | 0 | 25.0 | 25.0 | 0 | 25.0 | 0 | 25.0 |

*Neoplasms (Cont'd)*
*Malignant Neoplasms (Cont'd)*

| | | | | | | | | | |
|---|---|---|---|---|---|---|---|---|---|
| Lymphosarcoma | 100.0 | 0 | 0 | 0 | 0 | 0 | 25.0 | 25.0 | 0 |
| Hodgkin's Disease | 125.0 | 0 | 0 | 0 | 125.0 | 125.0 | 25.0 | 25.0 | 0 |
| Other Lymphoma | 150.0 | 50.0 | 0 | 0 | 0 | 16.7 | 66.7 | 33.4 | 33.3 |
| Multiple Myeloma | 0 | 350.0 | 0 | 0 | 0 | 0 | 100.0 | 0 | 100.0 |
| Leukemia | 190.0 | 260.0 | 20.0 | 30.0 | 30.0 | 370.0 | 40.0 | 0 | 40.0 |
| Not Elsewhere Classfied | 81.1 | 24.4 | 24.3 | 5.4 | 8.1 | 2.7 | 16.2 | 10.8 | 5.4 |
| Benign Neoplasms | 37.6 | 0 | 42.6 | 8.0 | 4.8 | 18.2 | 24.9 | 22.1 | 2.8 |
| Mouth | 63.2 | 15.8 | 29.0 | 7.9 | 0 | 2.6 | 26.3 | 23.7 | 2.6 |
| Rectum | 6.5 | 6.5 | 93.5 | 0 | 12.9 | 25.8 | 41.9 | 29.0 | 12.9 |
| Breast | 33.8 | 54.4 | 5.9 | 5.9 | 1.4 | 10.3 | 42.6 | 39.7 | 2.9 |
| Female Genital Organs | 52.4 | 42.3 | 16.7 | 9.8 | 2.8 | 35.0 | 39.4 | 36.9 | 2.5 |
| Skin | 31.6 | 22.9 | 67.7 | 6.2 | 2.6 | 9.8 | 13.5 | 11.6 | 1.9 |
| Other | 31.6 | 33.5 | 34.9 | 10.8 | 11.5 | 16.4 | 21.2 | 17.8 | 3.4 |
| Unspecified Neoplasms | 41.0 | 34.9 | 14.5 | 14.5 | 10.8 | 24.1 | 16.9 | 12.1 | 4.8 |
| Rectum | 40.0 | 0 | 60.0 | 0 | 0 | 0 | 20.0 | 20.0 | 0 |
| Breast | 23.1 | 15.4 | 0 | 15.4 | 0 | 0 | 7.7 | 7.7 | 0 |
| Female Genital Organs | 0 | 83.3 | 0 | 16.7 | 0 | 0 | 33.3 | 33.3 | 0 |
| Other | 49.2 | 37.3 | 15.2 | 15.2 | 15.3 | 33.9 | 16.9 | 10.1 | 6.8 |

*Allergic, Endocrine System, Metabolic and Nutritional Diseases*

| | | | | | | | | | |
|---|---|---|---|---|---|---|---|---|---|
| (Total) | 313.1 | 21.4 | .9 | 3.9 | 4.7 | 50.7 | 3.0 | .5 | 2.5 |
| Hay Fever | 312.1 | 9.2 | 1.1 | 7.6 | 1.3 | 14.1 | 0 | 0 | 0 |
| Asthma | 215.3 | 72.6 | .5 | 4.0 | 6.3 | 12.2 | 4.0 | 0 | 4.0 |
| Other Allergic Diseases | 226.1 | 16.1 | 0 | 5.9 | .9 | 7.6 | .5 | .2 | .3 |
| Diseases of Thyroid Gland | 304.5 | 6.7 | 1.1 | 4.3 | 7.0 | 85.8 | 6.5 | 3.8 | 2.7 |
| Diabetes Mellitus | 323.0 | 39.9 | 2.0 | 2.3 | 10.6 | 232.8 | 14.4 | 0 | 14.4 |
| Obesity (Not Otherwise Specified) | 429.5 | 3.7 | .9 | .9 | 3.3 | 36.8 | .5 | 0 | .5 |
| Other | 280.2 | 16.3 | 2.1 | 2.4 | 10.8 | 64.9 | 2.4 | .7 | 1.7 |

*Diseases of Blood and Blood Forming Organs*

| | | | | | | | | | |
|---|---|---|---|---|---|---|---|---|---|
| (Total) | 187.2 | 13.0 | 2.0 | 1.7 | 6.6 | 95.4 | 4.2 | .7 | 3.5 |
| Anemia | 191.4 | 12.3 | 1.3 | 1.3 | 6.9 | 84.7 | 2.8 | .2 | 2.6 |
| Other | 145.5 | 20.0 | 9.1 | 5.5 | 3.6 | 200.0 | 18.2 | 5.5 | 12.7 |

* † See footnotes at end of table.

## TABLE 134. (Cont'd)  Utilization of Principal Types of Service, by Diagnosis

| DIAGNOSIS | NUMBER OF SPECIFIED OUT-OF-HOSPITAL SERVICES PER 100 CASES | | | | | | | HOSPITAL ADMISSIONS PER 100 CASES | | |
|---|---|---|---|---|---|---|---|---|---|---|
| | OFFICE VISITS* | | Home Visits | Surgical Procedures | Consultations | Diagnostic x-rays | Laboratory Tests† | TOTAL† | Surgical | Medical |
| | G.P. | Spec. | | | | | | | | |
| *Mental, Psychoneurotic and Personality Disorders* | 60.6 | 33.2 | 8.2 | .6 | 26.5 | 4.1 | 34.1 | 6.5 | — | — |
| Chronic Brain Disorders | 23.1 | 23.1 | 15.4 | 0 | 46.1 | 46.2 | 176.9 | 7.7 | — | — |
| Psychoses | 35.7 | 19.0 | 2.4 | 2.4 | 26.2 | 0 | 0 | 9.5 | — | — |
| Psychophysiologic, Autonomic and Visceral Disorders | 100.0 | 25.0 | 0 | 0 | 12.5 | 0 | 12.5 | 0 | — | — |
| Psychoneuroses | 71.1 | 33.5 | 7.9 | .4 | 26.0 | 3.3 | 36.4 | 6.2 | — | — |
| Personality Disorders | 17.9 | 57.1 | 21.4 | 0 | 28.6 | 0 | 10.7 | 7.1 | — | — |
| Mental Deficiency | 42.9 | 42.8 | 0 | 0 | 14.3 | 0 | 14.3 | 0 | — | — |
| *Diseases of the Nervous System* | 160.1 | 52.3 | 40.1 | .6 | 9.2 | 6.9 | 18.8 | 8.6 | 2.3 | 6.3 |
| Multiple Sclerosis | 215.4 | 100.0 | 407.7 | 0 | 15.4 | 23.0 | 115.4 | 46.2 | 0 | 46.2 |
| Migraine | 111.9 | 31.5 | 62.2 | 0 | 11.9 | 1.4 | 11.9 | .7 | 0 | .7 |
| Epilepsy | 58.3 | 83.3 | 29.2 | 0 | 8.3 | 0 | 79.2 | 4.2 | 0 | 4.2 |
| Sciatica | 209.6 | 40.1 | 43.7 | 1.2 | 1.8 | 3.6 | 7.8 | 4.8 | 0 | 4.8 |
| Other | 160.6 | 57.7 | 28.0 | .6 | 10.4 | 8.8 | 19.0 | 10.6 | 3.5 | 7.1 |
| *Diseases of the Eye* | 46.4 | 66.1 | 4.1 | 7.9 | 30.5 | .5 | 2.3 | 4.3 | 3.9 | .4 |
| Conjunctivitis and Ophthalmia | 71.8 | 47.4 | 7.5 | .8 | 23.1 | 0 | 1.3 | .1 | 0 | .1 |
| Strabismus | 11.9 | 95.4 | .4 | 0 | 46.8 | .5 | 0 | 12.4 | 12.4 | 0 |
| Cataract | 6.2 | 87.5 | 0 | 0 | 30.0 | 1.3 | 1.3 | 45.0 | 43.8 | 1.2 |
| Glaucoma | 13.8 | 221.8 | 2.3 | 0 | 26.4 | 1.2 | 9.2 | 10.3 | 9.2 | 1.1 |
| Detachment of Retina | 0 | 166.7 | 0 | 0 | 0 | 0 | 0 | 66.7 | 50.0 | 16.7 |
| Other | 33.8 | 60.9 | 1.8 | 19.7 | 35.4 | .8 | 3.6 | 2.0 | 1.4 | .6 |
| *Diseases of the Ear* | 106.2 | 50.0 | 46.5 | 2.4 | 6.0 | .6 | 7.0 | 1.6 | 1.0 | .6 |
| Otitis Externa | 99.2 | 44.0 | 14.6 | 6.7 | 8.6 | 0 | 2.1 | .5 | 0 | .5 |
| Otitis Media | 112.3 | 51.3 | 63.8 | 1.6 | 3.5 | .2 | 3.3 | .7 | .4 | .3 |
| Deafness | 22.2 | 122.2 | 0 | 0 | 33.3 | 6.7 | 51.1 | 0 | 0 | 0 |
| Other | 96.8 | 44.5 | 13.5 | 2.6 | 10.3 | 2.0 | 18.5 | 5.2 | 3.5 | 1.7 |

340

| | 200.8 | 74.9 | 40.0 | 7.8 | 3.8 | 9.7 | 74.2 | 11.1 | 3.7 | 7.4 |
|---|---|---|---|---|---|---|---|---|---|---|
| *Diseases of the Circulatory System* | | | | | | | | | | |
| Rheumatic Fever without Mention of Heart | 154.5 | 104.5 | 95.5 | 0 | 4.6 | 13.6 | 95.5 | 18.2 | 0 | 18.2 |
| Diseases of the Heart | 197.3 | 104.4 | 70.8 | .9 | 5.5 | 16.1 | 131.1 | 16.2 | 1.3 | 14.9 |
| Rheumatic Heart Disease | 240.7 | 164.4 | 113.6 | 1.7 | 11.9 | 32.2 | 164.4 | 22.9 | 7.6 | 15.3 |
| Arteriosclerotic Heart Disease | 201.3 | 150.2 | 75.9 | .7 | 8.0 | 16.4 | 188.0 | 14.7 | .3 | 14.4 |
| Acute Coronary Occlusion | 134.1 | 97.7 | 107.7 | 0 | 3.1 | 7.8 | 138.8 | 40.3 | 1.5 | 38.8 |
| Coronary Insufficiency | 215.5 | 67.9 | 95.9 | 1.5 | 1.9 | 18.5 | 150.9 | 17.7 | .4 | 17.3 |
| Angina Pectoris | 207.3 | 54.3 | 40.2 | .9 | 2.7 | 12.8 | 102.3 | 6.4 | 0 | 6.4 |
| Hypertensive Heart Disease | 204.7 | 101.7 | 41.3 | 0 | 1.2 | 9.3 | 61.0 | 6.4 | 0 | 6.4 |
| Other | 177.0 | 107.9 | 51.4 | 1.3 | 9.1 | 17.0 | 103.1 | 16.1 | 2.2 | 13.9 |
| Diseases of Veins and Arteries (Other than the Heart) | 203.1 | 58.3 | 22.5 | 11.6 | 2.8 | 6.2 | 42.4 | 8.2 | 5.0 | 3.2 |
| Hypertensive Diseases | 303.0 | 71.4 | 20.4 | 1.1 | 1.9 | 7.8 | 64.2 | 2.4 | .3 | 2.1 |
| Hypotension | 223.9 | 36.3 | 18.6 | 0 | 0 | .9 | 15.0 | 0 | 0 | 0 |
| Hemorrhoids | 69.6 | 28.3 | 5.0 | 56.3 | 1.7 | 6.5 | 33.5 | 16.7 | 16.3 | .4 |
| General Arteriosclerosis | 100.0 | 148.8 | 25.6 | 0 | 7.0 | 0 | 27.9 | 7.0 | 7.0 | 0 |
| Varicose Veins of Lower Extremities | 96.4 | 35.2 | 2.7 | 25.2 | 7.2 | 1.8 | 6.3 | 27.0 | 26.1 | .9 |
| Pulmonary Embolism and Infarction | 100.0 | 45.4 | 27.3 | 0 | 9.1 | 27.3 | 72.7 | 36.4 | 9.1 | 27.3 |
| Lymphadenitis | 89.0 | 24.1 | 36.9 | 1.8 | 2.4 | 0 | 9.5 | 5.7 | 1.8 | 3.9 |
| Other | 154.8 | 85.2 | 47.0 | 2.9 | 7.3 | 9.0 | 24.3 | 17.4 | 5.5 | 11.9 |
| *Diseases of the Respiratory System* | 107.4 | 28.4 | 72.2 | .7 | .9 | 3.1 | 5.8 | 2.5 | 1.7 | .8 |
| Acute Nasopharyngitis | 106.7 | 23.1 | 44.8 | .2 | .8 | 1.0 | 2.1 | .3 | 0 | .3 |
| Pharyngitis | 95.5 | 25.1 | 72.5 | .1 | .6 | .4 | 5.7 | .3 | 0 | .3 |
| Tonsillitis | 84.8 | 23.8 | 99.9 | .4 | .7 | .4 | 2.8 | 1.0 | .7 | .3 |
| Hypertrophy of Tonsils | 22.1 | 32.0 | 7.0 | 6.3 | 6.7 | .4 | 5.1 | 64.8 | 64.8 | 0 |
| Laryngitis and Tracheitis | 83.4 | 23.3 | 62.8 | .8 | 4.4 | .8 | 3.2 | 1.0 | .1 | .9 |
| Sinusitis | 126.3 | 51.2 | 32.1 | 7.7 | 4.0 | 7.0 | 11.7 | 1.0 | .6 | .4 |
| Influenza | 75.5 | 22.1 | 119.8 | 0 | 0 | .5 | 5.5 | .2 | 0 | .2 |
| Pneumonia | 132.3 | 32.3 | 215.4 | 0 | 1.1 | 25.1 | 9.7 | 19.2 | .4 | 18.8 |
| Bronchitis | 128.9 | 31.3 | 90.1 | 0 | .3 | 8.2 | 9.8 | .8 | .2 | .6 |
| Other Diseases of Upper Respiratory Tract | 119.1 | 27.9 | 69.0 | .5 | .4 | 1.2 | 4.3 | .7 | .5 | .2 |
| Diseases of Lungs | 126.5 | 74.5 | 53.4 | .4 | 4.3 | 33.7 | 24.4 | 14.0 | 3.2 | 10.8 |

TABLE 134 (*Cont'd*)  Utilization of Principal Types of Service, by Diagnosis

| DIAGNOSIS | NUMBER OF SPECIFIED OUT-OF-HOSPITAL SERVICES PER 100 CASES | | | | | | | HOSPITAL ADMISSIONS PER 100 CASES | | |
|---|---|---|---|---|---|---|---|---|---|---|
| | OFFICE VISITS* | | Home Visits | Surgical Procedures | Consultations | Diagnostic x-rays | Laboratory Tests† | TOTAL† | Surgical | Medical |
| | G.P. | Spec. | | | | | | | | |
| *Diseases of the Digestive System* | | | | | | | | | | |
| Stomatitis | 109.0 | 33.7 | 45.5 | 5.4 | 1.8 | 12.7 | 23.3 | 12.0 | 6.8 | 5.2 |
| | 110.6 | 14.2 | 22.7 | 2.1 | 2.9 | 0 | 7.1 | .7 | 0 | .7 |
| Other Diseases of Buccal Cavity and Esophagus | 82.0 | 28.5 | 19.0 | 3.5 | 3.5 | 4.0 | 13.5 | 3.5 | 1.5 | 2.0 |
| Ulcers | 232.7 | 81.9 | 26.3 | 4.0 | 2.6 | 44.0 | 63.1 | 23.1 | 5.9 | 17.2 |
| Gastritis and Duodenitis | 123.4 | 28.8 | 32.1 | 1.9 | 1.4 | 11.6 | 22.2 | 3.6 | .3 | 3.3 |
| Other Diseases of Stomach and Duodenum | 85.2 | 24.4 | 18.6 | 0 | 1.4 | 13.9 | 35.4 | 2.4 | .5 | 1.9 |
| Appendicitis | 45.4 | 9.2 | 20.4 | 0 | 2.8 | .9 | 2.8 | 78.7 | 70.4 | 8.3 |
| Hernia of Abdominal Cavity | 66.2 | 41.8 | 6.9 | 2.1 | 5.8 | 17.5 | 23.7 | 53.8 | 49.1 | 4.7 |
| Gastroenteritis and Colitis (Except Ulcerative) | 91.8 | 23.3 | 71.8 | 1.7 | .3 | 2.9 | 8.5 | 2.0 | 0 | 2.0 |
| Other Diseases of Intestines and Peritoneum | 102.3 | 37.2 | 18.6 | 30.5 | 3.4 | 20.1 | 32.2 | 17.3 | 9.0 | 8.3 |
| Diseases of Liver, Gall Bladder and Pancreas | 128.8 | 60.5 | 53.9 | 1.8 | 3.5 | 33.2 | 60.0 | 33.0 | 19.4 | 13.6 |
| Diseases of the Liver | 223.5 | 90.1 | 79.0 | 0 | 2.5 | 14.8 | 161.8 | 30.9 | 1.3 | 29.6 |
| Diseases of the Gall Bladder | 108.8 | 47.5 | 52.8 | 1.7 | 3.8 | 38.5 | 28.3 | 33.2 | 25.1 | 8.1 |
| Diseases of the Pancreas | 105.9 | 120.6 | 5.9 | 5.9 | 3.0 | 23.5 | 138.2 | 35.3 | 5.9 | 29.4 |
| *Diseases of the Urinary System* | 132.3 | 54.4 | 38.1 | 18.3 | 3.7 | 9.1 | 23.8 | 14.3 | 6.9 | 7.4 |
| Nephritis and Nephrosis | 190.0 | 85.0 | 60.0 | 0 | 5.0 | 2.5 | 67.5 | 15.0 | 0 | 15.0 |
| Cystitis | 153.9 | 48.6 | 33.1 | 9.0 | 2.6 | 3.8 | 18.5 | 7.5 | 3.3 | 4.2 |
| Other | 103.0 | 58.8 | 42.3 | 30.4 | 5.0 | 15.6 | 26.7 | 22.1 | 11.5 | 10.6 |
| *Diseases of the Male Genital Organs* | 144.9 | 87.3 | 11.0 | 12.8 | 11.3 | 10.7 | 28.7 | 20.3 | 18.8 | 1.5 |

| | | | | | | | | | |
|---|---|---|---|---|---|---|---|---|---|
| *Diseases of the Female Genital Organs and Breast* | 95.1 | 57.5 | 6.3 | 17.2 | 6.4 | 2.3 | 34.4 | 9.4 | 8.4 | 1.0 |
| Diseases of the Breast | 80.4 | 58.7 | 7.8 | 10.6 | 11.2 | 5.6 | 17.3 | 19.6 | 18.5 | 1.1 |
| Diseases of the Ovaries, Fallopian Tubes and Parametrium | 201.7 | 73.9 | 16.5 | 2.6 | 6.1 | 7.0 | 23.5 | 13.0 | 6.9 | 6.1 |
| Cervicitis | 60.8 | 38.2 | 3.0 | 59.0 | 3.5 | 1.5 | 44.1 | 7.1 | 6.6 | .5 |
| Vaginitis and Vulvitis | 113.6 | 75.3 | 3.7 | 6.1 | 5.9 | 0 | 28.1 | 1.1 | .4 | .7 |
| Menstrual Disorders | 85.1 | 56.0 | 8.1 | 1.5 | 6.6 | 1.0 | 24.1 | 10.0 | 9.5 | .5 |
| Menopausal Symptoms | 166.1 | 52.3 | 7.6 | 1.0 | 4.3 | 4.3 | 61.8 | 0 | 0 | 0 |
| Other | 60.8 | 69.5 | 7.1 | 8.4 | 10.6 | 3.8 | 31.6 | 23.7 | 21.5 | 2.2 |
| *Deliveries and Complications of Pregnancy, Childbirth and Puerperium* | 0 | 0 | 0 | .2 | .4 | .7 | 4.0 | 95.5 | — | — |
| Normal Deliveries | 0 | 0 | 0 | .1 | 0 | .6 | 3.9 | 97.6 | — | — |
| Complicated Deliveries | 0 | 0 | 0 | 0 | 15.4 | 0 | 0 | 30.8 | — | — |
| Abortion | 0 | 0 | 0 | 1.0 | 0 | 0 | 0 | 96.0 | — | — |
| Ectopic Pregnancy | 0 | 0 | 0 | 0 | 25.0 | 0 | 0 | 50.0 | — | — |
| Other | 0 | 0 | 0 | 0 | 0 | 16.7 | 50.0 | 50.0 | — | — |
| *Diseases of Skin and Subcutaneous Tissues* | 97.7 | 50.9 | 9.2 | 34.3 | 5.7 | 1.2 | 6.0 | 1.8 | .9 | .9 |
| Boil and Carbuncle | 118.5 | 35.2 | 12.6 | 39.6 | 1.8 | .2 | 2.6 | 1.6 | .8 | .8 |
| Cellulitis | 104.1 | 23.7 | 13.5 | 52.2 | 1.3 | 1.8 | 5.1 | 2.8 | .8 | 2.0 |
| Impetigo | 111.0 | 27.4 | 9.8 | .8 | 2.0 | .4 | 3.3 | 0 | 0 | 0 |
| Infectious Wart | 22.1 | 18.4 | 1.5 | 101.3 | 1.8 | 1.1 | .7 | 1.1 | .7 | .4 |
| Dermatitis | 120.8 | 73.5 | 9.8 | .6 | 9.8 | .3 | 6.1 | .2 | 0 | .2 |
| Acne | 75.2 | 117.3 | .5 | 96.2 | 15.4 | .5 | 2.8 | 0 | 0 | 0 |
| Sebaceous Cyst | 55.3 | 20.9 | 0 | 72.1 | 2.1 | .8 | 2.1 | 6.1 | 5.7 | .4 |
| Other | 99.8 | 62.7 | 10.5 | 18.9 | 7.2 | 2.3 | 11.4 | 3.0 | 1.5 | 1.5 |
| *Diseases of Bones and Organs of Movement* | 146.9 | 49.4 | 18.2 | 8.3 | 6.4 | 24.6 | 20.6 | 4.2 | 2.6 | 1.6 |
| Arthritis and Rheumatism | 190.0 | 59.6 | 21.8 | 3.8 | 2.7 | 24.4 | 37.7 | 1.5 | .3 | 1.2 |
| Osteomyelitis and Other Diseases of Bones and Joints | 105.8 | 56.8 | 18.7 | 5.5 | 16.5 | 46.8 | 16.8 | 17.1 | 8.6 | 8.5 |
| Synovitis, Bursitis and Tenosynovitis | 163.7 | 53.6 | 19.8 | 17.5 | 4.2 | 22.7 | 12.6 | 4.1 | 3.3 | .8 |
| Infective Myositis | 134.0 | 27.0 | 16.9 | 1.7 | 2.7 | 10.8 | 19.2 | .3 | 0 | .3 |
| Muscular Dystrophy | 0 | 100.0 | 0 | 0 | 20.0 | 20.0 | 0 | 40.0 | 20.0 | 20.0 |
| Scoliosis | 31.3 | 33.3 | 4.2 | 0 | 14.6 | 85.4 | 8.3 | 4.2 | 4.2 | 0 |
| Other Deformities | 22.8 | 58.9 | 5.5 | 13.9 | 26.1 | 28.9 | 1.1 | 7.2 | 7.2 | 0 |
| Other Diseases of Musculoskeletal System | 77.4 | 28.8 | 7.5 | 8.2 | 13.7 | 25.4 | 2.7 | 5.5 | 4.1 | 1.4 |

| DIAGNOSIS | NUMBER OF SPECIFIED OUT-OF-HOSPITAL SERVICES PER 100 CASES | | | | | | | HOSPITAL ADMISSIONS PER 100 CASES | | |
|---|---|---|---|---|---|---|---|---|---|---|
| | OFFICE VISITS * | | Home Visits | Surgical Procedures | Consultations | Diagnostic x-rays | Laboratory Tests † | TOTAL‡ | Surgical | Medical |
| | G.P. | Spec. | | | | | | | | |
| *Injuries and Adverse Effects of External Causes* | 119.2 | 34.7 | | 18.6 | | 20.6 | | 5.1 | 2.6 | 2.5 |
| Fractures | 47.6 | 35.4 | 13.8 | 50.5 | 2.8 | 70.7 | 3.5 | 19.9 | 15.7 | 4.2 |
| Skull and Face | 63.1 | 24.6 | 11.3 | 28.1 | 1.4 | 40.4 | 2.2 | 40.4 | 24.6 | 15.8 |
| Torso | 111.1 | 57.2 | 15.8 | 25.4 | 7.0 | 49.2 | 14.0 | 15.9 | 6.4 | 9.5 |
| Spine (Vertebral Column) | 122.2 | 66.7 | 33.3 | 5.6 | 0 | 44.4 | 3.2 | 50.0 | 16.7 | 33.3 |
| Ribs, Sternum and Larynx | 106.7 | 53.3 | 55.5 | 33.3 | 0 | 51.1 | 0 | 2.2 | 2.2 | 0 |
| Upper Extremities | 42.0 | 28.1 | 24.4 | 59.9 | 1.6 | 78.2 | 4.5 | 16.7 | 15.1 | 1.6 |
| Clavicle | 32.4 | 17.6 | 1.6 | 64.7 | 3.0 | 79.4 | .6 | 14.7 | 8.8 | 5.9 |
| Scapula | 0 | 125.0 | 8.8 | 25.0 | 0 | 75.0 | 0 | 25.0 | 25.0 | 0 |
| Humerus | 30.8 | 96.2 | 0 | 50.0 | 3.8 | 84.6 | 0 | 30.8 | 30.8 | 0 |
| Radius and Ulna | 21.3 | 26.6 | 3.8 | 60.6 | 1.1 | 86.2 | 0 | 29.8 | 28.7 | 1.1 |
| Wrist | 42.9 | 14.3 | 1.1 | 51.4 | 0 | 71.4 | 1.0 | 8.6 | 8.6 | 0 |
| Hand—Finger | 63.7 | 18.6 | 0 | 63.7 | 1.6 | 72.6 | 0 | 6.5 | 4.9 | 1.6 |
| Lower Extremities | 32.5 | 41.0 | 18.5 | 49.5 | 0 | 75.0 | .8 | 20.5 | 17.0 | 3.5 |
| Pelvis | 0 | 25.0 | 650.0 | 0 | 0 | 75.0 | 1.0 | 50.0 | 0 | 50.0 |
| Femur | 8.3 | 91.7 | 8.3 | 0 | 0 | 33.3 | 50.0 | 75.0 | 58.3 | 16.7 |
| Patella | 0 | 37.5 | 0 | 12.5 | 0 | 75.0 | 0 | 0 | 0 | 0 |
| Tibia and Fibula | 68.7 | 29.4 | 13.7 | 39.2 | 0 | 86.3 | 0 | 31.4 | 29.4 | 2.0 |
| Ankle | 6.5 | 74.2 | 0 | 54.8 | 0 | 71.0 | 0 | 25.8 | 22.6 | 3.2 |
| Foot—Toe | 28.7 | 30.9 | 3.2 | 64.9 | 0 | 75.5 | 0 | 6.4 | 5.3 | 1.1 |
| Late Effects of Fractures | 0 | 250.0 | 0 | 100.0 | 0 | 0 | 0 | 0 | 0 | 0 |
| Dislocations | 70.4 | 19.8 | 8.6 | 29.6 | 8.6 | 27.2 | 0 | 18.5 | 13.6 | 4.9 |
| Sprains and Strains | 162.9 | 38.4 | 18.0 | 1.6 | 4.0 | 22.7 | 4.9 | 2.7 | .1 | 2.6 |
| Head Injuries (Other than Fractures) | 96.6 | 24.0 | 16.7 | 27.8 | 3.0 | 12.0 | 5.1 | 8.8 | 1.1 | 7.7 |
| Internal Injuries | 33.3 | 33.3 | 8.4 | 0 | 0 | 0 | 33.3 | 41.7 | 41.7 | 0 |
| Lacerations and Open Wounds | 107.7 | 24.6 | 7.1 | 39.0 | 1.6 | 3.8 | .1 | 3.0 | 2.6 | .4 |
| Superficial Injury | 106.7 | 28.4 | 9.3 | 5.0 | 1.5 | 13.1 | 4.0 | 1.3 | .4 | .9 |
| Foreign Body | 38.4 | 18.6 | 1.8 | 61.0 | 5.8 | 8.1 | 0 | 2.9 | 1.7 | 1.2 |

*Injuries (Cont'd)*

| | | | | | | | | | | |
|---|---|---|---|---|---|---|---|---|---|---|
| Contusion | 135.1 | 30.6 | 17.4 | 5.6 | 1.8 | 24.3 | 1.7 | 3.0 | .5 | 2.5 |
| Complications of Surgical and Medical Procedures | 73.5 | 102.5 | 12.5 | 9.7 | 5.0 | 10.4 | 21.2 | 1.8 | 1.1 | .7 |
| Other | 135.9 | 46.8 | 23.6 | 4.6 | 3.0 | 1.7 | 1.3 | 6.3 | 1.3 | 5.0 |
| *Congenital Malformations* | 38.6 | 82.9 | 1.9 | 5.7 | 29.1 | 13.3 | 5.7 | 22.2 | 19.0 | 3.2 |
| *Certain Diseases of Early Infancy* | 48.7 | 53.9 | 20.5 | 0 | 5.1 | 5.1 | 51.3 | 56.4 | 7.7 | 48.7 |
| *Symptoms, Senility and Ill-Defined Conditions* | | | | | | | | | | |
| Symptoms Referrable to Nervous System | 84.0 | 33.4 | 19.1 | 6.5 | 8.3 | 11.3 | 37.4 | 1.4 | .3 | 1.1 |
| Symptoms Referrable to Cardiovascular System | 91.5 | 35.2 | 19.7 | .3 | 11.8 | 3.0 | 27.0 | 3.9 | .3 | 3.6 |
| Symptoms Referrable to Respiratory System | 112.3 | 34.3 | 24.3 | 1.5 | 3.0 | 8.2 | 66.8 | 3.0 | 0 | 3.0 |
| Symptoms Referrable to Upper and Lower Gastrointestinal System | 70.4 | 32.2 | 17.2 | 28.7 | 4.8 | 17.4 | 47.7 | 3.9 | .8 | 3.1 |
| Symptoms Referrable to Urinary System | 77.8 | 38.7 | 33.5 | 2.4 | 3.7 | 14.0 | 32.3 | 4.9 | .2 | 4.7 |
| Pain in Back | 58.8 | 34.5 | 37.8 | 5.0 | 8.4 | 11.8 | 21.8 | 15.1 | 5.0 | 10.1 |
| Other Referrable Symptoms, N.E.C. | 87.7 | 30.2 | 7.1 | 2.4 | 4.7 | 32.5 | 16.5 | 1.4 | 0 | 1.4 |
| Headache | 85.0 | 28.0 | 16.1 | 2.4 | 5.9 | 5.6 | 22.3 | 6.5 | 1.9 | 4.6 |
| Other Ill-Defined Diseases | 82.7 | 31.6 | 8.5 | .3 | 27.4 | 4.9 | 26.7 | 0 | 0 | 0 |
| | 92.2 | 35.0 | 10.8 | .7 | 7.4 | 6.7 | 63.3 | 1.4 | .7 | .7 |
| *Supplementary Classifications* | | | | | | | | | | |
| General Medical Care (Including Immunizations) | .2 | 1.4 | — | 9.1 | .5 | 16.4 | 142.3 | — | — | — |
| Well Baby and Child Care (Including Immunizations) | 0 | 0 | 0 | 2.0 | .2 | 5.3 | 35.8 | — | — | — |
| | 0 | 0 | 0 | — | .1 | .2 | 6.5 | — | — | — |
| Diagnostic Screening | 1.3 | 12.5 | 0 | 74.5 | 2.7 | 122.9 | 1096.5 | — | — | — |
| Other | 4.5 | 1.1 | 1.1 | 0 | 6.8 | 18.0 | 153.9 | — | — | — |
| *Undetermined Classifications* | 25.5 | 15.7 | 5.6 | 2.8 | 3.1 | 40.5 | 109.9 | 2.6 | 1.5 | 1.1 |

* Excluding visits made in connection with surgical and obstetrical care.

† Excluding routine urinalysis and hemoglobin tests.

‡ Including surgical, medical, obstetrical and psychiatric.

## Comparison of Treatment for Cases with
## Same Diagnosis

In the second type of patient care studies, the retrieval process adopts a personalized approach to data analysis, operating as case-finder-recorder and becoming in effect an electronic method of composing individual (or family) insured-medical-care histories.

Theoretically, the method can be applied to longitudinal studies extending back over the years of the patient's insurance coverage. The program employed here retrieved only data recorded during the study year.

A number of diagnoses were selected for the experiment (ulcer, cystitis, gastroenteritis-colitis, sciatica, diabetes, hay fever, asthma, obesity, anemia, arthritis, arteriosclerotic heart disease, hypertensive heart disease).

A few patients per each of these diagnoses were electronically selected from the 10 per cent of the study sample which accounted for 39 per cent of all claims. Their records for the year, and those for other members of their families, were then compiled by computer.

Information was retrieved as to patient age, sex, relationship, family size, subscriber occupation, year of enrollment; all diagnoses recorded during the year; type, number and date of services rendered; procedures performed (where type of service was surgical, diagnostic x-ray or laboratory procedure); and identity, type, field of practice and qualifications of treating physician(s).

With its individual patient orientation, this substudy was the only one of the project series to permit examination of the number, sequence and association of diagnoses reported for the individual, as well as the number and types of physicians performing the various services listed.

This approach clearly has intrinsic advantages for patient-oriented medical care studies. In addition to serving as a case-finder for studies of patients with specified diagnoses, it demonstrates its superiority over the household interview with respect to reporting of clinical medical terminology, continuity, and identification of service sources. In comparison with studies of individual physician practices, it follows the patient in his travels from one physician to another—an important aspect of the data (evidenced by the frequent physician-shifting listed) in the accompanying histories. Each source—insurance records, interviews with patients and physicians' records—has its unique attributes and each can supplement the others to produce a more complete understanding of the medical processes in which patients engage.

The retrieval program achieved the immediate substudy objective of demonstrating the feasibility of this approach to patient care analysis, electronically speaking. As for substantive usefulness of results, this would depend on reviewer orientation. Etiologists should find interest, or support for existing theories, in combinations of diseases reported for individual patients. Medical care planners and medical insurers seeking evidence of underuse or overuse can probably detect some of each. Information on ambulatory care could serve as a starting point for qualitative studies.

The advantages of retrieving integrated pictures of individual patient care and illness over periods of a year or more exact their price in the form of necessarily cumbersome presentations. These require, in turn, a long, analytic review to determine the presence or absence of significant patterns. The cases selected for presentation in the following pages, from several hundred originally sampled, are believed sufficient to demonstrate both the advantages and the limitations of this approach.

## Examples of Individual Utilization Histories Recorded During Study Year, Showing All Diagnoses, Services, and Treating Physicians Reported for Patients with Selected Diagnoses

DIAGNOSIS SELECTOR: **ANEMIA** — Female Subscriber
RELATIONSHIP AND SEX:
AGE: 34
SUBSCRIBER OCCUPATION: Professional
FAMILY SIZE: 2
YEAR OF ENROLLMENT: 1961

| Diagnosis | Type of Service | Procedure Description | Visits: Office | Visits: Home | Physician No.[1] | Physician Practice[2] | Physician Qual.[3] | FDS[4] | LDS[4] |
|---|---|---|---|---|---|---|---|---|---|
| Anemia | Medical | General Medical Care | 3 | | 1 | Pulm. Dis. | F | 1/3 | 1/20 |
| | Laboratory | EKG | | | | | | | |
| Other Ill-Defined Diseases (Debility and Undue Fatigue) | Medical | General Medical Care | 1 | | | | | 1/31 | |
| Hypotension | Laboratory | Blood, Complete Count | | | | | | | |
| Anemia | Medical | General Medical Care | 6 | | | | | 2/7 | 3/19 |
| | Medical | Injections of Vitamins or Hormones | 1 | | | | | 4/7 | |
| Other Diseases of Upper Respiratory Tract | Medical | General Medical Care | 2 | | | | | 9/10 | 9/12 |
| | Laboratory | Blood, Complete Count | | | | | | | |
| | Laboratory | Blood, Red Cell Count | | | | | | | |
| Anemia | Medical | General Medical Care | 3 | | | | | 9/15 | 10/1 |
| | Laboratory | Blood, Complete Count | | | | | | | |
| | Laboratory | Blood, Sedimentation Rate | | | | | | | |
| | Laboratory | Blood, White Cell Count | | | | | | | |
| | Medical | Injection of Vitamins and Hormones | 1 | | | | | 10/15 | 11/12 |

[1] Each different physician is listed with a different number.

[2] GPMD = General Practitioner M.D.; GPDO = Doctor of Osteopathy.

[3] Highest Qualification: D = Diplomate of Specialty Board, F = Fellow of Specialty College, S = State Workmen's Compensation Specialty Rating.

[4] First date of service, last date of service. Includes service rendered previous year when claim received during study year.

Note: Where physician information and service dates are omitted, previous entry applies.

## Examples of Individual Utilization Histories Recorded During Study Year, Showing All Diagnoses, Services, and Treating Physicians Reported for Patients with Selected Diagnoses

| | | |
|---|---|---|
| DIAGNOSIS SELECTOR: ANEMIA | AGE: 50 | FAMILY SIZE: 2 |
| RELATIONSHIP AND SEX: Female Spouse | SUBSCRIBER OCCUPATION: Executive | YEAR OF ENROLLMENT: 1959 |

| Diagnosis | Type of Service | Procedure Description | Visits — Office | Visits — Home | Physician No.[1] | Physician Practice[2] | Physician Qual.[3] | FDS[4] | LDS[4] |
|---|---|---|---|---|---|---|---|---|---|
| Benign Neoplasm of Female Genital Organs | Medical | General Medical Care | 1 | | 1 | Gyn. and Obst. | S | 5/24 | 5/26 |
| | Anesthesia | D and C | | | 2 | Anesthesiology | F | | |
| | Surgery in Hospital | D and C | | | 1 | Gyn. and Obst. | S | | |
| | Anesthesia | Panhysterectomy | | | 2 | Anesthesiology | F | | |
| | Surgery in Hospital | Panhysterectomy | | | 1 | Gyn. and Obst. | S | | |
| Anemia | Medical in Hospital | General Medical Care | 3 | | 3 | GPMD | | 5/24 | 6/11 |
| | Medical | General Medical Care | | | | | | 6/19 | 7/3 |
| | Laboratory | Blood, Complete Count | | | | | | | |
| | Laboratory | Blood, Sedimentation Rate | | | | | | | |
| | Laboratory | Blood, Serum Iron and Iron Binding Capacity (Twice) | | | | | | | |
| | Medical | General Medical Care | 2 | | | | | 7/31 | 8/21 |
| | Laboratory | Blood, Sedimentation Rate | | | | | | | |
| | Laboratory | Blood, Complete Count | | | | | | | |
| | Laboratory | Blood, Serum Iron and Iron Binding Capacity | | | | | | | |
| Sprains and Strains | Medical | General Medical Care | 1 | | | | | 9/25 | |
| | X-ray | Ribs | | | | | | | |
| | Laboratory | EKG | | | | | | | |
| Anemia | Medical | General Medical Care | 1 | | | | | 10/9 | |
| | Medical | General Medical Care | 1 | | | | | 11/13 | |
| | Laboratory | Blood, Sedimentation Rate | | | | | | | |
| | Laboratory | Blood, Complete Count | | | | | | | |
| Diseases of Thyroid Gland | Medical | General Medical Care | 1 | | | | | 12/11 | |
| | Laboratory | Basal Metabolic Rate | | | | | | | |

Examples of Individual Utilization Histories Recorded During Study Year, Showing All Diagnoses, Services, and Treating Physicians Reported for Patients with Selected Diagnoses

| | | |
|---|---|---|
| DIAGNOSIS SELECTOR: | ARTERIOSCLEROTIC HEART DISEASE | FAMILY SIZE: 2 |
| RELATIONSHIP AND SEX: | Female Spouse | YEAR OF ENROLLMENT: 1962 |
| AGE: | 57 | |
| SUBSCRIBER OCCUPATION: | Blue-Collar | |

| Diagnosis | Type of Service | Procedure Description | Visits | | Physician | | | FDS[4] | LDS[4] |
|---|---|---|---|---|---|---|---|---|---|
| | | | Office | Home | No.[1] | Practice[2] | Qual.[3] | | |
| Bronchitis | Medical | General Medical Care | 7 | | 1 | GPMD | | 11/14 | 1/16 |
| Dermatitis | Radiation Therapy | Superficial X-ray Therapy (4 Treatments) | | | 2 | Dermatology | D | 2/4 | 5/19 |
| Arteriosclerotic Heart Disease | Medical | General Medical Care | 1 | | 3 | Internal Med. | D | 5/19 | |
| | Laboratory | Basal Metabolic Rate | | | | | | | |
| | Laboratory | EKG | | | | | | | |
| | Laboratory | Blood, Sugar | | | | | | | |
| | Laboratory | Blood, Protein-Bound Iodine | | | | | | | |
| | Laboratory | Blood, Complete Count | | | | | | | |
| | Laboratory | Blood, Cholesterol | | | | | | | |
| Dermatitis | Medical | Foot Care | 2 | | 2 | Dermatology | D | 5/22 | 5/26 |
| | Radiation Therapy | Superficial X-ray Therapy | | | | | | 6/3 | 6/21 |
| Arteriosclerotic Heart Disease | Medical in Hospital | General Medical Care | | | 3 | Internal Med. | D | 6/9 | |
| | Medical | General Medical Care | 7 | | | | | 6/30 | 9/9 |
| Dermatitis | Radiation Therapy | Superficial X-ray Therapy (3 Treatments) | | | 2 | Dermatology | D | 7/20 | 9/9 |
| Angina Pectoris | Medical | General Medical Care | 1 | | 3 | Internal Med. | D | 9/28 | |
| Arteriosclerotic Heart Disease | Medical | General Medical Care | 2 | | | | | 9/28 | 10/13 |
| | Laboratory | Blood, Icterus Index | | | | | | 9/28 | |
| | Medical in Hospital | General Medical Care | | | | | | 10/13 | 10/21 |
| | Medical | General Medical Care | 2 | | | | | 10/27 | 11/6 |
| Diseases of Gall Bladder | Anesthesia | Biliary Tract, Cholecystectomy | | | 4 | GPMD | | 11/13 | |
| | Surgery in Hospital | Biliary Tract, Cholecystectomy | | | 5 | General Surg. | D | 11/13 | 11/23 |

## Examples of Individual Utilization Histories Recorded During Study Year, Showing All Diagnoses, Services, and Treating Physicians Reported for Patients with Selected Diagnoses

| DIAGNOSIS SELECTOR: | ARTHRITIS | | AGE: | 49 | FAMILY SIZE: | 2 |
|---|---|---|---|---|---|---|
| RELATIONSHIP AND SEX: | Female Subscriber | | SUBSCRIBER OCCUPATION: | Other White-Collar | YEAR OF ENROLLMENT: | 1959 |

| Diagnosis | Type of Service | Procedure Description | Visits | | PHYSICIAN | | | FDS[4] | LDS[4] |
|---|---|---|---|---|---|---|---|---|---|
| | | | Office | Home | No.[1] | Practice[2] | Qual.[3] | | |
| Arthritis | Medical | General Medical Care | 3 | | 1 | Cardiology | F | 3/17 | 4/3 |
| | X-ray | Spine, Lumbo-Sacro, Including Pelvis | | | | | | | |
| | Laboratory | Blood, Complete Count | | | | | | | |
| | Laboratory | Blood, Uric Acid | | | | | | | |
| | Laboratory | Blood, Sedimentation Rate | | | | | | | |
| | Laboratory | Blood, C-Reactive Protein | | | | | | | |
| | Laboratory | EKG | | | | | | | |
| | Laboratory | Blood, Latex Immobilization | | | | | | | |
| | Laboratory | Blood, Antistreptolysin Titer | | | | | | | |
| | Laboratory | Blood, Differential Count | | | | | | | |
| | X-ray | Spine, Lumbar | | | 2 | Radiology | S | 3/26 | |
| Other Diseases of the Eye (Retina, Optic Nerve and Blindness) | Medical | General Medical Care | 1 | | 3 | Ophthalmology | D | 3/31 | 4/4 |
| | Specialist Consultation | Ophthalmology | | | | | | | |
| Arthritis | Medical | General Medical Care | 3 | | 1 | Cardiology | F | 4/9 | 4/18 |
| Other Diseases of the Eye (Retina, Optic Nerve and Blindness) | Medical | General Medical Care | 3 | | 3 | Ophthalmology | D | 4/21 | 7/13 |
| Menstrual Disorders | Medical | General Medical Care | 1 | | 4 | GPMD | D | 9/4 | |

Examples of Individual Utilization Histories Recorded During Study Year,
Showing All Diagnoses, Services, and Treating Physicians
Reported for Patients with Selected Diagnoses

| DIAGNOSIS SELECTOR: | ASTHMA | AGE: | 13 | | FAMILY SIZE: | 5 |
| RELATIONSHIP AND SEX: | Son | SUBSCRIBER OCCUPATION: | Executive | | YEAR OF ENROLLMENT: | 1959 |

| | | | Visits | | Physician | | | | |
| Diagnosis | Type of Service | Procedure Description | Office | Home | No.[1] | Practice [2] | Qual.[3] | FDS [4] | LDS [4] |
|---|---|---|---|---|---|---|---|---|---|
| Infectious Wart | Surgery out of Hospital | Electro-Cauterization or Fulguration of Local Lesion, Large | | | | | | | |
| Asthma | Medical | General Medical Care | | 4 | 1 | GPMD | | 10/21 | 12/4 |
| | Medical | Allergy Care | 1 | | 2 | Allergy | F | 2/21 | 2/28 |
| | Specialist Consultation | Allergy | | | | | | | |
| Other Diseases of Upper Respiratory Tract | Medical | General Medical Care | | 1 | 1 | GPMD | | 3/12 | 3/30 |
| Hay Fever | Medical | Allergy Care | 2 | | | | | 3/23 | 4/25 |
| Other Allergic Diseases | Medical | General Medical Care | 4 | | | | | 4/6 | 5/29 |
| Hay Fever | Medical | Allergy Care | 5 | | | | | 5/2 | 6/29 |
| Other Allergic Diseases | Medical | Allergy Care | 2 | | | | | 6/1 | 6/29 |
| | Laboratory | Blood, Sugar | | | | | | | |
| General Medical Examination | Preventive | Immunization, NEC | 1 | | | | | 10/8 | |
| | Laboratory | Blood, Complete Count | | | | | | | |

352

## Examples of Individual Utilization Histories Recorded During Study Year, Showing All Diagnoses, Services, and Treating Physicians Reported for Patients with Selected Diagnoses

| | | |
|---|---|---|
| DIAGNOSIS SELECTOR: | DIABETES MELLITUS | FAMILY SIZE: 4 |
| RELATIONSHIP AND SEX: | Female Spouse | |
| AGE: | 40 | YEAR OF ENROLLMENT: 1960 |
| SUBSCRIBER OCCUPATION: | Blue-Collar | |

| Diagnosis | Type of Service | Procedure Description | Visits Office | Visits Home | Physician No.[1] | Physician Practice[2] | Physician Qual.[3] | FDS[4] | LDS[4] |
|---|---|---|---|---|---|---|---|---|---|
| Bronchitis | Medical | General Medical Care | 4 | 3 | 1 | GPMD | | 3/10 | 4/24 |
| Conjunctivitis | Specialist Consultation | Ophthalmology | | | 2 | Ophthalmology | D | 4/17 | 9/30 |
| Diseases of Thyroid Gland | Medical | General Medical Care | 8 | | 1 | GPMD | | 5/7 | 11/25 |
| Diabetes Mellitus | Medical | General Medical Care | 8 | | | | | 10/7 | |
| | X-ray | Chest, Single PA | | | | | | | |
| | Laboratory | Blood, Alkaline | | | | | | | |
| | Laboratory | Blood, Uric Acid | | | | | | | |
| | Laboratory | Blood, Thymol Turbidity | | | | | | | |
| | Laboratory | Blood, Cephalin Flocculation | | | | | | | |
| | Laboratory | Blood, Bilirubin | | | | | | | |
| | Laboratory | Blood, Sedimentation Rate | | | | | | | |
| | Laboratory | EKG | | | | | | | |
| | Laboratory | Blood, Cholesterol | | | | | | | |
| | Laboratory | Blood, Albumin/Globulin Ratio | | | | | | | |
| | Laboratory | Blood, Protein-Bound Iodine | | | | | | | |
| | Laboratory | Blood, Sugar | | | | | | | |
| | Laboratory | Blood, Non-Protein Nitrogen or B.U.N. | | | | | | | |
| | Laboratory | Blood, Protein-Bound Idoine | | | 3 | Pathology | D | 11/2 | |
| | Laboratory | Blood, Alkaline | | | | | | | |
| | Laboratory | Blood, Calcium | | | | | | | |
| | Laboratory | Blood, Phosphorus | | | | | | | |
| | Laboratory | Blood, Sugar Tolerance 5 Hours | | | | | | | |
| Diseases of Thyroid Gland | Laboratory | Scintiscanning Studies | | | 4 | Radiology | D | 11/11 | 11/12 |
| | Laboratory | Radioactive Iodine Uptake Test | | | | | | | |

353

Examples of Individual Utilization Histories Recorded During Study Year,
Showing All Diagnoses, Services, and Treating Physicians
Reported for Patients with Selected Diagnoses

| DIAGNOSIS SELECTOR: | DIABETES MELLITUS | | AGE: | 58 | | FAMILY SIZE: | 3 | | |
| RELATIONSHIP AND SEX: | Female Spouse | | SUBSCRIBER OCCUPATION: | Blue-Collar | | YEAR OF ENROLLMENT: | 1962 | | |

| Diagnosis | Type of Service | Procedure Description | Visits | | PHYSICIAN | | | FDS [4] | LDS [4] |
| | | | Office | Home | No.[1] | Practice [2] | Qual.[3] | | |
|---|---|---|---|---|---|---|---|---|---|
| Diabetes Mellitus | Medical | General Medical Care | 3 | 3 | 1 | GPMD | | 1/29 | 3/6 |
| Hypertensive Heart Disease | Specialist Consultation | Internal Medicine | | | 2 | Internal Med. | D | 2/28 | 4/15 |
| Diabetes Mellitus | Medical | General Medical Care | 4 | | 1 | GPMD | | 3/13 | 4/1 |
| | Laboratory | Blood, Sugar | | | 3 | GPMD | | 3/24 | 7/2 |
| Rheumatic Heart Disease | Medical | General Medical Care | 6 | 2 | 1 | GPMD | | 4/26 | 7/25 |
| Diabetes Mellitus | Medical | General Medical Care | 1 | 1 | 4 | GPMD | | 7/22 | |
| | Laboratory | Blood, Sugar | | | 5 | GMPD | | 7/28 | |
| | Medical | General Medical Care | 1 | | 6 | GPMD | | 8/1 | |
| | Laboratory | Blood, Sugar | | | 3 | GPMD | | 9/21 | |
| Diabetes Mellitus | Medical | General Medical Care | 3 | | 1 | GPMD | | 9/23 | 10/17 |

Showing All Diagnoses, Services, and Treating Physicians During Study Year,
Reported for Patients with Selected Diagnoses

| DIAGNOSIS SELECTOR: | GASTROENTERITIS AND COLITIS | | AGE: | 22 | | FAMILY SIZE: | 2 |
|---|---|---|---|---|---|---|---|
| RELATIONSHIP AND SEX: | Female Spouse | | SUBSCRIBER OCCUPATION: | Other White-Collar | | YEAR OF ENROLLMENT: | 1962 |

| Diagnosis | Type of Service | Procedure Description | Visits | | Physician | | | FDS [4] | LDS [4] |
|---|---|---|---|---|---|---|---|---|---|
| | | | Office | Home | No.[1] | Practice [2] | Qual.[3] | | |
| Normal Delivery | Anesthesia | Normal Delivery | | | 1 | GPMD | | 6/10 | |
| | Maternity | Normal Delivery | | | 2 | Gyn. and Obst. | D | | |
| Cervicitis | Surgery out of Hospital | Electro-Cauterization of Cervix | | | | | | 8/7 | |
| Gastroenteritis and Colitis | Medical | General Medical Care | 1 | 1 | 3 | GPMD | | 8/19 | 8/20 |
| Diseases of Gall Bladder (Cholelithiasis) | Medical | General Medical Care | 1 | | 4 | Internal Med. | D | 8/24 | |
| | X-ray | Chest, Single PA | | | | | | | |
| | X-ray | Plain Film Study of Abdomen | | | | | | | |
| | Laboratory | Blood, Complete Count | | | | | | | |
| Diseases of Gall Bladder (Cholecystitis and Cholangiatis without Calculi) | Medical | General Medical Care | 1 | | | | | 8/31 | |
| | X-ray | Upper Gastrointestinal Tract | | | | | | | |
| | X-ray | Gall Bladder, Cholecystography | | | | | | | |
| Other Disease of Intestines and Peritoneum (Mucous Colitis) | Laboratory | Blood, Complete Count | | | | | | 9/24 | |
| | Surgery out of Hospital | Proctoscopy, Diagnostic without Biopsy | | | | | | | |
| Gastroenteritis and Colitis | Medical | General Medical Care | 3 | 2 | | | | 9/28 | 10/2 |
| | Laboratory | Blood, Complete Count | | | | | | | |
| | Laboratory | Blood, Non-Protein Nitrogen or B.U.N. | | | | | | | |
| | Surgery out of Hospital | Sigmoidoscopy, Diagnostic, Initial | | | | | | | |

## Examples of Individual Utilization Histories Recorded During Study Year, Showing All Diagnoses, Services, and Treating Physicians Reported for Patients with Selected Diagnoses

| DIAGNOSIS SELECTOR: | GASTROENTERITIS AND COLITIS | | FAMILY SIZE: | 4 |
|---|---|---|---|---|
| RELATIONSHIP AND SEX: | Male Subscriber | AGE: | 40 | |
| | | SUBSCRIBER OCCUPATION: | Blue-Collar | |
| | | | YEAR OF ENROLLMENT: | 1959 |

| Diagnosis | Type of Service | Procedure Description | Visits | | Physician | | | FDS[4] | LDS[4] |
|---|---|---|---|---|---|---|---|---|---|
| | | | Office | Home | No.[1] | Practice[2] | Qual.[3] | | |
| General Medical Exam. | Preventive | Immunization, NEC | 1 | | 1 | GPMD | | 4/22 | |
| Gastroenteritis and Colitis | Medical | General Medical Care | 3 | | | | | 5/11 | 5/15 |
| | X-ray | Plain Film Study of Abdomen | | 1 | | | | | |
| | Laboratory | Blood, Sugar | | | | | | | |
| | Laboratory | Blood, Cholesterol | | | | | | | |
| | Laboratory | Blood, Hematocrit | | | | | | | |
| | Laboratory | Blood, White Cell Count | | | | | | | |
| | Laboratory | Blood, Sedimentation Rate | | | | | | | |
| | Laboratory | Blood, Uric Acid | | | | | | | |
| General Medical Exam. | Preventive | Immunization, NEC | 1 | | | | | 6/22 | |
| Contusion | Medical | General Medical Care | 1 | | 2 | GPMD | | 7/5 | |
| | X-ray | Elbow | | | | | | | |
| Sprains and Strains | Medical | General Medical Care | 2 | | 1 | GPMD | | 7/6 | 7/7 |
| | X-ray | Elbow | | | | | | | |
| Synovitis, Bursitis and Tensoynovitis | Surgery out of Hospital | Arthrocentesis (Puncture for Aspiration of Joint) | | | | | | 7/9 | |
| General Medical Exam. | Preventive | General Medical Care | 1 | | | | | 9/8 | |
| | X-ray | Chest, Single PA | | | | | | | |
| | Laboratory | Blood, Hematocrit | | | | | | | |
| | Laboratory | Blood, White Cell Count | | | | | | | |
| | Laboratory | Blood, Flocculation Test | | | | | | | |
| Bronchitis | Medical | General Medical Care | 1 | | | | | 9/10 | |
| Otitis Externa | Surgery out of Hospital | Drainage of External Auditory Canal | | | | | | 10/12 | |
| Otitis Media | Medical | General Medical Care | 2 | | | | | 11/7 | 11/14 |

## Examples of Individual Utilization Histories Recorded During Study Year, Showing All Diagnoses, Services, and Treating Physicians Reported for Patients with Selected Diagnoses

DIAGNOSIS SELECTOR: HAY FEVER  
RELATIONSHIP AND SEX: Female Spouse  
AGE: 52  
SUBSCRIBER OCCUPATION: Blue-Collar  
FAMILY SIZE: 2  
YEAR OF ENROLLMENT: 1962

| Diagnosis | Type of Service | Procedure Description | Visits Office | Home | PHYSICIAN No.[1] | Practice [2] | Qual.[3] | FDS [4] | LDS [4] |
|---|---|---|---|---|---|---|---|---|---|
| Other Diseases of Intestines and Peritoneum (Diverticulitis) | Medical | General Medical Care | | 1 | 1 | GPMD | | 1/8 | |
| | Medical | General Medical Care | 1 | | | | | 1/18 | 1/22 |
| | X-ray | Abdomen, Colon by Barium Enema | | | | | | | |
| | Laboratory | Blood, Alkaline | | | 2 | Pathology | D | 1/20 | |
| | Laboratory | Blood, Transaminase | | | | | | | |
| | Laboratory | Blood, Cephalin Flocculation | | | | | | | |
| | Laboratory | Blood, Cholesterol | | | | | | | |
| | Laboratory | Blood, Bilirubin | | | | | | | |
| Hernia of Abdominal Cavity | Medical | General Medical Care | 1 | | 1 | GPMD | | 1/27 | |
| Anemia | Medical | Injection of Vitamins or Hormones | | | | | | 1/27 | |
| Other Allergic Diseases | Medical | Allergy Care | 3 | | | | | 1/31 | 3/6 |
| Hay Fever | Medical | General Medical Care | 1 | 1 | | | | 3/27 | |
| Other Allergic Diseases | Medical | Allergy Care | 7 | | | | | 4/27 | 7/13 |
| Hay Fever | Medical | Allergy Care | 1 | | | | | 8/11 | |
| Hay Fever | Medical | Allergy Care | 2 | | | | | 9/9 | 10/9 |
| General Medical Exam. | Preventive | Immunization, NEC | 1 | | | | | 10/26 | |
| Hay Fever | Medical | Allergy Care | 2 | | | | | 11/7 | 12/7 |

357

Examples of Individual Utilization Histories Recorded During Study Year,
Showing All Diagnoses, Services, and Treating Physicians
Reported for Patients with Selected Diagnoses

| DIAGNOSIS SELECTOR: | HYPERTENSIVE HEART DISEASE | AGE: | 51 | FAMILY SIZE: | 5 |
| RELATIONSHIP AND SEX: | Male Subscriber | SUBSCRIBER OCCUPATION: | Blue-Collar | YEAR OF ENROLLMENT: | 1958 |

| | | Visits | | | PHYSICIAN | | | | |
| Diagnosis | Type of Service | Office | Home | Procedure Description | No.[1] | Practice[2] | Qual.[3] | FDS[4] | LDS[4] |
|---|---|---|---|---|---|---|---|---|---|
| Malignant Neoplasm of Male Genital Organs (Prostate) | Surgery in Hospital | 1 | | Cystoscopy, with Biopsy | 1 | Urology | D | 11/20 | 11/23 |
| Hypertensive Heart Disease | Medical | | | General Medical Care | 2 | Internal Med. | S | 1/8 | |
| | X-ray | | | Chest, Single PA | | | | | |
| | X-ray | | | Bone, Survey | | | | | |
| | Laboratory | | | Blood, Complete Count | | | | | |
| | Laboratory | | | Blood, Urea | | | | | |
| | Laboratory | | | Blood, Sugar | | | | | |
| | Laboratory | | | Blood, Phosphatase, Acid | | | | | |
| | Laboratory | | | Blood, Alkaline | | | | | |
| | Laboratory | | | Blood, Complement Fixation Tests | | | | | |
| | Laboratory | | | Blood, Cholesterol | | | | | |
| | Laboratory | | | EKG | | | | | |
| Malignant Neoplasm of Male Genital Organs (Prostate) | Anesthesia | | | Orchiectomy, Bilateral | 3 | Anesthesiology | S | 2/3 | |
| | Surgery in Hospital | | | Orchiectomy, Bilateral | 4 | Urology | D | 2/3 | 2/6 |
| Other Diseases of the Ear | Medical | 1 | | General Medical Care | 5 | GPDO | | 4/1 | |
| Malignant Neoplasm of Male Genital Organs (Prostate) | Medical | 1 | | General Medical Care | 4 | Urology | D | 6/9 | |
| Otitis Media | Medical | 1 | | General Medical Care | 5 | GPDO | | 7/25 | |
| Malignant Neoplasm of Male Genital Organs (Prostate) | Medical | 1 | | General Medical Care | 6 | Urology | S | 9/8 | |
| Acute Nasopharyngitis | Medical | 1 | | General Medical Care | 5 | GPDO | | 12/2 | |
| Malignant Neoplasm of Male Genital Organs | Medical | 1 | | General Medical Care | 6 | Urology | S | 12/8 | |
| | X-ray | | | Plain Film Study of Abdomen | | | | | |

## Examples of Individual Utilization Histories Recorded During Study Year, Showing All Diagnoses, Services, and Treating Physicians Reported for Patients with Selected Diagnoses

| DIAGNOSIS SELECTOR: | HYPERTENSIVE HEART DISEASE | AGE: | 59 | FAMILY SIZE: | 2 |
| RELATIONSHIP AND SEX: | Male Subscriber | SUBSCRIBER OCCUPATION: | Blue-Collar | YEAR OF ENROLLMENT: | 1961 |

| Diagnosis | Type of Service | Procedure Description | Visits | | PHYSICIAN | | | FDS [4] | LDS [4] |
|---|---|---|---|---|---|---|---|---|---|
| | | | Office | Home | No.[1] | Practice [2] | Qual.[3] | | |
| Hypertensive Diseases | Medical | General Medical Care | 3 | | 1 | GPDO | | 11/16 | 2/15 |
| | Laboratory | Blood, Potassium (Twice) | | | | | | | |
| | Laboratory | Blood, Sodium (Twice) | | | | | | | |
| | Laboratory | Blood, Cholesterol (Twice) | | | | | | | |
| Other Diseases of Upper Respiratory Tract | Medical | General Medical Care | 1 | | | | | | |
| Sprains and Strains | Medical | General Medical Care | 1 | | | | | | |
| Hypertensive Heart Disease | Medical | General Medical Care | 1 | | | | | 4/18 | |
| | Laboratory | Blood, Cholesterol | | | | | | | |
| | Laboratory | Blood, Sodium | | | | | | | |
| | Laboratory | Blood, Potassium | | | | | | | |
| | Laboratory | Blood, Non-Protein Nitrogen or B.U.N. | | | | | | | |
| | Laboratory | Blood, Creatinine | | | | | | | |
| Other Diseases of Upper Respiratory Tract | Medical | General Medical Care | 1 | | | | | 5/23 | |
| Hypertensive Diseases | Medical | General Medical Care | 2 | | | | | 7/25 | 8/22 |
| | Laboratory | Blood, Cholesterol (Twice) | | | | | | | |
| | Laboratory | Blood, Potassium (Twice) | | | | | | | |
| | Laboratory | Blood, Sodium (Twice) | | | | | | | |
| Other Diseases of Upper Respiratory Tract | Medical | General Medical Care | 1 | 1 | 2 | GPMD | | 11/20 | |
| Respiratory Tract | Medical | General Medical Care | 1 | | 1 | GPDO | | 11/21 | |
| | Medical | General Medical Care | 1 | | 3 | GPMD | | 12/11 | |

359

## Examples of Individual Utilization Histories Recorded During Study Year, Showing All Diagnoses, Services, and Treating Physicians Reported for Patients with Selected Diagnoses

DIAGNOSIS SELECTOR: OBESITY    AGE: 40    FAMILY SIZE: 4

RELATIONSHIP AND SEX: Male Subscriber    SUBSCRIBER OCCUPATION: Blue-Collar    YEAR OF ENROLLMENT: 1959

| Diagnosis | Type of Service | Procedure Description | Visits | | PHYSICIAN | | | FDS [4] | LDS [4] |
| | | | Office | Home | No.[1] | Practice [2] | Qual.[3] | | |
| --- | --- | --- | --- | --- | --- | --- | --- | --- | --- |
| Obesity (Limited to 12 Office Visits every 3 Months, 24 per year) | Medical | General Medical Care | 1 | | 1 | Internal Med. | D | 12/24 | |
| | Laboratory | Blood, Flocculation Test | | | | | | | |
| | Laboratory | Blood, Cephalin Flocculation | | | | | | | |
| | Laboratory | Blood, Creatinine | | | | | | | |
| | Laboratory | Blood, Sedimentation Rate | | | | | | | |
| | Laboratory | Blood, Prothrombin Time | | | | | | | |
| | Laboratory | Blood, Bilirubin | | | | | | | |
| | Laboratory | Blood, Urea | | | | | | | |
| | Laboratory | Blood, Thymol Turbidity | | | | | | | |
| | Laboratory | Blood, Complete Count | | | | | | | |
| | Laboratory | Urine, Concentration and Dilution Tests | | | | | | | |
| | Laboratory | Blood, Total Protein | | | | | | | |
| | Laboratory | Feces, Occult Blood | | | | | | | |
| | Laboratory | Blood, Cholesterol | | | | | | | |
| | Laboratory | Blood, Sugar | | | | | | | |
| | Laboratory | Blood, Alkaline | | | | | | | |
| | Laboratory | Skin Tests with Bacterial Extracts | | | | | | | |
| | X-ray | Chest, Single PA | | | | | | | |
| | X-ray | Abdomen, Upper Gastro-intestinal Tract | | | | | | | |
| | Surgery out of Hospital | Rectum, Sigmoidoscopy, Diagnostic, Initial | | | | | | | |

| Condition | Service Type | Service / Test | No. | No. | Provider | D | Date(s) |
|---|---|---|---|---|---|---|---|
| **Hypertensive Diseases** | Specialist Consultation | Internal Medicine | | 2 | Internal Med. | D | 1/16, 1/23 |
| **Coronary Insufficiency** | Medical | General Medical Care | 1 | 1 | Internal Med. | D | 2/6 |
| | Medical | General Medical Care | 1 | | | | |
| | Laboratory | Blood, Creatinine | | | | | |
| | Laboratory | Blood, Prothrombin Time | | | | | |
| | Laboratory | Blood, Sugar | | | | | |
| | Laboratory | Feces, Occult Blood | | | | | |
| | Laboratory | Blood, Cholesterol | | | | | |
| | Laboratory | Blood, Non-Protein Nitrogen or B.U.N. | | | | | |
| | Laboratory | EKG | | | | | |
| | Laboratory | Blood, Sedimentation Rate | | | | | |
| **Diabetes Mellitus** | Medical | General Medical Care | 1 | 3 | GPMD | | 2/15, 2/16, 3/11, 2/21 |
| | Medical in Hospital | General Medical Care | 1 | | | | |
| | Medical | Blood, Sugar | | | | | |
| | Laboratory | Blood, Complete Count | | | | | |
| | Laboratory | Blood, Sedimentation Rate | | | | | |
| | Laboratory | Blood, Non-Protein Nitrogen or B.U.N. | | | | | |
| | Medical | General Medical Care | 1 | | | | 7/21 |
| | Laboratory | Blood, Sugar | | | | | |

## Examples of Individual Utilization Histories Recorded During Study Year, Showing All Diagnoses, Services, and Treating Physicians Reported for Patients with Selected Diagnoses

| | | | | | | | | | |
|---|---|---|---|---|---|---|---|---|---|
| DIAGNOSIS SELECTOR: | OBESITY | | | AGE: | 44 | | FAMILY SIZE: | 4 | |
| RELATIONSHIP AND SEX: | Female Spouse | | | SUBSCRIBER OCCUPATION: | Blue-Collar | | YEAR OF ENROLLMENT: | 1959 | |

| Diagnosis | Type of Service | Procedure Description | Visits Office | Visits Home | No.[1] | Practice [2] | Qual.[3] | FDS [4] | LDS [4] |
|---|---|---|---|---|---|---|---|---|---|
| Obesity (Limited to 12 Office Visits every 3 Months, 24 per year) | Medical | General Medical Care | 6 | | 1 | GPMD | | 9/30 | 12/24 |
| | Medical | General Medical Care | 1 | | 2 | GPMD | | 1/27 | |
| | X-ray | Chest, Single PA | | | | | | | |
| | X-ray | Spine, Lumbo-Sacro, Including Pelvis | | | | | | | |
| | Laboratory | Tissues, Cytologic Study | | | | | | | |
| | Laboratory | Blood, Sugar | | | | | | | |
| | Laboratory | Blood, Calcium | | | | | | | |
| | Laboratory | Culture for Bacteria | | | | | | | |
| | Laboratory | Blood, Urea | | | | | | | |
| | Laboratory | EKG | | | | | | | |
| | Laboratory | Blood, Complement Fixation Tests | | | | | | | |
| | Laboratory | Blood, Phosphorus | | | | | | | |
| | Laboratory | Blood, Complete Count | | | | | | | |
| | Laboratory | Blood, Protein-Bound Iodine | | | | | | | |
| | Laboratory | Blood, Alkaline | | | | | | | |
| | Laboratory | Blood, Carbon Dioxide Combining Power | | | | | | | |
| | Laboratory | Blood, Potassium | | | | | | | |
| | Laboratory | Blood, Sodium | | | | | | | |
| | Laboratory | Blood, Sedimentation Rate | | | | | | | |
| | Laboratory | Blood, Cholesterol | | | | | | | |
| Other Diseases of Female Genital Organs (Disease of Uterus) | Specialist Consultation | Gynecology and Obstetrics | | | 3 | Gyn. and Obst. | D | 2/1 | |
| | Laboratory | Tissues, Cytologic Study | 14 | | | | | | |
| Obesity | Medical | General Medical Care | | | 1 | GPMD | | 2/7 | 7/17 |
| Other Diseases of Intestines and Peritoneum (Diverticulitis) | Surgery in Hospital | Intestines, Large Bowel Resection | | | 4 | General Surg. | D | 11/21 | |
| Other Diseases of Intestines and Peritoneum (Intestinal Obstruction) | Ambulance Service | Paramedical Services | | 1 | 5 | | | | |
| | Medical | General Medical Care | | | | GPMD | | 11/24 | |

362

## Examples of Individual Utilization Histories Recorded During Study Year, Showing All Diagnoses, Services, and Treating Physicians Reported for Patients with Selected Diagnoses

| DIAGNOSIS SELECTOR: | SCIATICA | AGE: | 43 | FAMILY SIZE: | 3 |
|---|---|---|---|---|---|
| RELATIONSHIP AND SEX: | Female Spouse | SUBSCRIBER OCCUPATION: | Executive | YEAR OF ENROLLMENT: | 1959 |

| Diagnosis | Type of Service | Procedure Description | Visits Office | Visits Home | No.[1] | Physician Practice [2] | Qual.[3] | FDS [4] | LDS [4] |
|---|---|---|---|---|---|---|---|---|---|
| Other Diseases of Nervous System (Neuritis and Neuralgia) | Medical | General Medical Care | | 3 | 1 | GPMD | | 1/31 | 2/8 |
| Ulcers | Medical | General Medical Care | | 14 | 2 | GPMD | | 2/11 | 9/11 |
| | Medical in Hospital | General Medical Care | | | | | | | |
| Other Diseases of Nervous System (Neuritis and Neuralgia) | Medical | General Medical Care | 4 | 9 | 3 | Neurology | D | 2/14 | 3/7 |
| Sciatica | Medical | General Medical Care | | | | | | 2/28 | 3/10 |
| | Laboratory | Blood, Sedimentation Rate | | | | | | | |
| | Laboratory | Blood, Flocculation Test | | | | | | | |
| | Laboratory | Blood, Complete Count | | | | | | | |
| Other Diseases of Nervous System | Specialist Consultation | Neurological Surgery | | | 4 | Neurology Surg. | S | 3/14 | |
| Other Ill-Defined Diseases (Nervousness) | Consultation in Hospital | Psychiatry | | | 5 | Psychiatry | D | 4/7 | 4/10 |
| Symptoms Referrable to Upper and Lower Gastrointestinal System (Abdominal Pain) | Medical | General Medical Care | 1 | | 6 | GPMD | | 9/16 | |
| Ulcers | Medical | General Medical Care | 1 | | | | | 10/1 | |

363

Examples of Individual Utilization Histories Recorded During Study Year, Showing All Diagnoses, Services, and Treating Physicians Reported for Patients with Selected Diagnoses

| DIAGNOSIS SELECTOR: | SCIATICA | | FAMILY SIZE: | 1 |
|---|---|---|---|---|
| RELATIONSHIP AND SEX: | Male Subscriber | | | |
| AGE: | 46 | | | |
| SUBSCRIBER OCCUPATION: | Blue-Collar | | YEAR OF ENROLLMENT: | 1959 |

| Diagnosis | Type of Service | Procedure Description | Visits Office | Visits Home | No.[1] | Practice[2] | Qual.[3] | FDS[4] | LDS[4] |
|---|---|---|---|---|---|---|---|---|---|
| Benign Neoplasm of Skin | Medical | General Medical Care | 1 | | 1 | General Surg. | D | 3/2 | 3/16 |
| Sciatica | Medical | General Medical Care | 4 | | 2 | GPDO | | 3/9 | 3/20 |
| Influenza | Medical | General Medical Care | 3 | 3 | | | | 3/18 | 4/2 |
| Sciatica | Medical | General Medical Care | 3 | | | | | 3/21 | |
| | Medical | Physiotherapy | 6 | | | | | 4/3 | 4/15 |
| Streptococcal Sore Throat | Medical | General Medical Care | | 3 | | | | 4/17 | 4/19 |
| Sciatica | Medical | General Medical Care | 5 | | | | | 4/20 | 4/30 |
| Streptococcal Sore Throat | Medical | General Medical Care | 1 | | | | | 5/15 | 5/18 |
| Sciatica | Medical | General Medical Care | 1 | | | | | 5/28 | 6/5 |
| | Medical | Osteopathic Manipulation | 2 | 2 | | | | 6/22 | 6/25 |
| Bronchitis | Medical | General Medical Care | | 3 | | | | 7/6 | 7/8 |
| Streptococcal Sore Throat | Medical | General Medical Care | 5 | | | | | 7/13 | 7/24 |
| Dermatitis | Medical | General Medical Care | 1 | 2 | | | | 8/6 | 8/10 |
| Influenza | Medical | General Medical Care | | | | | | | |
| Gastroenteritis and Colitis | Medical | General Medical Care | 3 | 3 | | | | 8/24 | 8/26 |
| Synovitis, Bursitis and Tenosynovitis | Medical | General Medical Care | 4 | | | | | 9/4 | 9/14 |
| Other Injuries and Adverse Effects of External Causes (Adverse Effects of Chemical Substances) | Medical | General Medical Care | 4 | | | | | 9/18 | 9/24 |

Examples of Individual Utilization Histories Recorded During Study Year,
Showing All Diagnoses, Services, and Treating Physicians
Reported for Patients with Selected Diagnoses

| DIAGNOSIS SELECTOR: | ULCERS (G.I. Tract) | AGE: | 53 | FAMILY SIZE: | 2 |
| RELATIONSHIP AND SEX: | Female Subscriber | SUBSCRIBER OCCUPATION: | Blue-Collar | YEAR OF ENROLLMENT: | 1956 |

| Diagnosis | Type of Service | Procedure Description | Visits Office | Visits Home | PHYSICIAN No.[1] | PHYSICIAN Practice [2] | PHYSICIAN Qual.[3] | FDS [4] | LDS [4] |
|---|---|---|---|---|---|---|---|---|---|
| Ulcers | Medical | General Medical Care | 2 | | 1 | General Surg. | D | 11/1 | 12/3 |
| | Anesthesia | Subtotal, Gastrectomy, Partial | | | 2 | GPMD | | 12/3 | |
| | | Gastrojejunostomy | | | | | | | |
| | Surgery in Hospital | Subtotal, Gastrectomy, Partial | | | 1 | General Surg. | D | | |
| | Surgery in Hospital | Gastrojejunostomy | | | | | | | |
| Symptoms Referrable to Cardiovascular System (Acute Heart Failure) | Medical in Hospital | General Medical Care | | | 3 | Internal Med. | D | 12/10 | 1/17 |
| Complications of Surgical or Medical Procedures | Medical | General Medical Care | 2 | | 1 | General Surg. | D | 1/22 | 2/5 |
| | Surgery out of Hospital | Drainage of Small Subcutaneous Abscess | | | | | | 2/12 3/20 | |
| | Medical | General Medical Care | | | | | | | |
| | Surgery out of Hospital | Local Excision of Small Benign Neoplasm | 1 | | | | | 3/30 | |
| Other Diseases of Skin and Subcutaneous Tissues (Alopecia) | Specialist Consultation | Dermatology | | | 4 | Dermatology | D | 4/20 | |
| Complications of Surgical or Medical Procedures | Medical | General Medical Care | 1 | | 1 | General Surg. | D | 5/20 | |
| Gastritis and Duodenitis | Medical | General Medical Care | 1 | | | | | 11/10 | |

365

Examples of Individual Utilization Histories Recorded During Study Year,
Showing All Diagnoses, Services, and Treating Physicians
Reported for Patients with Selected Diagnoses

| DIAGNOSIS SELECTOR: | ULCERS (G.I. Tract) | AGE: | 50 | | FAMILY SIZE: | 5 |
| RELATIONSHIP AND SEX: | Male Subscriber | SUBSCRIBER OCCUPATION: | Blue-Collar | | YEAR OF ENROLLMENT: | 1958 |

| | | Visits | | | PHYSICIAN | | | |
| Diagnosis | Type of Service | Procedure Description | Office | Home | No.[1] | Practice [2] | Qual.[3] | FDS [4] | LDS [4] |
|---|---|---|---|---|---|---|---|---|---|
| Ulcers Other Diseases of Stomach and Duodenum | Medical | General Medical Care | 2 | | 1 | GPMD | | 1/15 | 3/16 |
| | X-ray | Abdomen, Upper Gastro-intestinal Tract | | | 2 | Radiology | D | 3/23 | |
| Ulcers | Medical | General Medical Care | 1 | | 1 | GPMD | | 5/12 | |
| | Medical | General Medical Care | 3 | | 3 | GPMD | | 6/17 | 6/26 |
| | Medical in Hospital | Repair of Diaphragmatic Hernia | | | | | | 6/27 | |
| | Anesthesia | | | | 4 | Anesthesiology | | | |
| | Surgery in Hospital | Repair of Diaphragmatic Hernia | | | | | D | 7/10 | |
| | Medical in Hospital | General Medical Care | | | 5 | GPMD | | | |
| | | | | | 3 | GPMD | | 7/26 | |

# HOSPITALIZATION STUDIES

# Chapter 18
# HOSPITALIZATION STUDIES

Although GHI was not responsible for hospital bills incurred by the study population, its coverage of private physician services rendered in hospitals provided access to data on hospital utilization by GHI members.* Since such information was not available from the hospitalization insurers, it was decided to include hospital data in "input" plans. The material produced by this decision proved of practical value when GHI took steps to formulate its own hospitalization insurance program.

Records available on hospitalization (in addition to data on physician services rendered in hospitals, shown previously) included characteristics of the population at risk; hospital identity and characteristics; physician identity and characteristics; patient identity, characteristics, and type of insurance coverage; type of case, diagnosis, type of accommodation; dates of admission and discharge. Data were not available as to other-than-bed facilities used or services performed by hospital employees, such as laboratory and x-ray tests.

Hospitalization analyses are classified under two general

---

* The utilization count thus excludes cases hospitalized in municipal or other government institutions except where a private physician billed GHI for medical services. It is believed that such exclusions involve mainly care in psychiatric or veteran facilities, since people with hospital and medical insurance probably try to avoid municipal hospitals.

headings: those relating experience to the population at risk; and those confined to the hospitalized population. Within each category, the range of GHI analysis conducted thus far represents an initial program feasible for development under a limited budget. The potential for multivariate and detailed analysis implicit in the scope of retrieved data is of course much greater.

In relating utilization to the population at risk, frequencies were derived using as numerators the number of medical, surgical, and obstetrical patients, admissions, and days; and as denominators the number of exposure years of population subgroups classified according to type of GHI coverage, age, sex, marital status, family size, relationship to subscriber, subscriber occupation class, duration of medical insurance coverage, and area of residence.

A diagnostic frequency index for admissions and hospital days was also derived; in this instance the sample population as a whole, rather than its subgroups, was used as the denominator in calculation of rates.

Data in the first section of this chapter were derived from the resulting indices. They illustrate how the records of a medical insurance plan can contribute to hospital utilization questions of special interest, such as the influence of comprehensiveness of medical coverage, before introducing the series of tabulations showing utilization variance associated with measured characteristics of the eligible membership and with diagnosis.

The second section of data presented consists of tabulations analyzing variations in hospital admission experience by type of hospital, area, type of case, month of year, diagnostic category, and length of stay. These non-population-related analyses are all of the type which, coordinated by area, should be readily available from hospital statistics. The advantage of retrieving such data from insurance records is in providing source data for comparing the experience of the insured vs. the general population, or of one prepayment plan with another. The disadvantage in the present case is data gaps resulting from non-responsibility for payment—e.g., number of days for surgical and obstetrical cases may be understated because GHI lump-sum payment of physicians did not require knowledge of number of days in hospital. Missing information in such cases was inferred from data supplied on other surgical and obstetrical cases.

## Hospital Use Under Comprehensive vs. Limited Physician Insurance Coverage

Nearly all of the utilization data presented in previous chapters refers to experience under the "Family Doctor Plan" —i.e. to that section of the membership covered for physician services in office and home as well as in hospital.

The separate consideration of hospitalization experience offers an opportunity to explore the differences between hospital use by members with comprehensive coverage and by those whose physician coverage excluded most or all office and home treatment.

It has often been assumed, without definitive evidence, that one way to decrease the use of hospitals is by providing out-of-hospital medical insurance. The opposite hypothesis, also unproven, poses the possibility that comprehensive coverage, by encouraging early attention, may increase hospitalization through the disclosure of conditions which might otherwise have been neglected.

In exploring these conflicting hypotheses, it is desirable to control other factors influencing hospital use such as the form of organization under which medical care is delivered, the composition of the populations whose experience is being compared, and the hospital facilities available. Hospital use under comprehensive coverage arranged through closed-panel or group practice prepayment plans is generally reportedly lower than under the limited coverage provided through open fee-for-service community plans, but the reasons have not been investigated. In the type of comparison cited, lower use under comprehensive prepayment is not necessarily attributable to comprehensiveness of coverage; the method of delivering service, the composition of the population, the geographic location of the plan and consequent access to hospital facilities may be more important factors.

Control of such extraneous considerations which may distort the coverage factor is implicit under the GHI situation where, irrespective of degree of physician coverage, members with known demographic characteristics use the same community medical resources, distributed under the same system.

### Results of the Analyses

*Admission Rates.* The possibility of fallacious conclusions resulting from comparing the hospitalization experience of two populations of unknown sex-age composition is well demonstrated by the GHI data.

Observation of unadjusted data seems to bear out the hypothesis that comprehensive coverage will lead to fewer admissions. GHI members with limited coverage had 127 admissions per thousand exposure years, as compared with 114 admissions for those with comprehensive coverage of physician services (Table 135).

TABLE 135. Hospital Admission Rates Under Two Types of GHI Coverage *

| | ADMISSIONS PER 1000 EXPOSURE YEARS | |
| --- | --- | --- |
| | *Comprehensive Plan* | *Limited Plan* |
| All Members | 113.9 | 127.4 |
| Males | 91.3 | 110.8 |
| Females | 137.2 | 143.4 |
| All Members, excluding obstetrics | 94.8 | 108.7 |
| Females, excluding obstetrics | 98.4 | 106.8 |

* The term coverage applies to physician services, not to hospitalization.

It is known, however, that the limited plan attracts fewer young people and more older people, proportionately; and each of these operates to produce the lower overall rates shown for the comprehensive plan. If the admission rates under each plan were adjusted to the age-sex composition of the other plan's membership, the picture would be reversed.

In order to rule out the effect of age-sex disparities between the two populations, the experience of each is adjusted below to the composition of the same population—in this case the general population of the New York-Northeast New Jersey metropolitan area (Table 136).

TABLE 136.  Admission Rates Under Two Types of Medical Coverage, Adjusted to Age-Sex Composition of Metropolitan New York-Northeast New Jersey Population

|  | ADMISSIONS PER 1000 EXPOSURE YEARS | |
|---|---|---|
|  | Comprehensive Plan | Limited Plan |
| All Members | 127.7 | 122.3 |
| Males | 96.3 | 103.3 |
| Females | 152.0 | 140.0 |
| All Members, excluding obstetrics | 102.9 | 100.0 |
| Females, excluding obstetrics | 106.0 | 100.0 |

With these adjustments, admission rates for the two types of membership tend to converge, strikingly so when maternity care is excluded. Although the overall convergence is achieved by averaging the male and female divergencies, and although the reasons for the divergencies are not known, it may be concluded that extent of medical coverage was not a factor affecting hospital admission rates among the GHI membership studied.

*Length of Stay.*  In the final analysis, however, it is not only admission rates but also length of stay which determines the total number of hospital days charged; and here there appears to be evidence of consistent differences in experience under the two types of coverage which persist even when age-sex composition is taken into account.

The membership with narrower medical coverage stayed longer, on the average, once admitted. For every thousand admissions, those with limited coverage actually used 1,900 more days of hospitalization, representing an increase of 26 percent, than accrued from a like number of admissions of comprehensive-coverage members. If both groups were distributed by age and sex as the general population of the area, the difference would have been reduced to 900 days, or 11.5 percent.

In terms of the entire eligible membership, the increased length of stay averaged by limited-coverage patients, applied to the admission rates for this segment, produce an actual liability of 344 more hospital days per year per thousand limited-coverage members, and an age-sex-adjusted liability of 57 more days, than that incurred by the comprehensive-coverage membership (Table 137).

TABLE 137. Number of Hospital Days Per Stay and Per 1000 Exposure Years, Among Members with Comprehensive vs. Limited GHI Coverage, Unadjusted and Adjusted to Age-Sex Composition of Metropolitan New York-Northeast New Jersey Population

| | DAYS PER STAY | | | | DAYS PER 1000 EXPOSURE YEARS | | | |
|---|---|---|---|---|---|---|---|---|
| | UNADJUSTED | | ADJUSTED | | UNADJUSTED | | ADJUSTED | |
| | Comp. Plan | Lim. Plan | Comp. Plan | Lim. Plan | Comp. Plan | Lim. Plan | Comp. Plan | Lim. Plan |
| TOTAL POPULATION | 7.4 | 9.3 | 7.8 | 8.7 | 843 | 1187 | 1001 | 1058 |
| Males | 7.9 | 10.2 | 8.4 | 9.3 | 719 | 1125 | 809 | 960 |
| Females | 7.1 | 8.4 | 7.7 | 8.3 | 971 | 1246 | 1163 | 1162 |
| Total excluding maternity care | 8.0 | 10.1 | 8.7 | 9.5 | 759 | 1102 | 893 | 964 |
| Females excluding maternity care | 8.1 | 10.1 | 9.1 | 9.8 | 800 | 1080 | 961 | 981 |

*Observations*

The evidence from one year's experience supports the hypothesis that office-home care coverage can be a factor in reducing hospital utilization. In the population studied, savings resulted not from keeping members out of the hospital but from discharging them sooner.

The reasons for longer average stays by patients without office-home coverage can only be conjectured: They may wait longer to seek care, they may be admitted for more serious conditions, they may require more hospitalized time for diagnostic determinations performed on an ambulatory basis in the case of those with office coverage, or they may remain longer because medical benefits cease when they leave the hospital. Probably all of these are factors.

It should be remembered that the economies in hospital charges and hospital insurance premiums indicated in the experience described, while substantial, constitute only a fraction of the additional premiums required for comprehensive coverage.

## Inter-County Differences in Bed Ratios as a Factor in Hospital Use

The applicability of Parkinson's Law to hospital economics—i.e. the tendency for hospital use rates to rise with the level of bed availability—is one of the hypotheses proposed by economists to explain geographic variations, or trends over time, in hospital utilization.

The hypothesis finds an apparent degree of support in the GHI data. Although the population studied is concentrated in a relatively small area, wide variations in hospitalization indices are seen among area subdivisions, only part of which can be explained by inter-area differences in member age distribution.

When the available indices are juxtaposed for six selected

counties, it becomes necessary to differentiate between the two basic indices of hospital use—admission rates, and length of stay—in judging the possible influence of bed ratios (Table 138).

It will be observed that both bed ratios and admission rates were roughly 50 per cent higher in Westchester-Richmond than in the other four counties listed. On the basis of age distribution, Westchester and Richmond would be expected to experience admission rates between those of the Bronx-Queens and Nassau-Suffolk areas. Bronx and Queens, with the lowest proportions under age 19 and the highest proportions over age 55, would be expected to have the highest utilization, but their admission rates were the lowest, and only the length-of-stay index reflects their high percentage of membership over age 55. Suffolk and Nassau, with bed ratios and admission rates at levels comparable to Bronx and Queens, incurred far fewer days per thousand members because of relatively short average stays, which in turn were related to their comparatively youthful populations.

It may thus be inferred, pending study of further experi-

TABLE 138.   Hospital Bed Ratios and Hospital Utilization
by GHI Membership in Six Counties of
New York Metropolitan Area

| AREA OF MEMBER RESIDENCE | General Private Beds per 1000 Population [1] | NON-MATERNITY HOSPITAL UTILIZATION, GHI MEMBERSHIP | | | AGE DISTRIBUTION | |
|---|---|---|---|---|---|---|
| | | Adm. Rates per 1000 Members | Days per Stay | Days per 1000 Members | Per Cent of GHI Membership * | |
| | | | | | 19 or under | 55 or over |
| Bronx | 2.18 | 91.1 | 8.8 | 804 | 33.6 | 17.2 |
| Queens | 2.30 | 94.0 | 8.6 | 804 | 33.9 | 17.2 |
| Suffolk | 2.33 | 97.8 | 5.8 | 572 | 45.2 | 7.7 |
| Nassau | 2.37 | 98.5 | 7.2 | 711 | 42.5 | 10.1 |
| Richmond | 3.44 | 151.6 | 8.4 | 1269 | 38.4 | 14.5 |
| Westchester | 3.46 | 137.2 | 8.3 | 1144 | 37.3 | 12.7 |

[1] Derived from Census Data and *Hospital Statistics of Southern New York, 1964,* published by Hospital Review and Planning Council.

* Practical data-processing considerations (time and cost) precluded adjusting each variable for age, but it is believed this method of assessing age data in relation to the other indices presented is sufficient for purposes of the present analysis.

ence, that in the areas listed * the decision to hospitalize a GHI member was influenced by the number of beds available, while other factors were more likely determinants of length of stay, once the patient was admitted.

None of the above can be interpreted as indicating over-use or under-use in any area. The definition of adequacy remains as the perennial question.

## Hospital Use Indices

The indices employed to describe hospital use overall and by demographic subgroups include number of admissions and hospital days per year per thousand members, by type of case, plus days per admission, plus number of individual persons hospitalized.

This last index, permitting calculations of number of admissions for the same person, also allows flexibility for purposes of comparison with other studies, some of which present only total admission rates (including readmissions) while some list only first-admission, or person, rates.

Demographic indices selected for presentation apply to the combined GHI population covered for the full study year, irrespective of type of GHI coverage. The diagnostic index applies only to those with comprehensive coverage.

Hospital day rates among the GHI population as a whole totaled 896.5 per thousand members for the year (compared with 1,119.4, reported national average [1]), of which 812.7 represent non-maternity care. Although surgical patients and admissions outnumbered medical patients and admissions, medical cases accounted for more hospital days used because the aver-

---

* The two metropolitan areas not listed, Manhattan and Brooklyn, do not fit the pattern described. Admission rates were lower and show no comparable relationship to bed availability, while average length of stay was significantly higher, probably reflecting the interference of complicating factors such as medical schools.

[1] *Hospital Discharges and Length of Stay: Short-Stay Hospitals, United States, July 1963–June 1964.* Publication Series 10, Number 30, National Center for Health Statistics, Washington, D.C., June 1966.

age medical case remained half again as long as the average surgical case (10.4 vs. 6.9 days per admission). The average obstetrical case involved 4.4 days of hospitalization, as against 8.4 days for non-maternity cases and 7.7 days for all cases (Table 139).

TABLE 139.   Hospital Utilization Indices,
by Type of Admission

| | NUMBER PER 1000 EXPOSURE YEARS [*] | | | Average Number of Days Per Admission |
|---|---|---|---|---|
| TYPE OF CASE | Members Admitted | Admissions | Hospital Days | |
| All Cases | 102.6 | 116.0 | 896.5 | 7.7 |
| Non-Maternity | 84.1 | 97.0 | 812.7 | 8.4 |
| Surgical | 48.9 | 55.1 | 378.7 | 6.9 |
| Medical | 35.2 | 41.9 | 434.0 | 10.4 |
| Maternity | 18.5 | 19.0 | 83.8 | 4.4 |

[*] Comprehensive and Limited Plan samples.

The average stay of 7.7 days for GHI patients compares with averages of 8.1 nationally and 9.2, northeastern United States, reported by the National Center for Health Statistics.[1] The discrepancy in data coming from the two different types of sources may be related to age distribution differences as well as to the fact that insurance figures, by their nature, exclude most of the care rendered in government hospitals, where stays tend to be much longer than in voluntary or proprietary hospitals. Blue Cross experience, not regularly published, happens to be available for 1964. When Blue Cross data rather than national health survey data are used as the basis of comparison, it is found that the GHI experience conformed rather closely: the GHI average stay for members under age 65 was 7.3 days, as against the Blue Cross figure of 7.6 in the Northeast, and 13.2 days for members aged 65 and over as against the Blue Cross figure of 13.4 in the Northeast, for the same period.[2]

---

[1] *Op. cit.*
[2] Passman, Mary Jane, *Hospitalization by Blue Cross Members in 1964,* "Inquiry," Blue Cross Association, May 1966.

# HOSPITAL UTILIZATION
## ADMISSIONS AND DAY-RATES
## BY AGE AND SEX

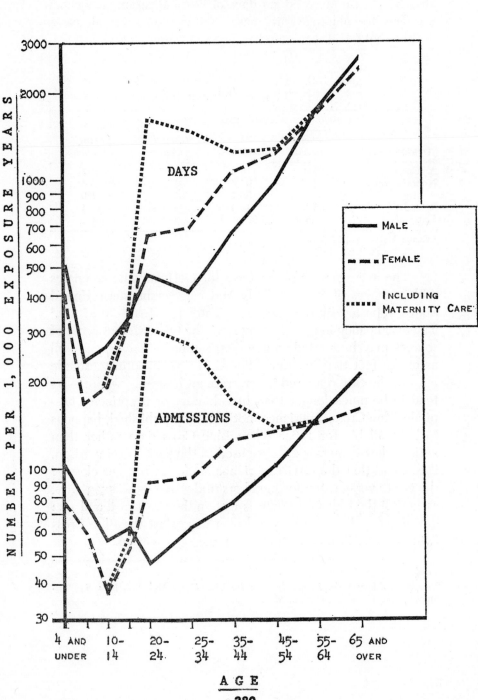

HOSPITAL UTILIZATION OF ADULTS: PERSONS ADMITTED
ONCE OR MORE, ADMISSIONS, AND DAY-RATES,
PER 1,000 EXPOSURE YEARS, BY TYPE OF ADMISSION,
BY MARITAL STATUS AND RELATIONSHIP

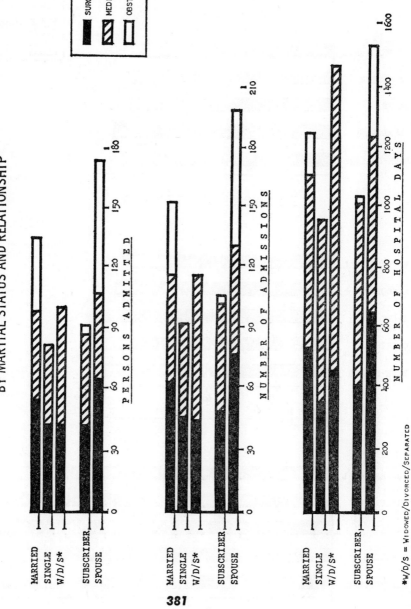

381

*W/D/S = WIDOWED/DIVORCED/SEPARATED

# HOSPITAL UTILIZATION: PERSONS ADMITTED ONCE OR MORE, ADMISSIONS AND DAY-RATES, PER 1,000 EXPOSURE YEARS, BY TYPE OF ADMISSION, BY OCCUPATION CLASS OF SUBSCRIBER*

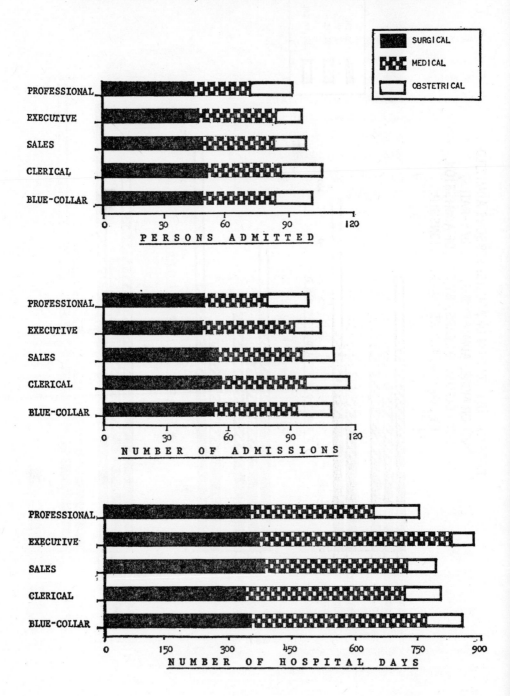

*INCLUDING DEPENDENTS

# HOSPITAL UTILIZATION: PERSONS ADMITTED ONCE OR MORE, ADMISSIONS, AND DAY-RATES, PER 1,000 EXPOSURE YEARS BY TYPE OF ADMISSION, BY AREA OF SUBSCRIBER RESIDENCE

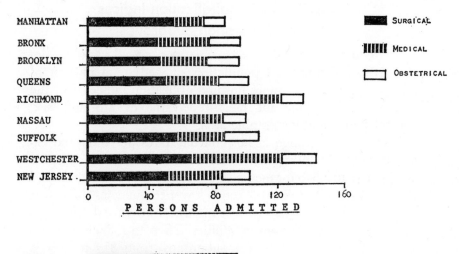

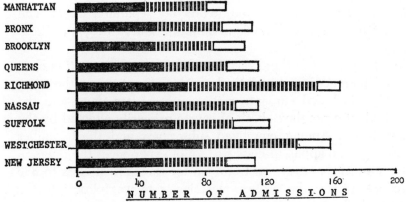

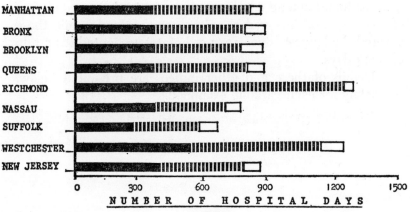

## Variations in Hospitalization Indices
## Among Population Subgroups

Except for occupation class of subscriber, all variables descriptive of the insured population showed some pattern of relationship to one or more hospital utilization indices; but the independently significant measured variables are age, sex, marital status, and geographic area.

The age-sex range in hospital day rates per thousand exposure years, including maternity care, was from 171 for girls aged 5 to 9, to 2,678 for men past 65. Subscribers, both male and female, were hospitalized at much lower frequencies than their spouses. For family-size subgroups, the rate varied from 476 days per thousand persons in families of five, to 1,599 in families of two; for marital status-sex subgroups, from 817 for single males to 1,653 for widowed-divorced-or-separated males. The area variation was from 664 in Suffolk County to 1,303 in Richmond.

In contrast to these very broad variations, occupation-class rate differences were relatively minor except when the comparison included students, with a rate of 427 days, and the retired, at 2,742 days—both of course primarily affected by the age factor. Among employed subscribers and their families there was no apparent class pattern of experience: the range in the annual day rate was from 740 for the clerical class to 886 for executives; the professional class rate was closest to the clerical, the blue-collar group to the executive.

As for duration of GHI membership, the lowest hospital use was found among enrollees who were in their second year of coverage and incurred 522 days per thousand, while those covered the longest (since 1957 or before) accounted for a rate of 1,104 days.

Details of these and other indices are presented below, separately for each variable examined.

VARIATIONS ASSOCIATED WITH RELATIONSHIP TO SUBSCRIBER

Utilization indices for subscribers (policyholders), spouses and dependent children probably are the most easily retrieved, or at least most likely to be available, from insurance records. When the data for each subgroup are further subdivided by sex, the resulting indices for male subscribers, female spouses, and dependent children provide a good introductory view of the large utilization differences characterizing the major segments of the insured population.

There were ten admissions during the year for every hundred male subscribers, and twenty for every hundred female spouses. Much of the difference is accounted for by maternity admissions. The latter, because of their relative brevity, were also a factor in bringing the average length of stay for all female spouse admissions to 7.5, as against 9.8 for male subscriber admissions. The surgical admission rate for female spouses, which was two-thirds higher than for male subscribers, was another contributor to the lower overall average stays of this group, since surgical stays were generally much shorter. Lower average stays of female spouses as compared with male subscribers offset a good portion of the 102 per cent differential in the admission rates of these two major subgroups; in the annual day-rate index, the differential was reduced to 54 per cent.

Utilization by female subscribers was closer to that of male subscribers than to female spouses because of their much lower maternity rate. When obstetrical admissions are excluded, the female subscriber utilization rate is closer to that of female spouses with respect to number of persons admitted, but closer to male subscribers with respect to hospital-day rates. Their surgical admission rate was midway between the rates of male subscribers and female spouses.

The remaining adult subgroup, male spouses, experienced far higher hospital use than other adult males. Their hospital-day rate was in fact greater than that of female spouses, even when maternity care for the latter is included. Furthermore, their average length of stay per admission was higher than that of any other subscriber-relationship subgroup.

The reasons for this high rate of hospital use by male spouses are not known. It is conceivable that enough married female subscribers (who by definition must have been employed to become subscribers) may have been working because of the illness of their spouses, to overweight the small male spouse group with high hospitalization utilizers. It is also notable that this same group of male spouses experienced generally low rates of ambulatory service utilization. Any suggestion of a possible pattern, however, would require study of further experience.

Table 140 shows in broad perspective the pattern of utilization among children which is detailed in the next section under "Age". The hospitalization pattern for boys to age 19 was significantly higher than for girls, on all indices except days per admission. Length of stay among girls admitted as medical cases averaged nearly 20 per cent longer than among boys. Surgical stays were about the same for both sexes. But admission rates, both medical and surgical, were a third higher for boys.

The annual hospital day rate for children averaged 0.3 days per capita as compared with 1 day per subscriber and 1.55 days per spouse. For the combined membership, the average of 7.7 days per hospital stay including maternity and 8.4 days excluding maternity care, rises to 9.7 days exclusive of both maternity and children's admissions (Table 140).

It is apparent that attempts to compare hospitalization experience under different types of insurance plans must take into account differences in family composition of the eligible memberships, especially if data on age distribution are unavailable.

TABLE 140. Hospital Utilization: User Rates, Admission Rates, Day Rates, Length of Stay, by Type of Admission, by Relationship to Subscriber and Sex

| INDEX AND TYPE OF ADMISSION | ALL MEMBERS | | | SUBSCRIBERS | | | SPOUSES | | | CHILDREN TO AGE 19 | | |
|---|---|---|---|---|---|---|---|---|---|---|---|---|
| | All | Male | Female | All | Male | Female | All | Male | Female | All | Male | Female |
| | NUMBER PER 1,000 EXPOSURE YEARS * | | | | | | | | | | | |
| *Members Admitted* | 102.6 | 81.6 | 124.1 | 93.3 | 86.5 | 121.0 | 176.2 | 119.5 | 182.0 | 61.3 | 69.4 | 53.0 |
| Non-Maternity | 84.1 | 81.6 | 86.7 | 89.7 | 86.5 | 102.9 | 109.8 | 119.5 | 108.8 | 61.3 | 69.4 | 53.0 |
| Surgical | 48.9 | 43.8 | 54.1 | 45.1 | 42.3 | 56.7 | 68.3 | 56.9 | 69.4 | 39.3 | 44.6 | 33.9 |
| Medical | 35.2 | 37.8 | 32.6 | 44.6 | 44.2 | 46.2 | 41.5 | 62.6 | 39.4 | 22.0 | 24.8 | 19.1 |
| *Admissions* | 116.0 | 94.3 | 138.3 | 108.0 | 101.3 | 135.2 | 200.9 | 163.2 | 204.8 | 65.9 | 75.1 | 56.4 |
| Non-Maternity | 97.0 | 94.3 | 99.8 | 104.4 | 101.3 | 116.9 | 132.5 | 163.2 | 129.4 | 65.9 | 75.1 | 56.4 |
| Surgical | 55.1 | 49.4 | 61.0 | 51.5 | 48.3 | 64.0 | 79.6 | 73.4 | 80.2 | 41.9 | 47.7 | 35.8 |
| Medical | 41.9 | 44.9 | 38.8 | 52.9 | 53.0 | 52.9 | 52.9 | 89.8 | 49.2 | 24.0 | 27.4 | 20.6 |
| *Hospital Days* | 896.5 | 780.8 | 1015.2 | 1048.5 | 1002.1 | 1237.0 | 1551.3 | 1663.6 | 1539.8 | 308.8 | 341.1 | 275.5 |
| Non-Maternity | 812.7 | 780.8 | 845.4 | 1033.4 | 1002.1 | 1160.5 | 1248.3 | 1663.6 | 1205.8 | 308.8 | 341.1 | 275.5 |
| Surgical | 378.7 | 330.2 | 428.5 | 431.6 | 414.6 | 500.1 | 668.2 | 731.2 | 661.8 | 132.4 | 154.6 | 109.6 |
| Medical | 434.0 | 450.6 | 416.9 | 601.8 | 587.5 | 660.4 | 580.1 | 932.4 | 544.0 | 176.4 | 186.5 | 165.9 |
| | AVERAGE NUMBER OF DAYS PER ADMISSION | | | | | | | | | | | |
| *Length of Stay* | 7.7 | 8.3 | 7.3 | 9.8 | 9.8 | 9.2 | 7.7 | 10.2 | 7.5 | 4.7 | 4.5 | 4.9 |
| Non-Maternity | 8.4 | 8.3 | 8.5 | 9.9 | 9.9 | 9.9 | 9.4 | 10.2 | 9.3 | 4.7 | 4.5 | 4.9 |
| Surgical | 6.9 | 6.7 | 7.0 | 8.4 | 8.6 | 7.7 | 8.4 | 10.0 | 8.3 | 3.2 | 3.2 | 3.1 |
| Medical | 10.4 | 10.0 | 10.7 | 11.4 | 11.1 | 12.5 | 11.0 | 10.4 | 11.1 | 7.3 | 6.8 | 8.1 |

* Comprehensive and Limited Plan samples.

387

VARIATIONS BY AGE AND SEX

Ten per cent of the eligible population were hospitalized during the year. Repeated admissions for some brought the admission rate for the population as a whole to 116, with the range from 37 among girls aged 10–14, to 217 among men past 65 (Table 141).

For both sexes combined, the expected accelerating age curve of hospital use was reflected in all indices—most clearly with maternity care excluded. After age 4, the annual day rate showed a steadily upward trend: the rate for those over 65 was nearly thirteen times that for the lowest group, reflecting increases not only in admission rates but in length of stay per admission. The interaction of these two rising indices—admission rates from 47 to 196, days per stay from 2.9 to 13.2—produced an annual day rate of 2,572 for those past 65, as against 738 non-maternity (or 825 including maternity) for the rest of the population.

The acceleration in hospital day rates is of course not a sudden happening at age 65. The non-maternity hospitalization day rate of those aged 20 to 34 represented an increase of about 70 per cent over the rate of those aged 19 or under. At ages 35 to 44, the rate increased, over the 20-to-34-year level, by another 54 per cent—and so on, with another 30 per cent increment at ages 45 to 54, followed by a 53 per cent increase at ages 55 to 64.

The gap between proportion of individual members admitted, and admission rates, also broadened with increasing age, reflecting a greater tendency toward multiple admissions among older patients.

Although the rising age pattern of hospital use was characteristic of both sexes, deviations from the combined averages overall and at various age levels were of significance. At two age levels—15 to 19 and 55 to 64—the annual day rate for males and females was almost the same; at all other age levels, the differences were pronounced. Males to age 14 used nearly 13 days for every 10 used by females, most of the excess coming from surgical admissions. Among males past 65, the rate of both surgical and medical admissions was substantially higher than among females. But females from age 20 through 54, especially those aged 35 to 44, accounted for far higher day rates, even disregarding maternity care. The differences are attributable largely to the much higher surgical admission rates of females, although from ages 25 through 54 their medical day rates were also higher than those of males.

The effect of maternity care on hospital use is seen mainly at ages 20 to 34. One of every five women aged 20 to 24 was hospitalized for maternity care. Since the average maternity stay lasted only 4.4 days, however, the impact on the annual day rate was of less consequence than on the admission rate: women in all the child-bearing years had higher admission rates than any other female age group, whereas their annual day rate, including maternity care, was surpassed by women of 55 and over.

VARIATIONS ASSOCIATED WITH MARITAL STATUS

The influence of marital status on hospital utilization (Table 142), while diluted somewhat by the age composition of each marital subgroup, emerged in the data on length of stay per admission.

All spouseless categories showed substantially longer stays for medical admissions. Surgical stays of single males and females were shorter than those of the married, reflecting the younger age composition of the single group and thus the likelihood that type of surgery permitted earlier discharge. But medical admissions of this group averaged far longer stays (13.3 days) than the medical admissions of the married (10.8 days), and in fact approached more closely the record of 14.3 days per average medical admission achieved by the widowed-divorced-separated category.

The latter group also incurred substantially longer surgical stays—10.1 days vs. 8.4 for married and 7.7 for single adults. As a result, their hospital day rate of 1,494 was sub-

TABLE 141. Hospital Utilization: User Rates, Length of Stay, by Type of Admission,

NUMBER PER 1,000

| AGE AND SEX | MEMBERS ADMITTED | | | | ADMISSIONS | | | |
|---|---|---|---|---|---|---|---|---|
| | | Non-Maternity | | | | Non-Maternity | | |
| | Total | Total | Sur-gical | Med-ical | Total | Total | Sur-gical | Med-ical |
| All Persons | 102.6 | 84.1 | 48.9 | 35.2 | 116.0 | 97.0 | 55.1 | 41.9 |
| 4 and Under | 84.3 | 84.3 | 47.1 | 37.2 | 92.1 | 92.1 | 49.5 | 42.6 |
| 5–9 | 65.2 | 65.2 | 51.6 | 13.6 | 69.0 | 69.0 | 54.4 | 14.6 |
| 10–14 | 44.2 | 44.2 | 26.7 | 17.5 | 47.3 | 47.3 | 29.4 | 17.9 |
| 14 and Under | 63.7 | 63.7 | 41.7 | 22.0 | 68.5 | 68.5 | 44.3 | 24.2 |
| 15–19 | 57.7 | 55.2 | 33.1 | 22.1 | 61.3 | 58.7 | 35.1 | 23.6 |
| 20–24 | 196.7 | 68.3 | 46.8 | 21.5 | 206.2 | 73.4 | 50.6 | 22.8 |
| 25–34 | 161.3 | 70.1 | 44.0 | 26.1 | 174.6 | 80.2 | 50.3 | 29.9 |
| 35–44 | 112.9 | 90.4 | 54.7 | 35.7 | 126.0 | 103.4 | 61.6 | 41.8 |
| 45–54 | 100.0 | 99.3 | 55.8 | 43.5 | 121.1 | 120.4 | 66.8 | 53.6 |
| 55–64 | 122.4 | 122.4 | 59.3 | 63.1 | 149.1 | 149.1 | 70.2 | 78.9 |
| 65 and Over | 158.7 | 158.7 | 70.8 | 87.9 | 195.5 | 195.5 | 79.1 | 116.4 |
| TOTAL EXCL. 65 AND OVER | 100.2 | 81.0 | 48.0 | 33.0 | 112.6 | 92.8 | 54.1 | 38.7 |
| Males | 81.6 | 81.6 | 43.8 | 37.8 | 94.2 | 94.2 | 49.3 | 44.9 |
| 4 and Under | 96.1 | 96.1 | 55.1 | 41.0 | 106.2 | 106.2 | 58.8 | 47.4 |
| 5–9 | 73.0 | 73.0 | 57.7 | 15.3 | 77.7 | 77.7 | 61.0 | 16.7 |
| 10–14 | 52.7 | 52.7 | 34.0 | 18.7 | 56.7 | 56.7 | 37.3 | 19.4 |
| 14 and Under | 72.9 | 72.9 | 48.7 | 24.2 | 79.0 | 79.0 | 52.1 | 26.9 |
| 15–19 | 59.9 | 59.9 | 31.0 | 28.9 | 63.5 | 63.5 | 32.5 | 31.0 |
| 20–24 | 45.9 | 45.9 | 30.1 | 15.8 | 47.4 | 47.4 | 31.6 | 15.8 |
| 25–34 | 51.7 | 51.7 | 29.5 | 22.2 | 63.7 | 63.7 | 37.1 | 26.6 |
| 35–44 | 69.1 | 69.1 | 34.4 | 34.7 | 78.0 | 78.0 | 37.3 | 40.7 |
| 45–54 | 87.2 | 87.2 | 41.5 | 45.7 | 104.5 | 104.5 | 49.4 | 55.1 |
| 55–64 | 124.4 | 124.4 | 57.7 | 66.7 | 150.1 | 150.1 | 68.7 | 81.4 |
| 65 and Over | 174.5 | 174.5 | 77.9 | 96.6 | 216.8 | 216.8 | 86.9 | 129.9 |
| TOTAL EXCL. 65 AND OVER | 76.9 | 76.9 | 42.2 | 34.7 | 88.0 | 88.0 | 47.4 | 40.6 |
| Females | 124.1 | 86.7 | 54.1 | 32.6 | 138.3 | 99.8 | 61.0 | 38.8 |
| 4 and Under | 72.0 | 72.0 | 38.9 | 33.1 | 77.4 | 77.4 | 39.8 | 37.6 |
| 5–9 | 57.2 | 57.2 | 45.3 | 11.9 | 60.1 | 60.1 | 47.5 | 12.6 |
| 10–14 | 35.3 | 35.3 | 19.0 | 16.3 | 37.3 | 37.3 | 21.0 | 16.3 |
| 14 and Under | 54.2 | 54.2 | 34.4 | 19.8 | 57.5 | 57.5 | 36.1 | 21.4 |
| 15–19 | 55.6 | 50.6 | 35.1 | 15.5 | 59.1 | 54.0 | 37.5 | 16.5 |
| 20–24 | 297.2 | 83.3 | 58.0 | 25.3 | 311.9 | 90.6 | 63.2 | 27.4 |
| 25–34 | 260.2 | 86.8 | 57.2 | 29.6 | 274.6 | 95.0 | 62.1 | 32.9 |
| 35–44 | 156.7 | 111.7 | 75.0 | 36.7 | 173.8 | 128.6 | 85.8 | 42.8 |
| 45–54 | 112.6 | 111.2 | 69.9 | 41.3 | 137.5 | 136.1 | 83.9 | 52.2 |
| 55–64 | 119.8 | 119.8 | 61.4 | 58.4 | 147.9 | 147.9 | 72.2 | 75.7 |
| 65 and Over | 135.1 | 135.1 | 60.3 | 74.8 | 164.1 | 164.1 | 67.6 | 96.5 |
| TOTAL EXCL. 65 AND OVER | 123.8 | 85.1 | 53.9 | 31.2 | 137.4 | 97.6 | 60.8 | 36.8 |

* Comprehensive and Limited Plan samples.

# Admission Rates, Day Rates, by Age and Sex

| HOSPITAL DAYS | | | | DAYS PER ADMISSION | | | | |
|---|---|---|---|---|---|---|---|---|
| | Non-Maternity | | | | Non-Maternity | | | |
| Total | Total | Sur-gical | Med-ical | Total | Total | Sur-gical | Med-ical | Obstet-rical |
| 896.5 | 812.7 | 378.7 | 434.0 | 7.7 | 8.4 | 6.9 | 10.4 | 4.4 |
| 500.2 | 500.2 | 123.0 | 377.2 | 5.4 | 5.4 | 2.5 | 8.9 | — |
| 202.8 | 202.8 | 110.2 | 92.6 | 2.9 | 2.9 | 2.0 | 6.3 | — |
| 229.9 | 229.9 | 132.9 | 97.0 | 4.9 | 4.9 | 4.5 | 5.4 | — |
| 301.6 | 301.6 | 121.9 | 179.7 | 4.4 | 4.4 | 2.8 | 7.4 | — |
| 349.3 | 335.3 | 178.4 | 156.9 | 5.7 | 5.7 | 5.1 | 6.6 | 5.5 |
| 1166.4 | 579.4 | 392.2 | 187.2 | 5.7 | 7.9 | 7.8 | 8.2 | 4.4 |
| 981.2 | 557.9 | 300.8 | 257.1 | 5.6 | 7.0 | 6.0 | 8.6 | 4.5 |
| 964.3 | 869.4 | 447.7 | 421.7 | 7.7 | 8.4 | 7.3 | 10.1 | 4.2 |
| 1134.9 | 1132.8 | 567.2 | 565.6 | 9.4 | 9.4 | 8.5 | 10.6 | 2.8 |
| 1727.6 | 1727.6 | 710.8 | 1016.8 | 11.6 | 11.6 | 10.1 | 12.9 | 0 |
| 2572.1 | 2572.1 | 1002.4 | 1569.7 | 13.2 | 13.2 | 12.7 | 13.5 | 0 |
| 825.2 | 737.8 | 352.2 | 385.6 | 7.3 | 8.0 | 6.5 | 10.0 | 4.4 |
| 780.8 | 780.8 | 330.2 | 450.6 | 8.3 | 8.3 | 6.7 | 10.0 | — |
| 544.2 | 544.2 | 168.0 | 376.2 | 5.1 | 5.1 | 2.9 | 7.9 | — |
| 233.6 | 233.6 | 130.8 | 102.8 | 3.0 | 3.0 | 2.1 | 6.2 | — |
| 264.8 | 264.8 | 164.2 | 100.6 | 4.7 | 4.7 | 4.4 | 5.2 | — |
| 338.0 | 338.0 | 153.7 | 184.4 | 4.3 | 4.3 | 2.9 | 6.9 | — |
| 332.6 | 332.6 | 142.0 | 190.6 | 5.2 | 5.2 | 4.4 | 6.2 | — |
| 463.6 | 463.6 | 256.3 | 207.3 | 9.8 | 9.8 | 8.1 | 13.1 | — |
| 416.5 | 416.5 | 194.4 | 222.1 | 6.5 | 6.5 | 5.2 | 8.4 | — |
| 662.4 | 662.4 | 266.6 | 395.8 | 8.5 | 8.5 | 7.1 | 9.7 | — |
| 987.7 | 987.7 | 430.8 | 556.9 | 9.5 | 9.5 | 8.7 | 10.1 | — |
| 1732.6 | 1732.6 | 714.2 | 1018.4 | 11.5 | 11.5 | 10.4 | 12.5 | — |
| 2677.8 | 2677.8 | 1038.1 | 1639.7 | 12.4 | 12.4 | 12.0 | 12.6 | — |
| 684.9 | 684.9 | 294.4 | 390.5 | 7.8 | 7.8 | 6.2 | 9.6 | — |
| 1015.2 | 845.3 | 428.4 | 416.9 | 7.3 | 8.5 | 7.0 | 10.7 | 4.4 |
| 454.3 | 454.3 | 76.0 | 378.3 | 5.9 | 5.9 | 1.9 | 10.1 | — |
| 171.2 | 171.2 | 89.2 | 82.0 | 2.8 | 2.8 | 1.9 | 6.5 | — |
| 192.9 | 192.9 | 99.7 | 93.2 | 5.2 | 5.2 | 4.8 | 5.7 | — |
| 263.7 | 263.7 | 88.8 | 174.9 | 4.6 | 4.6 | 2.5 | 8.2 | — |
| 365.4 | 337.8 | 213.7 | 124.1 | 6.2 | 6.3 | 5.7 | 7.5 | 5.5 |
| 1634.4 | 656.5 | 482.6 | 173.9 | 5.2 | 7.2 | 7.6 | 6.3 | 4.4 |
| 1490.8 | 685.6 | 396.8 | 288.8 | 5.4 | 7.2 | 6.4 | 8.8 | 4.5 |
| 1265.5 | 1075.9 | 628.4 | 447.5 | 7.3 | 8.4 | 7.3 | 10.5 | 4.2 |
| 1279.6 | 1275.5 | 701.3 | 574.2 | 9.3 | 9.4 | 8.4 | 11.0 | 2.8 |
| 1721.1 | 1721.1 | 706.4 | 1014.7 | 11.6 | 11.6 | 9.8 | 13.4 | 0 |
| 2415.0 | 2415.0 | 949.3 | 1465.7 | 14.7 | 14.7 | 14.1 | 15.2 | 0 |
| 967.0 | 791.4 | 410.5 | 380.9 | 7.0 | 8.1 | 6.7 | 10.3 | 4.4 |

stantially higher than that of married members (1,126, non-maternity) although the non-maternity admission rates of the two classes were practically identical.

With the data further subdivided by sex, it was found that the admission rate of widowed-divorced-separated males (126) was far higher than those of married (109) or single (83) males, higher than for widowed-divorced-separated females (114), and nearly as high as the non-maternity rate for married females (129). Whereas the latter rate was caused largely by surgical admissions, however, the opposite is true of widowed-divorced-separated males, who incurred a lower surgical admission rate (39) than either married (52) or single (43) males, while showing an extraordinary rate of 87 medical admissions per thousand compared with 53 for the population as a whole. This high rate of medical admissions, combined with an average stay of 13.5 days, produced an annual medical-hospitalization rate for the group of 1,180 days, vs. 614 for married men.

It may also be of significance that widowed-divorced-or-separated males incurred more multiple admissions than married males—a ratio of five admissions to every four patients, as against six admissions to five married male patients.

In the absence of age-adjusted data and separate indices for the widowed, divorced, and separated, it would be unfair to ascribe the hospital experience of the combined group to their marital status. Undoubtedly age is a stronger factor among the widowed than among the divorced or separated. On the other hand, the longer stays of this group and of the younger, single group tend to separate the spouseless from the married, bolstering the hypothesis that practical considerations (i.e. unavailability of care at home) rather than medical need may frequently have postponed the date of discharge.

VARIATIONS BY FAMILY SIZE

The size of the enrolled family is one of the least useful of the variables available for analysis of insured hospital utilization. Other factors affect the data—primarily the age composition of families of different size; also marital status; and the fact

## TABLE 142. Hospital Utilization: User Rates, Admission Rates, Day Rates, Length of Stay, by Type of Admission, by Marital Status and Sex

| INDEX AND TYPE OF ADMISSION | ALL ADULTS | | | MARRIED | | | SINGLE | | | WIDOWED-DIVORCED-SEPARATED | | |
|---|---|---|---|---|---|---|---|---|---|---|---|---|
| | All | Male | Female | All | Male | Female | All | Male | Female | All | Male | Female |
| *NUMBER PER 1,000 EXPOSURE YEARS * | | | | | | | | | | | | |
| *Members Admitted* | 128.0 | 89.1 | 167.8 | 134.6 | 90.9 | 179.2 | 83.7 | 73.2 | 97.9 | 102.7 | 100.3 | 103.9 |
| Non-Maternity | 98.2 | 89.1 | 107.4 | 99.8 | 90.9 | 108.8 | 83.7 | 73.2 | 97.9 | 102.7 | 100.3 | 103.9 |
| Surgical | 54.8 | 43.4 | 66.4 | 56.6 | 44.3 | 69.2 | 44.0 | 37.9 | 52.2 | 44.0 | 38.6 | 46.8 |
| Medical | 43.4 | 45.7 | 41.0 | 43.2 | 46.6 | 39.6 | 39.7 | 35.3 | 45.7 | 58.7 | 61.7 | 57.1 |
| *Admissions* | 146.9 | 106.1 | 188.6 | 154.7 | 108.8 | 201.5 | 94.3 | 82.7 | 110.1 | 118.2 | 126.0 | 114.3 |
| Non-Maternity | 116.2 | 106.1 | 126.5 | 118.9 | 108.8 | 129.1 | 94.3 | 82.7 | 110.1 | 118.2 | 126.0 | 114.3 |
| Surgical | 63.3 | 50.3 | 76.4 | 65.8 | 51.7 | 80.1 | 48.5 | 42.7 | 56.5 | 47.5 | 38.6 | 51.9 |
| Medical | 52.9 | 55.8 | 50.1 | 53.1 | 57.1 | 49.0 | 45.8 | 40.0 | 53.6 | 70.7 | 87.4 | 62.4 |
| *Hospital Days* | 1258.7 | 1052.9 | 1469.4 | 1284.4 | 1068.3 | 1504.6 | 978.5 | 817.3 | 1197.3 | 1493.5 | 1653.0 | 1413.0 |
| Non-Maternity | 1123.2 | 1052.9 | 1195.3 | 1126.2 | 1068.3 | 1185.2 | 978.5 | 817.3 | 1197.3 | 1493.5 | 1653.0 | 1413.0 |
| Surgical | 530.4 | 439.0 | 624.2 | 552.8 | 454.2 | 653.3 | 371.7 | 318.6 | 443.9 | 479.7 | 473.0 | 483.1 |
| Medical | 592.8 | 613.9 | 571.1 | 573.4 | 614.1 | 531.9 | 606.8 | 498.7 | 753.4 | 1013.8 | 1180.0 | 929.9 |
| *AVERAGE NUMBER OF DAYS PER ADMISSION* | | | | | | | | | | | | |
| *Length of Stay* | 8.6 | 9.9 | 7.8 | 8.3 | 9.8 | 7.5 | 10.4 | 9.9 | 10.9 | 12.7 | 13.1 | 12.4 |
| Maternity† | 4.4 | — | 4.4 | 4.4 | — | 4.4 | — | — | — | — | — | — |
| Non-Maternity | 9.7 | 9.9 | 9.5 | 9.4 | 9.8 | 9.2 | 10.4 | 9.9 | 10.9 | 12.7 | 13.1 | 12.4 |
| Surgical | 8.4 | 8.6 | 8.2 | 8.4 | 8.8 | 8.2 | 7.7 | 7.5 | 7.9 | 10.1 | 12.3 | 9.0 |
| Medical | 11.2 | 11.0 | 11.4 | 10.8 | 10.8 | 10.9 | 13.3 | 12.5 | 14.1 | 14.3 | 13.5 | 14.9 |

* Comprehensive and Limited Plan samples.
† Including normal and Caesarian deliveries, abortions, miscarriages, and ectopic pregnancies.

393

that enrolled size of family may not coincide with actual size—
e.g. where a married member purchased a single-person contract.

In the GHI population, over half the subscribers enrolled
under single-person contracts were past age 50 (37 per cent) or
under age 25 (22 per cent). Two thirds of subscribers in two-
person families were aged 50 or more. In families with enrolled
children, subscribers tended to be younger. These facts, in
combination with utilization patterns previously shown for the
various age segments, led to an expectation of decreasing per
capita hospital use with increasing family size (starting with
families of 2). The expectation was generally substantiated by
the findings except for families of six or more, who used more
hospitalization per capita than families of five.

Presentation of data in terms of family size may generally
be characterized as superfluous when age-sex data are available
and of uncertain value when they are not. The influence of
family size is difficult to isolate. Since this variable is sometimes
encountered elsewhere, however, the GHI experience is given
to permit comparison.

Perhaps the most noteworthy finding in Table 143 concerns variations in length of stay per admission. The contrast is
between families of three or more and families of one or two.
The smaller units averaged about four to six days longer. This
is again assumed to be another way of stating the effects of age
and marital status, previously shown.

OCCUPATION CLASS VARIATIONS

Variations in experience among employed subscribers and
their dependents in different occupation classes were relatively
minor, as compared with those shown for other variables, and
showed no evidence of a descending or ascending curve related
to the occupational hierarchy.

Utilization rates of blue-collar class members were practically the same as those of the combined white-collar class,
with respect to number of members admitted and number of

TABLE 143.  Hospital Utilization: User Rates, Admission Rates, Day Rates, Length of Stay, by Type of Admission, by Family Size

| INDEX AND TYPE OF ADMISSION | FAMILY SIZE | | | | | |
|---|---|---|---|---|---|---|
| | 1 | 2 | 3 | 4 | 5 | 6 or more |
| | NUMBER PER 1,000 EXPOSURE YEARS * | | | | | |
| *Members Admitted* | 94.5 | 127.9 | 110.6 | 101.2 | 82.1 | 88.5 |
| Non-Maternity | 94.5 | 110.4 | 82.1 | 80.6 | 66.6 | 69.2 |
| Surgical | 47.7 | 58.5 | 49.0 | 49.1 | 42.7 | 43.0 |
| Medical | 46.8 | 51.9 | 33.1 | 31.5 | 23.9 | 26.2 |
| *Admissions* | 109.4 | 152.6 | 123.2 | 110.6 | 89.1 | 99.8 |
| Non-Maternity | 109.4 | 134.3 | 93.8 | 89.7 | 73.0 | 80.3 |
| Surgical | 52.7 | 69.0 | 54.9 | 54.3 | 46.6 | 48.4 |
| Medical | 56.7 | 65.3 | 38.9 | 35.4 | 26.4 | 31.9 |
| *Hospital Days* | 1242.1 | 1598.5 | 833.0 | 698.3 | 475.7 | 581.3 |
| Non-Maternity | 1242.1 | 1515.0 | 702.8 | 605.4 | 409.0 | 495.6 |
| Surgical | 452.3 | 703.3 | 356.3 | 296.3 | 186.4 | 259.7 |
| Medical | 789.8 | 811.7 | 346.5 | 309.1 | 222.6 | 235.9 |
| | AVERAGE NUMBER OF DAYS PER ADMISSION | | | | | |
| *Length of Stay* | 11.4 | 10.5 | 6.8 | 6.3 | 5.3 | 5.8 |
| Non-Maternity | 11.4 | 11.3 | 7.5 | 6.8 | 5.6 | 6.2 |
| Surgical | 8.6 | 10.2 | 6.5 | 5.5 | 4.0 | 5.4 |
| Medical | 13.9 | 12.4 | 8.9 | 8.7 | 8.4 | 7.4 |

* Comprehensive and Limited Plan samples.

admissions; their annual hospital day rate was higher than that of most white-collar subgroups but lower than the executive class rate; and their average length of stay per admission was the same as that of the professional class.

There is no class pattern here. Whatever the reasons for the variations shown in Table 144, it appears that other factors acted, in the presence of insurance, to level class differences in hospital utilization which might have occurred without insurance.

This conclusion, it is believed, would not be substantially modified by age-adjustment of the data, since the various indices of use within each occupation class do not consistently relate to each other, and to their comparable number in other

TABLE 144. Hospital Utilization: User Rates, Admission Rates, Day Rates, Length of Stay, by Type of Admission, by Occupation Class of Subscriber

| INDEX AND TYPE OF ADMISSION | Professional | Executive | Sales | Other White Collar | All White Collar | All Blue Collar | Retired | Student |
|---|---|---|---|---|---|---|---|---|
| | NUMBER PER 1,000 EXPOSURE YEARS * | | | | | | | |
| *Members Admitted* | 90.2 | 96.0 | 97.1 | 104.7 | 101.9 | 100.5 | 148.2 | 48.8 |
| Non-Maternity | 70.7 | 83.2 | 82.0 | 85.1 | 83.4 | 81.4 | 148.2 | 48.8 |
| Surgical | 44.2 | 46.1 | 47.9 | 50.8 | 49.5 | 47.7 | 64.3 | 24.4 |
| Medical | 26.5 | 37.1 | 34.1 | 34.3 | 33.9 | 33.7 | 83.9 | 24.4 |
| *Admissions* | 99.4 | 104.6 | 111.5 | 118.2 | 114.5 | 113.2 | 191.7 | 61.0 |
| Non-Maternity | 78.7 | 91.8 | 95.8 | 97.8 | 95.2 | 93.6 | 191.7 | 61.0 |
| Surgical | 50.0 | 49.0 | 56.4 | 57.6 | 55.8 | 53.8 | 69.4 | 24.4 |
| Medical | 28.7 | 42.8 | 39.4 | 40.2 | 39.4 | 39.8 | 122.3 | 36.6 |
| *Hospital Days* | 755.9 | 885.9 | 794.0 | 807.6 | 810.4 | 858.7 | 2742.0 | 426.8 |
| Non-Maternity | 646.2 | 835.5 | 723.8 | 720.1 | 726.3 | 772.4 | 2742.0 | 426.8 |
| Surgical | 351.5 | 375.4 | 384.5 | 341.6 | 349.5 | 366.7 | 1018.7 | 317.1 |
| Medical | 294.7 | 460.1 | 339.3 | 378.5 | 376.8 | 405.7 | 1723.3 | 109.7 |
| | AVERAGE NUMBER OF DAYS PER ADMISSION | | | | | | | |
| *Length of Stay* | 7.6 | 8.5 | 7.1 | 6.8 | 7.1 | 7.6 | 14.3 | 7.0 |
| Non-Maternity | 8.2 | 9.1 | 7.6 | 7.4 | 7.6 | 8.3 | 14.3 | 7.0 |
| Surgical | 7.0 | 7.7 | 6.8 | 5.9 | 6.3 | 6.8 | 14.7 | 13.0 |
| Medical | 10.3 | 10.8 | 8.6 | 9.4 | 9.6 | 10.2 | 14.1 | 3.0 |

* Comprehensive and Limited Plan samples, including dependents.

classes, in a pattern that would be expected if age distribution of various occupation classes were a primary differentiating influence.

In the case of students and the retired group, of course, the age factor was paramount.

VARIATIONS WITH DURATION OF COVERAGE

Unadjusted utilization data for the study year showed a general pattern of increased utilization with increased duration of coverage.

In the case of this variable, however, any conclusions to be drawn would require prior age-adjustment of the findings since, as previously mentioned, those with lengthier accrued periods of membership tended to be concentrated in the older, higher-utilizing age groups, to a greater extent than would have been expected merely on the basis of age increases paralleling increased intervals of coverage. Inasmuch as it was not possible to perform such multivariate analyses as part of the initial studies, the figures presented do not warrant inferences of a relationship between duration of coverage and hospital use.

The value of Table 145, in fact, may well be in its demonstration of how honestly-derived statistics, casually examined, can lead to erroneous impressions. In this case, it was the very tidiness of the decreasing admission-rate curve for those enrolling at different points between 1958 and 1964 which suggested the need to analyze the age composition of each year's

TABLE 145.  Hospital Utilization: User Rates, Admission Rates, Day Rates, Length of Stay, by Type of Admission, by Duration of Coverage

| INDEX AND TYPE OF ADMISSION | YEAR OF MEMBER ENTRY INTO GHI | | | | | | | |
|---|---|---|---|---|---|---|---|---|
| | 1957 and before | 1958 | 1959 | 1960 | 1961 | 1962 | 1963 | 1964 |
| NUMBER PER 1,000 EXPOSURE YEARS * | | | | | | | | |
| *Members Admitted* | 110.3 | 122.1 | 110.6 | 106.1 | 102.5 | 96.4 | 77.9 | 75.0 |
| Non-Maternity | 98.9 | 102.0 | 93.7 | 85.5 | 83.4 | 70.2 | 59.8 | 69.4 |
| Surgical | 55.0 | 57.9 | 52.0 | 53.1 | 47.7 | 43.6 | 35.4 | 44.4 |
| Medical | 43.9 | 44.1 | 41.7 | 32.4 | 35.7 | 26.6 | 24.4 | 25.0 |
| *Admissions* | 126.4 | 139.5 | 127.8 | 119.8 | 115.9 | 106.3 | 86.0 | 80.6 |
| Non-Maternity | 114.9 | 119.1 | 110.9 | 98.7 | 95.9 | 78.6 | 67.2 | 75.0 |
| Surgical | 62.3 | 66.2 | 60.3 | 59.2 | 54.9 | 47.4 | 38.7 | 48.6 |
| Medical | 52.6 | 52.9 | 50.6 | 39.5 | 41.0 | 31.2 | 28.5 | 26.4 |
| *Hospital Days* | 1154.4 | 1002.6 | 1061.7 | 886.0 | 829.7 | 727.0 | 605.2 | 752.8 |
| Non-Maternity | 1104.0 | 899.1 | 992.3 | 795.4 | 745.1 | 603.7 | 522.4 | 726.4 |
| Surgical | 514.7 | 394.9 | 432.7 | 403.5 | 331.9 | 301.4 | 251.8 | 348.6 |
| Medical | 589.3 | 504.2 | 559.6 | 391.9 | 413.2 | 302.3 | 270.6 | 377.8 |
| AVERAGE NUMBER OF DAYS PER ADMISSION | | | | | | | | |
| *Length of Stay* | 9.1 | 7.2 | 8.3 | 7.4 | 7.2 | 6.8 | 7.0 | 9.3 |
| Non-Maternity | 9.6 | 7.6 | 9.0 | 6.3 | 7.8 | 7.7 | 7.7 | 9.7 |
| Surgical | 8.3 | 6.0 | 7.2 | 6.8 | 6.0 | 6.4 | 6.5 | 7.2 |
| Medical | 11.2 | 9.5 | 11.1 | 9.9 | 10.1 | 9.7 | 9.4 | 14.3 |

* Comprehensive and Limited Plan samples.

enrollees; before the present studies were initiated, there was no reason to suspect the existence of major differences, and the original plan for demographic analysis of the membership made no provision for such a breakdown.

GEOGRAPHIC VARIATIONS

Variations in overall hospitalization rates of member subgroups living in different areas have already been described in connection with the discussion of bed ratios as a factor in hospital use. Table 146 presents the area utilization picture in greater detail, adding the "members admitted" index as well as a breakdown of each index by type of admission.

The number of individuals hospitalized once or more ranged from an annual rate of 82 per thousand members in Manhattan to 143 in Westchester; the admission rate from 93 in Manhattan to 166 in Richmond; the length of stay per admission from 5.5 in Suffolk to 9.4 in Manhattan; and the hospital day rate from 664 in Suffolk to 1,303 in Richmond.

Areas showing the highest day rates—Richmond, Westchester, and "other New York"—do so mainly because of high person- and admission-rates, rather than long stays per admission. Areas with lowest day rates (Nassau and Suffolk) had average or above-average admission rates but below-average length of stay (the latter because of their younger populations). Areas with near-average day rates achieved this through varying combinations: Manhattan's rate of admission was lowest but its average length of stay was highest; Brooklyn showed the next lowest admission rate (105) and the next highest average length of stay (8.4 days); but three other areas (Bronx, Queens, New Jersey) with day rates fairly similar to Manhattan and Brooklyn were also close to each other on most other indices. Of all areas, Queens most nearly approached the overall average for each index, but no area can be called "typical."

Within each utilization index, the type-of-case indices (medical or surgical) showed generally similar patterns of inter-area variation; that is, areas higher-than-average on the combined index usually were high on each component, and vice versa. In most areas, as in the overall pattern, surgical patients and admissions outnumbered medical patients and admissions, but the annual medical day rate topped the surgical day rate everywhere except in Nassau because of longer medical stays. Medical patients were also more likely than surgical patients to be readmitted, particularly in Richmond County where there were nearly four medical admissions for every three medical patients.

The wide inter-area range in both surgical and medical admission rates indicates the desirability of a membership-related, area-by-area breakdown of admissions by diagnosis, in future studies. Such analysis would presumably also help to explain variations in length of stay—for example, why medical cases in Manhattan, Brooklyn and Queens averaged over 11 days as compared with 8.7 days in Richmond. The inordinately high medical admission rate in Richmond (82 vs. 36 to 59 elsewhere) might conceivably be associated with admissions of less serious cases, of a type not ordinarily hospitalized in other areas, and this in turn would explain the relatively short average stays of Richmond medical cases (8.7 days vs. 10.4 overall). Even if the total incidence of treated illness (including ambulatory) of various categories varied insignificantly from one area to the next, the incidence of *hospitalized* illness of different types might show substantial variation, and the sources of variation would presumably provide clues to local differences in the practice of medicine.

The total geographic area included in the present study is not large, but the variety of medical circumstances in its component areas (e.g. bed supply, physician characteristics, the presence of medical schools, population density) probably represents a good cross section of the type of variations encountered in many parts of the country, and thus might provide a fruitful base for further investigation of variations in hospital utilization by insured populations.

TABLE 146. Hospital Utilization: User Rates, Admission Rates, Day Rates, Length of Stay, by Type of Admission, by Area of Subscriber Residence

| INDEX AND TYPE OF ADMISSION | NEW YORK CITY | | | | | Nassau | Suffolk | West-chester | Other New York | New Jersey | All Areas |
|---|---|---|---|---|---|---|---|---|---|---|---|
| | Manhattan | Bronx | Brooklyn | Queens | Richmond | | | | | | |
| | NUMBER PER 1,000 EXPOSURE YEARS * | | | | | | | | | | |
| *Members Admitted* | 81.7 | 96.0 | 94.7 | 101.5 | 135.4 | 99.6 | 107.7 | 143.2 | 128.6 | 102.3 | 102.6 |
| Non-Maternity | 71.8 | 77.4 | 74.8 | 82.0 | 121.5 | 84.5 | 85.9 | 121.4 | 103.3 | 84.6 | 84.1 |
| Surgical | 38.6 | 44.2 | 44.5 | 48.4 | 57.9 | 52.6 | 55.8 | 68.8 | 55.0 | 49.3 | 48.9 |
| Medical | 33.2 | 33.2 | 30.3 | 33.6 | 63.6 | 31.9 | 30.1 | 52.6 | 48.3 | 35.3 | 35.2 |
| *Admissions* | 93.1 | 110.2 | 105.0 | 114.2 | 165.5 | 114.1 | 121.0 | 159.5 | 146.1 | 112.1 | 116.0 |
| Non-Maternity | 82.2 | 91.1 | 84.7 | 94.0 | 151.6 | 98.5 | 97.8 | 137.2 | 120.3 | 94.2 | 97.0 |
| Surgical | 43.3 | 50.4 | 48.9 | 54.6 | 69.4 | 60.2 | 60.9 | 78.6 | 63.1 | 54.6 | 55.1 |
| Medical | 38.9 | 40.7 | 35.8 | 39.4 | 82.2 | 38.3 | 36.9 | 58.6 | 57.2 | 39.6 | 41.9 |
| *Hospital Days* | 874.5 | 892.2 | 883.2 | 887.2 | 1303.2 | 776.3 | 663.8 | 1258.0 | 1084.9 | 863.5 | 896.5 |
| Non-Maternity | 825.7 | 803.9 | 785.2 | 804.0 | 1268.5 | 711.2 | 571.7 | 1143.8 | 972.5 | 788.1 | 812.7 |
| Surgical | 362.7 | 372.9 | 372.0 | 365.6 | 556.7 | 370.7 | 267.6 | 539.0 | 387.9 | 391.2 | 378.7 |
| Medical | 463.0 | 431.0 | 413.2 | 438.4 | 711.8 | 340.5 | 304.1 | 604.8 | 584.6 | 396.9 | 434.0 |
| | AVERAGE NUMBER OF DAYS PER ADMISSION | | | | | | | | | | |
| *Length of Stay* | 9.4 | 8.1 | 8.4 | 7.8 | 7.9 | 6.8 | 5.5 | 7.9 | 7.4 | 7.7 | 7.7 |
| Maternity † | 4.5 | 4.6 | 4.8 | 4.1 | 2.5 | 4.2 | 4.0 | 5.1 | 4.4 | 4.2 | 4.4 |
| Non-Maternity | 10.4 | 8.8 | 9.3 | 8.6 | 8.4 | 7.2 | 5.8 | 8.3 | 7.7 | 8.4 | 8.4 |
| Surgical | 8.4 | 7.4 | 7.6 | 6.7 | 8.0 | 6.2 | 4.4 | 6.9 | 6.1 | 7.2 | 6.9 |
| Medical | 11.9 | 10.6 | 11.5 | 11.1 | 8.7 | 8.9 | 8.3 | 10.3 | 10.2 | 10.0 | 10.4 |

* Comprehensive and Limited Plan samples.
† Including normal and Caesarian deliveries, abortions, miscarriages, and ectopic pregnancies.

## Diagnosis

Up to this point, analysis of hospitalization experience has related utilization to characteristics of the membership. One further index based on the population at risk, offered below, assigns to each diagnosis listed as a cause of hospitalization its ascribed frequency of admissions and hospital days per thousand persons per year.

This is an example of the type of analysis which, with further breakdown of data for age-sex and residence subgroups, could be most helpful in tracing sources of utilization differences under different types of prepayment arrangements or in different areas. Such detailed analysis would require a much larger population base than the sample used for the present studies.

The data in Table 147 describe the experience of the "Family Doctor Plan" membership having comprehensive medical coverage, and the totals shown are therefore somewhat at variance with previous totals in this Chapter which included, in addition, the membership with limited coverage.

| DIAGNOSIS | Total Admissions Per 1,000 Exposure Years † | Total Days Per 1,000 Exposure Years † | TYPE OF ADMISSION | | | |
|---|---|---|---|---|---|---|
| | | | SURGICAL | | MEDICAL | |
| | | | Admissions Per 1,000 Exposure Years | Days Per 1,000 Exposure Years | Admissions Per 1,000 Exposure Years | Days Per 1,000 Exposure Years |
| Combined Total | 114.4 | 851.2 | 54.6 | 357.6 | 40.2 | 401.3 |
| | | | | | | |
| *Infective and Parasitic Diseases* | .9 | 8.8 | — | — | .9 | 8.8 |
| Streptococcal Sore Throat | .1 | .5 | — | — | .1 | .5 |
| Measles | 0 | 0 | — | — | 0 | 0 |
| Rubella (German Measles) | 0 * | .1 | — | — | 0 * | .1 |
| Chicken Pox | 0 | 0 | — | — | 0 | 0 |
| Mumps | 0 | 0 | — | — | 0 | 0 |
| Infectious Hepatitis | .1 | 2.1 | — | — | .1 | 2.1 |
| Glandular Fever (Infectious Mononucleosis) | .1 | 1.6 | — | — | .1 | 1.6 |
| Intestinal Virus | .4 | 2.4 | — | — | .4 | 2.4 |
| Dermatophytoses | 0 | 0 | — | — | 0 | 0 |
| Other | .2 | 2.1 | — | — | .2 | 2.1 |
| | | | | | | |
| *Neoplasms* | 10.6 | 93.0 | 8.9 | 73.3 | 1.7 | 19.7 |
| Malignant Neoplasms | 3.3 | 44.0 | 2.5 | 31.8 | .8 | 12.2 |
| Digestive System (Including Mouth) | .6 | 10.0 | .5 | 9.1 | .1 | .9 |
| Respiratory System | .6 | 7.2 | .4 | 5.4 | .2 | 1.8 |
| Breast | .5 | 7.0 | .4 | 6.4 | .1 | .6 |
| Female Genital Organs | .4 | 3.8 | .4 | 3.1 | 0 * | .7 |
| Male Genital Organs | .3 | 5.2 | .2 | 3.0 | .1 | 2.2 |
| Urinary System | .2 | 2.1 | .2 | 2.1 | 0 | 0 |
| Skin | .2 | .7 | .2 | .7 | 0 | 0 |
| Eye | 0 * | .2 | 0 * | .2 | 0 | 0 |
| Nervous System (Including Brain) | .1 | 1.1 | .1 | .4 | 0 * | .7 |
| Endocrine Glands | 0 | 0 | 0 | 0 | 0 | 0 |
| Bone | 0 * | .5 | 0 | 0 | 0 * | .5 |
| Connective Tissue | 0 | 0 | 0 | 0 | 0 | 0 |
| Lymphosarcoma | 0 * | .1 | 0 * | .1 | 0 | 0 |
| Hodgkin's Disease | 0 * | .2 | 0 * | .2 | 0 | 0 |
| Other Lymphoma | .1 | 2.1 | 0 * | .3 | .1 | 1.8 |
| Multiple Myeloma | .1 | 1.2 | 0 | 0 | .1 | 1.2 |
| Leukemia | .1 | 1.5 | 0 | 0 | .1 | 1.5 |
| N.E.C.‡ | .1 | 1.1 | .1 | .8 | 0 * | .3 |
| Benign Neoplasms | 7.0 | 47.2 | 6.2 | 40.8 | .8 | 6.4 |
| Mouth | .2 | .6 | .2 | .5 | 0 * | .1 |
| Rectum | .3 | 3.0 | .2 | 2.6 | .1 | .4 |
| Breast | .7 | 3.4 | .6 | 3.0 | .1 | .4 |
| Female Genital Organs | 2.9 | 27.2 | 2.7 | 25.5 | .2 | 1.7 |
| Skin | 1.5 | 6.2 | 1.3 | 4.5 | .2 | 1.7 |
| Other | 1.4 | 6.8 | 1.2 | 4.7 | .2 | 2.1 |

TABLE 147. *(Cont'd)*

| DIAGNOSIS | Total Admissions Per 1,000 Exposure Years † | Total Days Per 1,000 Exposure Years † | TYPE OF ADMISSION | | | |
|---|---|---|---|---|---|---|
| | | | SURGICAL | | MEDICAL | |
| | | | Admissions Per 1,000 Exposure Years | Days Per 1,000 Exposure Years | Admissions Per 1,000 Exposure Years | Days Per 1,000 Exposure Years |
| *Neoplasms (Cont'd)* | | | | | | |
| Unspecified Neoplasms | .3 | 1.8 | .2 | .7 | .1 | 1.1 |
| Rectum | 0 * | .2 | 0 * | .2 | 0 | 0 |
| Breast | 0 * | .1 | 0 * | .1 | 0 | 0 |
| Female Genital Organs | .1 | .1 | .1 | .1 | 0 | 0 |
| Other | .2 | 1.4 | .1 | .3 | .1 | 1.1 |
| *Allergic, Endocrine System, Metabolic and Nutritional Diseases* | 3.0 | 30.9 | .5 | 3.5 | 2.5 | 27.4 |
| Hay Fever | 0 | 0 | 0 | 0 | 0 | 0 |
| Asthma | .6 | 5.9 | 0 | 0 | .6 | 5.9 |
| Other Allergic Diseases | .1 | .5 | 0 * | .2 | .1 | .3 |
| Diseases of Thyroid Gland | .7 | 5.4 | .4 | 2.8 | .3 | 2.6 |
| Diabetes Mellitus | 1.3 | 15.4 | 0 | 0 | 1.3 | 15.4 |
| Obesity (N.O.S.) ‡ | .1 | 1.6 | 0 | 0 | .1 | 1.6 |
| Other | .2 | 2.1 | .1 | .5 | .1 | 1.6 |
| *Diseases of Blood and Blood-Forming Organs* | .6 | 5.5 | .1 | .2 | .5 | 5.3 |
| Anemias | .4 | 3.6 | 0 * | 0 * | .4 | 3.6 |
| Other | .2 | 1.9 | .1 | .2 | .1 | 1.7 |
| *Mental, Psychoneurotic and Personality Disorders* † | .5 | 8.6 | — | — | — | — |
| *Diseases of the Nervous System* | 2.1 | 18.4 | .6 | 3.1 | 1.5 | 15.3 |
| Stroke | .1 | .7 | 0 * | .1 | .1 | .6 |
| Multiple Sclerosis | .1 | 1.3 | 0 | 0 | .1 | 1.3 |
| Migraine | 0 * | .2 | 0 | 0 | 0 * | .2 |
| Epilepsy | 0 * | .1 | 0 | 0 | 0 * | .1 |
| Sciatica | .2 | 2.6 | 0 | 0 | .2 | 2.6 |
| Other | 1.7 | 13.5 | .6 | 3.0 | 1.1 | 10.5 |
| *Diseases of the Eye* | 2.2 | 12.4 | 2.0 | 10.9 | .2 | 1.5 |
| Conjunctivitis and Ophthalmia | 0 * | .2 | 0 | 0 | 0 * | .2 |
| Strabismus | .6 | 1.7 | .6 | 1.7 | 0 | 0 |
| Cataract | .9 | 6.3 | .8 | 6.2 | .1 | .1 |
| Glaucoma | .2 | .8 | .2 | .7 | 0 * | .1 |
| Detachment of Retina | .1 | 2.6 | .1 | 2.0 | 0 * | .6 |
| Other | .4 | .8 | .3 | .3 | .1 | .5 |

| DIAGNOSIS | Total Admissions Per 1,000 Exposure Years † | Total Days Per 1,000 Exposure Years † | SURGICAL Admissions Per 1,000 Exposure Years | SURGICAL Days Per 1,000 Exposure Years | MEDICAL Admissions Per 1,000 Exposure Years | MEDICAL Days Per 1,000 Exposure Years |
|---|---|---|---|---|---|---|
| *Diseases of the Ear* | 1.2 | 6.7 | .7 | 3.2 | .5 | 3.5 |
| Otitis Externa | 0 * | .2 | 0 | 0 | 0 * | .2 |
| Otitis Media | .4 | 1.7 | .2 | .5 | .2 | 1.2 |
| Deafness | 0 | 0 | 0 | 0 | 0 | 0 |
| Other | .8 | 4.8 | .5 | 2.7 | .3 | 2.1 |
| | | | | | | |
| *Diseases of the Circulatory System* | 11.1 | 133.6 | 3.6 | 30.9 | 7.5 | 102.7 |
| Rheumatic Fever without Mention of Heart | .1 | 2.0 | 0 | 0 | .1 | 2.0 |
| Diseases of the Heart | 5.8 | 84.7 | .4 | 8.7 | 5.4 | 76.0 |
| Rheumatic Heart Disease | .7 | 9.4 | .2 | 3.7 | .5 | 5.7 |
| Arteriosclerotic Heart Disease, So Described | 1.0 | 16.7 | 0 * | .1 | 1.0 | 16.6 |
| Acute Coronary Occlusion | 1.2 | 23.9 | 0 * | .3 | 1.2 | 23.6 |
| Coronary Insufficiency | 1.1 | 10.6 | 0 * | .1 | 1.1 | 10.5 |
| Angina Pectoris | .3 | 3.6 | 0 | 0 | .3 | 3.6 |
| Hypertensive Heart Disease | .3 | 2.3 | 0 | 0 | .3 | 2.3 |
| Other | 1.2 | 18.2 | .2 | 4.5 | 1.0 | 13.7 |
| Diseases of Veins and Arteries (Other than the Heart) | 5.2 | 46.9 | 3.2 | 22.2 | 2.0 | 24.7 |
| Hypertensive Diseases | .7 | 9.1 | .1 | .4 | .6 | 8.7 |
| Hypotension | 0 | 0 | 0 | 0 | 0 | 0 |
| Hemorrhoids | 1.8 | 11.7 | 1.8 | 11.3 | 0 * | .4 |
| General Arteriosclerosis | .1 | 1.1 | .1 | 1.1 | 0 | 0 |
| Varicose Veins of Lower Extremities | .7 | 4.1 | .7 | 4.0 | 0 * | .1 |
| Pulmonary Embolism and Infarction | .1 | 1.8 | 0 * | .2 | .1 | 1.6 |
| Lymphadenitis | .4 | 1.7 | .1 | .4 | .3 | 1.3 |
| Other | 1.4 | 17.4 | .4 | 4.8 | 1.0 | 12.6 |
| | | | | | | |
| *Diseases of the Respiratory System* | 14.5 | 59.2 | 9.9 | 17.5 | 4.6 | 41.7 |
| Acute Nasopharyngitis | .1 | .5 | 0 | 0 | .1 | .5 |
| Pharyngitis | .2 | 2.1 | 0 | 0 | .2 | 2.1 |
| Tonsillitis | .7 | 2.7 | .5 | 1.3 | .2 | 1.4 |
| Hypertrophy of Tonsils | 8.0 | 9.2 | 8.0 | 9.2 | 0 | 0 |
| Laryngitis and Tracheitis | .2 | 1.0 | 0 * | .2 | .2 | .8 |
| Sinusitis | .2 | 1.5 | .1 | .9 | .1 | .6 |
| Influenza | .1 | .2 | 0 | 0 | .1 | .2 |
| Pneumonia | 2.1 | 22.2 | .1 | 0 * | 2.0 | 22.2 |
| Bronchitis | .7 | 5.3 | .1 | .3 | .6 | 5.0 |
| Other Diseases of Upper Respiratory Tract | 1.3 | 5.2 | .9 | 3.3 | .4 | 1.9 |
| Diseases of Lungs | .9 | 9.3 | .2 | 2.3 | .7 | 7.0 |

TABLE 147. (Cont'd)

| DIAGNOSIS | Total Admissions Per 1,000 Exposure Years † | Total Days Per 1,000 Exposure Years † | TYPE OF ADMISSION | | | |
|---|---|---|---|---|---|---|
| | | | SURGICAL | | MEDICAL | |
| | | | Admissions Per 1,000 Exposure Years | Days Per 1,000 Exposure Years | Admissions Per 1,000 Exposure Years | Days Per 1,000 Exposure Years |
| *Diseases of the Digestive System* | 16.3 | 151.1 | 9.3 | 91.2 | 7.0 | 59.9 |
| Stomatitis | 0 * | .1 | 0 | 0 | 0 * | .1 |
| Other Diseases of Buccal Cavity and Esophagus | .2 | .7 | .1 | .2 | .1 | .5 |
| Ulcers | 2.3 | 26.6 | .6 | 10.1 | 1.7 | 16.5 |
| Gastritis and Duodenitis | .8 | 4.7 | .1 | .4 | .7 | 4.3 |
| Other Diseases of Stomach and Duodenum | .1 | .5 | 0 * | .1 | .1 | .4 |
| Appendicitis | 2.0 | 15.0 | 1.8 | 14.2 | .2 | .8 |
| Hernia of Abdominal Cavity | 3.5 | 28.7 | 3.2 | 26.5 | .3 | 2.2 |
| Gastroenteritis and Colitis (Except Ulcerative) | 1.1 | 7.3 | 0 | 0 | 1.1 | 7.3 |
| Other Diseases of Intestines and Peritoneum | 2.8 | 23.2 | 1.4 | 10.4 | 1.4 | 12.8 |
| Diseases of the Liver, Gall Bladder and Pancreas | 3.5 | 44.3 | 2.1 | 29.3 | 1.4 | 15.0 |
| Diseases of the Liver | .6 | 7.1 | 0 * | .1 | .6 | 7.0 |
| Diseases of the Gall Bladder | 2.6 | 34.9 | 2.0 | 28.9 | .6 | 6.0 |
| Diseases of the Pancreas | .3 | 2.3 | .1 | .3 | .2 | 2.0 |
| *Diseases of the Urinary System* | 4.0 | 31.6 | 1.9 | 13.9 | 2.1 | 17.7 |
| Nephritis and Nephrosis | .1 | 2.3 | 0 | 0 | .1 | 2.3 |
| Cystitis | 1.1 | 6.1 | .5 | 2.1 | .6 | 4.0 |
| Other | 2.8 | 23.2 | 1.4 | 11.8 | 1.4 | 11.4 |
| *Diseases of the Male Genital Organs* | 1.7 | 13.2 | 1.6 | 12.2 | .1 | 1.0 |
| *Diseases of the Female Genital Organs and Breast* | 5.8 | 36.4 | 5.1 | 31.8 | .7 | 4.6 |
| Diseases of the Breast | .8 | 3.3 | .8 | 2.8 | 0 * | .5 |
| Diseases of the Ovaries, Fallopian Tubes and Parametrium | .4 | 3.1 | .2 | 1.9 | .2 | 1.2 |
| Cervicitis | 1.0 | 7.1 | .9 | 6.6 | .1 | .5 |
| Vaginitis and Vulvitis | .1 | .8 | 0 * | .3 | .1 | .5 |
| Menstrual Disorders | 1.4 | 5.3 | 1.3 | 4.8 | .1 | .5 |
| Menopausal Symptoms | 0 | 0 | 0 | 0 | 0 | 0 |
| Other | 2.1 | 16.8 | 1.9 | 15.4 | .2 | 1.4 |
| *Deliveries and Complications of Pregnancy, Childbirth and Puerperium* † | 19.1 | 83.7 | — | — | — | — |

| DIAGNOSIS | Total Admissions Per 1,000 Exposure Years † | Total Days Per 1,000 Exposure Years † | SURGICAL | | MEDICAL | |
|---|---|---|---|---|---|---|
| | | | Admissions Per 1,000 Exposure Years | Days Per 1,000 Exposure Years | Admissions Per 1,000 Exposure Years | Days Per 1,000 Exposure Years |
| *Diseases of Skin and Subcutaneous Tissues* | 2.1 | 11.6 | 1.0 | 4.3 | 1.1 | 7.3 |
| Boil and Carbuncle | .1 | .8 | 0 * | .1 | .1 | .7 |
| Cellulitis | .6 | 4.8 | .2 | 1.8 | .4 | 3.0 |
| Impetigo | 0 | 0 | 0 | 0 | 0 | 0 |
| Infectious Wart | .1 | .7 | .1 | .2 | 0 * | .5 |
| Dermatitis | .1 | .9 | 0 | 0 | .1 | .9 |
| Acne | 0 | 0 | 0 | 0 | 0 | 0 |
| Sebaceous Cyst | .3 | .4 | .3 | .4 | 0 * | 0 * |
| Other | .9 | 4.0 | .4 | 1.8 | .5 | 2.2 |
| *Diseases of Bones and Organs of Movement* | 3.5 | 35.1 | 2.2 | 17.9 | 1.3 | 17.2 |
| Arthritis and Rheumatism | .4 | 5.8 | .1 | .8 | .3 | 5.0 |
| Osteomyelitis and Other Diseases of Bones and Joints | 1.5 | 20.8 | .8 | 10.6 | .7 | 10.2 |
| Synovitis, Bursitis and Tenosynovitis | 1.0 | 4.3 | .8 | 3.0 | .2 | 1.3 |
| Infective Myositis | 0 * | .4 | 0 | 0 | 0 * | .4 |
| Muscular Dystrophy | 0 * | .3 | 0 * | .1 | 0 * | .2 |
| Scoliosis | .1 | .4 | .1 | .4 | 0 | 0 |
| Other Deformities | .3 | 2.0 | .3 | 2.0 | 0 | 0 |
| Other Diseases of Musculoskeletal System | .2 | 1.1 | .1 | 1.0 | .1 | .1 |
| *Injuries and Adverse Effects of External Causes* | 8.1 | 54.1 | 4.1 | 22.0 | 4.0 | 32.1 |
| Fractures | 3.0 | 24.2 | 2.4 | 14.5 | .6 | 9.7 |
| Skull and Face | .5 | 3.6 | .3 | .7 | .2 | 2.9 |
| Torso | .2 | 3.3 | .1 | 1.0 | .1 | 2.3 |
| Spine (Vertebral Column) | .2 | 3.3 | .1 | 1.0 | .1 | 2.3 |
| Ribs, Sternum and Larynx | 0 * | 0 * | 0 * | 0 * | 0 | 0 |
| Upper Extremities | 1.3 | 6.1 | 1.2 | 5.3 | .1 | .8 |
| Clavicle | .1 | .9 | .1 | .4 | 0 * | .5 |
| Scapula | 0 * | .1 | 0 * | .1 | 0 | 0 |
| Humerus | .2 | 2.3 | .2 | 2.3 | 0 | 0 |
| Radius and Ulna | .7 | 2.0 | .7 | 1.9 | 0 * | .1 |
| Wrist | .1 | .4 | .1 | .4 | 0 | 0 |
| Hand-Finger | .2 | .4 | .1 | .2 | .1 | .2 |
| Lower Extremities | 1.0 | 11.2 | .8 | 7.5 | .2 | 3.7 |
| Pelvis | 0 * | .3 | 0 | 0 | 0 * | .3 |
| Femur | .2 | 4.6 | .2 | 2.4 | 0 * | 2.2 |
| Patella | 0 | 0 | 0 | 0 | 0 | 0 |
| Tibia and Fibula | .4 | 1.9 | .4 | 1.6 | 0 * | .3 |
| Ankle | .2 | 2.2 | .1 | 1.5 | .1 | .7 |
| Foot-Toe | .2 | 2.2 | .1 | 2.0 | .1 | .2 |
| Late Effects of Fractures | 0 | 0 | 0 | 0 | 0 | 0 |

TABLE 147. (Concluded)

| DIAGNOSIS | Total Admissions Per 1,000 Exposure Years † | Total Days Per 1,000 Exposure Years † | SURGICAL Admissions Per 1,000 Exposure Years | SURGICAL Days Per 1,000 Exposure Years | MEDICAL Admissions Per 1,000 Exposure Years | MEDICAL Days Per 1,000 Exposure Years |
|---|---|---|---|---|---|---|
| *Injuries (Cont'd)* | | | | | | |
| Dislocations | .3 | 1.6 | .2 | 1.1 | .1 | .5 |
| Sprains and Strains | 1.3 | 9.8 | .1 | .7 | 1.2 | 9.1 |
| Head Injuries (Other than Fractures) | 1.0 | 5.3 | .1 | .9 | .9 | 4.4 |
| Internal Injuries | .1 | .5 | .1 | .5 | 0 | 0 |
| Lacerations and Open Wounds | 1.0 | 3.5 | .8 | 2.7 | .2 | .8 |
| Superficial Injuries | .1 | .5 | 0 * | .2 | .1 | .3 |
| Foreign Body | .1 | .3 | .1 | .1 | 0 * | .2 |
| Contusions | .7 | 5.6 | .1 | .7 | .6 | 4.9 |
| Complications of Surgical or Medical Procedures | .1 | .5 | .1 | .2 | 0 * | .3 |
| Other | .4 | 2.3 | .1 | .4 | .3 | 1.9 |
| *Congenital Malformations* | .8 | 6.3 | .7 | 5.0 | .1 | 1.3 |
| *Certain Diseases of Early Infancy* | .5 | 5.4 | .1 | .5 | .4 | 4.9 |
| *Symptoms, Senility and Ill-Defined Conditions* | 2.6 | 18.7 | .5 | 3.8 | 2.1 | 14.9 |
| Symptoms Referrable to Nervous System | .3 | 1.9 | 0 * | .2 | .3 | 1.7 |
| Symptoms Referrable to Cardiovascular System | .2 | .7 | 0 | 0 | .2 | .7 |
| Symptoms Referrable to Respiratory System | .5 | 2.9 | .1 | .5 | .4 | 2.4 |
| Symptoms Referrable to Upper and Lower Gastro-intestinal System | .5 | 5.7 | 0 * | .4 | .5 | 5.3 |
| Symptoms Referrable to Urinary System | .4 | 2.7 | .1 | 1.0 | .3 | 1.7 |
| Pain in Back | .1 | .4 | 0 | 0 | .1 | .4 |
| Other Referrable Symptoms, N.E.C.‡ | .5 | 3.6 | .2 | 1.1 | .3 | 2.5 |
| Headache | 0 | 0 | 0 | 0 | 0 | 0 |
| Other Ill-Defined Diseases | .1 | .8 | .1 | .6 | 0 * | .2 |
| *Undetermined Classifications* | 3.3 | 28.5 | 1.8 | 12.4 | 1.4 | 14.5 |

1 Comprehensive Plan sample.

* Less than .05.

† Including in addition to surgical and medical admissions, 19.1 obstetrical admissions and 83.7 obstetrical days, and .5 psychiatric admissions and 8.6 psychiatric days, per 1,000 exposure years. Of the obstetrical admissions, 16.5 were for normal deliveries, 2.3 for abortions or miscarriages, .3 for complicated deliveries or ectopic pregnancies.

‡ Not elsewhere classified or otherwise specified.

# HOSPITALIZATION STUDIES NOT RELATED
# TO POPULATION AT RISK

As mentioned earlier, hospitalization studies have been categorized into those involving analyses of frequencies, expressed in terms of a number of indices related to the population at risk; and those involving only the hospitalized population. The remainder of this Chapter is devoted to a few examples of the latter category.

It is recognized that for non-population-related analyses, the hospitals themselves or their associations, rather than insurance plans (particularly those not covering hospitalization!) would be the preferable source of statistics on trends and local differences.

Characteristics recorded for each admission include diagnosis, type of admission, dates of admission and discharge, hospital identity, physician identity (specialty, qualifications, location, highest hospital staff affiliation, age), patient identity (all characteristics listed in previous section). The record thus provides the possibility of multivariate analyses involving about twenty variables.

The analyses actually performed are illustrative only. Findings as to physician characteristics associated with hospitalization have appeared previously (Chapter 6). Presentations below concern the distribution of admissions and/or aggregate days of hospitalization according to time of year, area location, type of hospital, type of case, length of stay, and diagnosis.

## Monthly Variations in Admissions

The proportion of admissions entering the hospital during the highest admission month, October, was 35 per cent greater than in the lowest month, August.

Throughout most of the year, admission rates varied generally within a range of only 15 per cent from month to month (Table 148). Except for January, the third highest month, the busiest times were fall (October-November) and spring (April, May, June). These six months accounted for 53.5 per cent of admissions. The fact that February was the second lowest month is not entirely explained by its comparative shortness.

TABLE 148.   Distribution of Hospital Admissions, by Month

| MONTH | Per Cent of Admissions |
|---|---|
| October | 9.3 |
| November | 9.1 |
| January | 9.0 |
| April | 8.9 |
| May | 8.7 |
| June | 8.5 |
| September | 8.2 |
| December | 8.2 |
| March | 8.1 |
| July | 7.9 |
| February | 7.2 |
| August | 6.9 |
| TOTAL | 100.0 |

The overall picture does not necessarily apply to the various types of admissions—surgical, medical, obstetrical. The leading month for medical and obstetrical cases was the same—October—but May was first in surgery.

The highest proportions of maternity admissions occurred in four successive months—October, November, December, January in that order. Next highest were April and July. There were apparently 50 per cent more such cases in October than in May, the low month.

Obstetrical cases are the only type in which December ranked as one of the three leading months.

Whereas surgical admission rates were most frequent in the spring months—April, May, June—medical cases reached their highest level in the fall—September, October, November—and in January, dropped to their lowest point in February, then maintained a fairly stationary level for the six-month period March through August. In general, medical rates tended to be steadier from month to month; the spread between the highest and lowest months was much smaller than between the corresponding figures for surgical cases, where May admissions outnumbered those in August with a ratio of five to three (Table 149).

TABLE 149. Distribution of Surgical, Medical, and Obstetrical Admissions, by Month

| MONTH | PER CENT OF ADMISSIONS | | | MONTH RANK | | |
|---|---|---|---|---|---|---|
| | Surgical | Medical | Obstetrical | Surgical | Medical | Obstetrical |
| January | 8.6 | 9.5 | 9.1 | 6 | 2 | 4 |
| February | 7.1 | 7.0 | 7.7 | 11 | 12 | 8–9 |
| March | 8.5 | 7.8 | 7.5 | 7 | 7–9 | 11 |
| April | 9.5 | 8.1 | 8.6 | 2 | 6 | 5–6 |
| May | 10.0 | 7.7 | 6.5 | 1 | 10 | 12 |
| June | 9.2 | 7.8 | 8.0 | 3 | 7–9 | 7 |
| July | 8.0 | 7.6 | 8.6 | 8 | 11 | 5–6 |
| August | 6.1 | 7.8 | 7.7 | 12 | 7–9 | 8–9 |
| September | 7.6 | 9.3 | 7.6 | 9–10 | 3 | 10 |
| October | 8.8 | 9.7 | 9.8 | 5 | 1 | 1 |
| November | 9.0 | 9.0 | 9.6 | 4 | 4 | 2 |
| December | 7.6 | 8.7 | 9.3 | 9–10 | 5 | 3 |
| | 100.0 | 100.0 | 100.0 | | | |

With reprogramming, the timing of hospital admissions could also, or alternatively, be retrieved on a day-of-the-week basis, for studies of week-end waste.

## Geographic Distribution of Admissions

The distribution of admissions among hospitals located in different areas corresponds fairly well with the home area listed for patients, when each distribution—that is, hospital address and patient home address—is analyzed separately. In other words, the proportion of admissions to hospitals in most geographic subdivisions tended to approximate the proportion of hospitalized patients listed as residing in these areas (Table 150).

TABLE 150.   Geographic Distribution of Admissions

|  | Area of Hospital | Area of Patient Residence |
|---|---|---|
|  | % | % |
| Manhattan | 11.9 | 6.5 |
| Bronx | 7.0 | 9.6 |
| Brooklyn | 17.3 | 19.7 |
| Queens | 13.0 | 16.0 |
| Richmond | 2.6 | 2.7 |
| Nassau | 10.9 | 11.4 |
| Suffolk | 10.3 | 8.1 |
| Westchester | 4.7 | 4.2 |
| Other New York | 8.1 | 11.3 |
| New Jersey | 7.8 | 8.0 |
| Other or Unknown | 6.4 | 2.5 |
|  | 100.0 | 100.0 |

The overall distributions fail to show the extent to which individual patients hospitalized in each area were out-of-area residents. Further analysis revealed apparent crossing of area lines on the part of a substantial minority. Although it is known that many patients do enter hospitals outside their home areas for a variety of reasons, it may be that a good portion of what is listed as area-shifting represents rather a lag in data recording; there is always the possibility that the patient had moved by the time of hospitalization. With this in mind, it would be desirable to spot-check patient addresses at time of hospitalization before accepting results of the type of analysis presented in Table 151.

## DISTRIBUTION OF HOSPITAL ADMISSIONS IN SUBDIVISIONS OF 8-COUNTY NEW YORK METROPOLITAN AREA, BY TYPE OF HOSPITAL

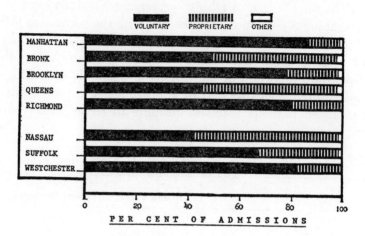

## VOLUNTARY BED RATIOS vs. PROPORTION OF CASES ADMITTED TO PROPRIETARY HOSPITALS, BY AREA

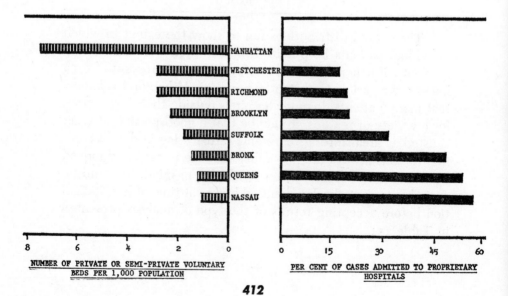

## TABLE 151. Distribution of Hospital Admissions in Each Area, by Residence of Patients

| AREA RECORDED AS PATIENT RESIDENCE | HOSPITAL AREA | | | | | | | | | |
|---|---|---|---|---|---|---|---|---|---|---|
| | Manhattan | Bronx | Brooklyn | Queens | Richmond | Nassau | Suffolk | West-chester | Other New York | New Jersey |
| | PER CENT OF ADMISSIONS | | | | | | | | | |
| TOTAL | 100.0 | 100.0 | 100.0 | 100.0 | 100.0 | 100.0 | 100.0 | 100.0 | 100.0 | 100.0 |
| Manhattan | 34.9 | 6.7 | 1.6 | 3.6 | .7 | .7 | .7 | 1.9 | 3.1 | 4.2 |
| Bronx | 16.7 | 77.3 | .7 | 2.9 | 2.1 | .7 | .8 | 14.9 | 2.2 | 3.2 |
| Brooklyn | 14.1 | 3.4 | 83.6 | 8.5 | 5.7 | 4.3 | 6.0 | 1.5 | 3.4 | 1.4 |
| Queens | 17.3 | 4.4 | 9.6 | 69.8 | 1.4 | 11.1 | 7.4 | 1.2 | 1.6 | .7 |
| Richmond | 2.3 | 0 | .7 | 0 | 87.3 | 0 | 0 | 0 | 0 | 0 |
| Nassau | 4.1 | .5 | 1.7 | 11.1 | 0 | 65.7 | 13.2 | 1.2 | 1.4 | .4 |
| Suffolk | 1.1 | 0 | .2 | 1.1 | 0 | 9.3 | 61.5 | 0 | 1.1 | .7 |
| Westchester | 2.7 | 4.6 | .1 | | 0 | .9 | 0 | 68.2 | .7 | 0 |
| Other New York | 3.3 | 1.3 | .5 | 1.8 | 1.4 | 6.3 | 8.8 | 9.2 | 85.8 | .7 |
| New Jersey | 2.4 | 1.3 | .1 | 1.0 | .7 | .2 | .2 | .8 | .2 | 88.5 |
| Other | .3 | .5 | .3 | .1 | .7 | 0 | 0 | .7 | .5 | 0 |
| Unknown | .8 | 0 | .9 | .1 | 0 | .8 | 1.4 | .4 | 0 | .2 |

413

## Type of Hospital Used *

Voluntary hospitals accounted for 68 per cent of all recorded admissions, proprietary hospitals for 28 per cent, and government hospitals for 4 per cent.

Of voluntary hospital admissions, half were in hospitals approved for training residents and interns, and one fifth in hospitals associated with medical schools.

These proportions generally obtained for the three principal types of admissions, with a slightly higher proportion of obstetrical cases going to voluntary hospitals (71 per cent, vs. 66 per cent of medical cases), and a compensatingly lower proportion to proprietary hospitals (24 per cent, vs. 29 per cent of medical cases).

TABLE 152.  Distribution of Hospital Admissions by Type of Hospital and Type of Admission

| TYPE OF HOSPITAL | TYPE OF ADMISSION | | | |
| --- | --- | --- | --- | --- |
| | All Types | Surgical | Medical | Obstetrical |
| | % | % | % | % |
| Voluntary | 68 | 69 | 66 | 71 |
| Affiliated * | 13 | 14 | 14 | 12 |
| Approved † | 34 | 34 | 33 | 37 |
| Other | 21 | 21 | 19 | 22 |
| Proprietary | 28 | 27 | 29 | 24 |
| Government | 4 | 4 | 5 | 5 |
| TOTAL | 100 | 100 | 100 | 100 |

* Affiliated with medical school.
† Approved for resident or intern training.

The various categories of non-government hospitals experienced practically no difference in their proportions of surgical admissions, which averaged 45 to 47 per cent of all GHI admissions in affiliated, approved, other voluntary, and proprietary hospitals. A departure from this pattern was found for

* See also Chapter 6, Tables 56 and 58.

government hospital admissions, of which 37 per cent were surgical, and 45 per cent medical. Within the voluntary and proprietary categories, the proportion of medical cases was less consistent than that found for surgery, ranging from 36 to 42 per cent. Somewhat surprisingly, the breakdown as to type of case in proprietary hospitals was about the same as in medical-school-affiliated voluntary hospitals. The other types of voluntary hospitals had more obstetrical and fewer medical cases, proportionately (Table 153).

TABLE 153.  Type of Admission, by Type of Hospital

| TYPE OF HOSPITAL | TYPE OF ADMISSION | | | |
|---|---|---|---|---|
| | *Total* | *Surgical* | *Medical* | *Obstetrical* |
| | % | % | % | % |
| Voluntary | 100 | 46 | 37 | 17 |
| Affiliated * | 100 | 45 | 41 | 14 |
| Approved † | 100 | 46 | 37 | 17 |
| Other | 100 | 47 | 36 | 17 |
| Proprietary | 100 | 45 | 42 | 13 |
| Government | 100 | 37 | 45 | 18 |
| All | 100 | 45 | 39 | 16 |

* Affiliated with medical school.
† Approved for resident or intern training.

### Local Variations in Type of Hospital Used

The proportionate use of different types of hospitals in different geographic subsections reflects local differences as to available facilities.

Areas such as Queens and Nassau, which are the least endowed with voluntary beds and have the most proprietary beds per thousand population, showed far higher proportions of cases—over half—entering proprietary hospitals.

At the other extreme, in Manhattan, with its concentration of medical-school-affiliated voluntary hospitals, 44 per cent of admissions were to such hospitals, as compared with the overall area average of 13 per cent, and only 12 per cent were to proprietary hospitals, as against 33 per cent of all admissions in the eight-county metropolitan area (Table 154).

TABLE 154. Distribution of Hospital Admissions in 8-County
New York Metropolitan Area, by Type
and Location of Hospital

| | | TYPE OF HOSPITAL | | | | | |
| | | VOLUNTARY | | | | | |
| HOSPITAL LOCATION | All Types | All | Affili- ated * | Ap- proved † | Other | Propri- etary | Other ‡ |
|---|---|---|---|---|---|---|---|
| | % | % | % | % | % | % | % |
| All Areas | 100 | 68 | 13 | 34 | 21 | 28 | 4 |
| 8–County Area | 100 | 66 | 16 | 33 | 17 | 33 | 1 |
| 5–County Area | 100 | 69 | 23 | 34 | 12 | 30 | 1 |
| Manhattan | 100 | 87 | 44 | 35 | 8 | 12 | 1 |
| Bronx | 100 | 50 | 13 | 32 | 5 | 48 | 2 |
| Brooklyn | 100 | 79 | 27 | 30 | 22 | 20 | 1 |
| Queens | 100 | 46 | 8 | 35 | 3 | 53 | 1 |
| Richmond | 100 | 81 | 0 | 60 | 21 | 19 | 0 |
| Nassau | 100 | 43 | 0 | 39 | 4 | 56 | 1 |
| Suffolk | 100 | 68 | 0 | 5 | 63 | 31 | 1 |
| Westchester | 100 | 83 | 1 | 68 | 14 | 17 | 0 |

* Affiliated with medical school.
† Approved for resident or intern training.
‡ Mainly county or state hospitals.

The tendency on the part of some analysts to treat the New York metropolitan area as though it were a homogeneous unit ignores the wide variations in local resources which cannot be ignored by those involved in day-to-day confrontations with problems of private patient placement.

In the interests of discouraging what is called unnecessary hospitalization, those responsible for assessing hospital needs have taken the position that although many hospitals are in deplorable condition there are enough beds in the New York metropolitan area as a whole, counting municipal hospital beds as fulfilling a substantial part of the (undefined) requirements.

At the same time, those interested in improved quality of care recommend hospitalization in medical school affiliates and avoidance of proprietary institutions.

The fact is, however, that the individual's chance of choosing the type of hospital he wishes to enter—assuming he knows —is generally limited by the facilities in his area, which in turn limit his physician's choice.

In areas with lowest private voluntary bed ratios, fewer than half of the practicing physicians have appointments on voluntary staffs. In all areas, even those with such appointments are not sure of a bed when requested. The primacy of the varying bed situations would hardly seem to require belaboring, but analysts rarely call attention to it.

GHI experience shows a marked inverse relationship between local voluntary bed-population ratios and proprietary hospital admissions: the higher the voluntary bed ratio, the lower the proportion of proprietary admissions (Table 155).

TABLE 155.   Voluntary Bed Ratios vs. Proportion of Cases Admitted to Proprietary Hospitals, by Area

| AREA | Number of Private Voluntary Beds Per 1000 Population | Per Cent of GHI Cases Admitted to Proprietary Hospitals |
|---|---|---|
| Manhattan | 7.40 | 12 |
| Westchester | 3.03 | 17 |
| Richmond | 2.97 | 19 |
| Brooklyn | 2.26 | 20 |
| Suffolk | 1.81 | 31 |
| Bronx | 1.44 | 48 |
| Queens | 1.20 | 53 |
| Nassau | 1.11 | 56 |

The ratio of proprietary beds to total private beds is highest, as would be expected, where voluntary beds are scarcest; but although the existence of proprietary beds is a prerequisite for high proportionate use of such beds, the percentage of cases admitted to proprietary hospitals in each area is more consistently related to voluntary bed ratios than to proprietary bed ratios.

Of GHI patients hospitalized in each area, the percentage entering proprietary hospitals was somewhat larger than the percentage of private beds accounted for by proprietary hospitals, but was generally much smaller than the percentage of physicians without voluntary hospital appointments (Table 156).

Thus, while there seems to be some margin to effectuate

TABLE 156. Proportion of Cases in Proprietary Hospitals vs.
Proportion of Proprietary Beds and Physician
Staff Appointments, by Area

| AREA | Per Cent of GHI Cases Admitted to Proprietary Hospitals | Per Cent of All Private Beds Represented by Proprietary Beds | Per Cent of Practicing Physicians Without Voluntary Staff Appointments |
|---|---|---|---|
| Manhattan | 12 | 5 | 47 |
| Westchester | 17 | 12 | 46 |
| Richmond | 19 | 14 | 42 |
| Brooklyn | 20 | 14 | 52 |
| Suffolk | 31 | 22 | 49 |
| Bronx | 48 | 34 | 67 |
| Queens | 53 | 48 | 61 |
| Nassau | 56 | 53 | 61 |

greater proportionate use of voluntary beds, other factors may
interfere; if the treating physician lacks the necessary staff
appointment or if no bed is available for his patient at the time
requested, use of a proprietary bed is the only alternative,
irrespective of patient or physician preference. In voluntary
bed shortage areas, the repetition of this situation for patient
after patient has led many a physician to the exclusive use of
proprietary hospitals.

### Local Variations in Type of Hospital Used
### for Different Types of Cases

As a rule, type of case had little effect on area patterns of
hospital use. In counties with relatively lower overall proportions of admissions going to voluntary hospitals, this tendency
generally applied to surgical, medical, and obstetrical admissions.

In Queens and Nassau, obstetrical cases entered voluntary
hospitals in greater proportions than did surgical or medical
cases; the latter were most likely to be sent to proprietary hospitals. The opposite situation prevailed in the Bronx, with the
majority of medical cases going to voluntary hospitals and
obstetrical cases to proprietaries. In Manhattan, Westchester,
Brooklyn and Richmond, the great majority of all types of cases
entered voluntary hospitals (Table 157).

TABLE 157. Distribution of Admissions by Type of Hospital and Type of Admission, by County, in 8-County New York Metropolitan Area

| COUNTY | TYPE OF ADMISSION | All | TYPE OF HOSPITAL | | | | Proprietary | Other ‡ |
|---|---|---|---|---|---|---|---|---|
| | | | VOLUNTARY | | | | | |
| | | | All | Affiliated * | Approved † | Other | | |
| | | % | % | % | % | % | % | % |
| Manhattan | Surgical | 100 | 87 | 44 | 36 | 7 | 13 | 0 |
| | Medical | 100 | 87 | 42 | 33 | 12 | 13 | 0 |
| | Obstetrical | 100 | 92 | 55 | 34 | 3 | 3 | 5 |
| Westchester | Surgical | 100 | 83 | 1 | 66 | 16 | 17 | 0 |
| | Medical | 100 | 81 | 1 | 70 | 10 | 19 | 0 |
| | Obstetrical | 100 | 89 | 0 | 67 | 22 | 11 | 0 |
| Richmond | Surgical | 100 | 82 | 0 | 60 | 22 | 18 | 0 |
| | Medical | 100 | 77 | 0 | 60 | 17 | 23 | 0 |
| | Obstetrical | 100 | 94 | 0 | 61 | 33 | 6 | 0 |
| Brooklyn | Surgical | 100 | 78 | 24 | 30 | 24 | 21 | 1 |
| | Medical | 100 | 78 | 31 | 27 | 20 | 21 | 1 |
| | Obstetrical | 100 | 83 | 26 | 35 | 22 | 17 | 0 |
| Suffolk | Surgical | 100 | 69 | 0 | 4 | 65 | 31 | 0 |
| | Medical | 100 | 59 | 0 | 8 | 51 | 38 | 3 |
| | Obstetrical | 100 | 81 | 0 | 4 | 77 | 19 | 0 |
| Bronx | Surgical | 100 | 50 | 17 | 24 | 9 | 49 | 1 |
| | Medical | 100 | 56 | 16 | 37 | 3 | 42 | 2 |
| | Obstetrical | 100 | 38 | 0 | 38 | 0 | 60 | 2 |
| Queens | Surgical | 100 | 47 | 7 | 37 | 3 | 52 | 1 |
| | Medical | 100 | 43 | 8 | 32 | 3 | 57 | 0 |
| | Obstetrical | 100 | 50 | 8 | 36 | 6 | 49 | 1 |
| Nassau | Surgical | 100 | 45 | 0 | 42 | 3 | 54 | 1 |
| | Medical | 100 | 33 | 0 | 28 | 5 | 65 | 2 |
| | Obstetrical | 100 | 55 | 0 | 54 | 1 | 45 | 0 |

* Affiliated with medical school.
† Approved for resident or intern training.
‡ Mainly county or state hospitals.

## Distribution of Cases and Aggregate Days
## Stayed, by Length of Stay *

As with all medical care, a relatively small portion of the hospitalized patients accounted for a large portion of services received, and vice versa. Thus, every fourth admission involved 10 or more days in the hospital, and these cases used 58 per cent of all days charged; while the 55 per cent of cases remaining 5 days or less used only 22 per cent of total days charged. The intermediate group of cases, those remaining 6 to 9 days, constituted one fifth of the admissions and also contributed one fifth of the aggregate days.

Two thirds of the medical cases remained in the hospital more than 5 days, as compared with 40 per cent of the surgical and 12.5 per cent of the obstetrical cases. Nearly half the surgical patients stayed only one, two, or three days; as a result, the 24 per cent of cases which involved stays of 10 days or more accounted for 60 per cent of all the surgical days. Comparatively few medical cases (17 per cent) were discharged within three days; 48 per cent stayed from 6 days to two weeks, as against 28 per cent of surgical admissions. Medical cases remaining longer than two weeks were the exception, 18.5 per cent of medical admissions—but they accounted for nearly half (45 per cent) of aggregate medical days (Table 158).

### Length of Stay in Different Types of Hospitals

The higher the hospital's rank in the hospital hierarchy, the longer was the average stay. For both medical and surgical admissions, voluntary hospitals affiliated with medical schools retained their patients for significantly longer periods than did other types of voluntary hospitals and proprietary institutions. (Government institutions, with generally highest average stays, are excluded from this analysis. They accounted for only 4 per cent of admissions.)

---

* The data presented in the remaining tables of this chapter are limited to the experience of the GHI membership covered by the "Family Doctor Plan," i.e. comprehensive physician coverage in office, home, hospital. As shown previously, the average length of hospital stays for these members was found to be somewhat shorter than for those with more limited physician coverage.

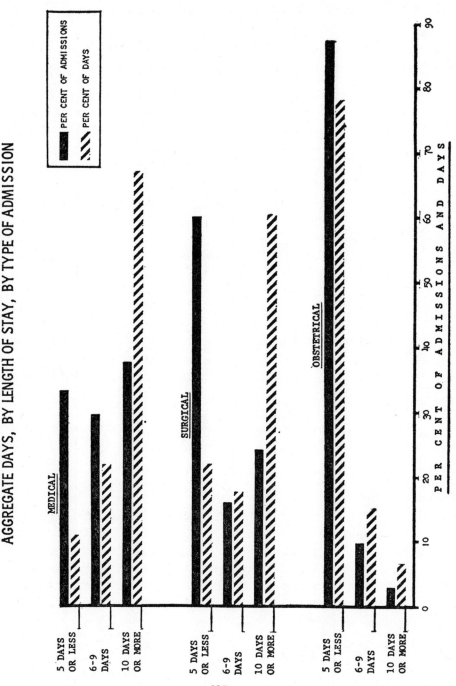

HOSPITALIZATION: DISTRIBUTION OF ADMISSIONS AND AGGREGATE DAYS, BY LENGTH OF STAY, BY TYPE OF ADMISSION

■ PER CENT OF ADMISSIONS
▨ PER CENT OF DAYS

MEDICAL

5 DAYS OR LESS
6-9 DAYS
10 DAYS OR MORE

SURGICAL

5 DAYS OR LESS
6-9 DAYS
10 DAYS OR MORE

OBSTETRICAL

5 DAYS OR LESS
6-9 DAYS
10 DAYS OR MORE

PER CENT OF ADMISSIONS AND DAYS

0   10   20   30   40   50   60   70   80   90

## TABLE 158. Distribution of Admissions and Aggregate Days, by Length of Stay and Type of Admission

### PER CENT OF ADMISSIONS AND AGGREGATE DAYS *

| LENGTH OF STAY (DAYS) | ALL | | MEDICAL | | SURGICAL | | OBSTETRICAL | |
|---|---|---|---|---|---|---|---|---|
| | Admissions | Days | Admissions | Days | Admissions | Days | Admissions | Days |
| | % | % | % | % | % | % | % | % |
| 1 | 11.7 | 1.6 | 4.0 | .4 | 20.7 | 3.2 | 2.4 | .6 |
| 2 | 10.1 | 2.7 | 6.4 | 1.3 | 14.2 | 4.3 | 6.5 | 3.0 |
| 3 | 10.0 | 4.0 | 6.4 | 1.9 | 11.7 | 5.3 | 12.8 | 8.7 |
| 4–5 | 23.2 | 14.0 | 16.3 | 7.4 | 13.4 | 9.1 | 65.8 | 65.9 |
| 6–9 | 19.8 | 19.5 | 29.5 | 21.8 | 16.0 | 17.8 | 9.8 | 15.3 |
| 10–14 | 12.8 | 20.3 | 18.9 | 22.5 | 11.9 | 21.1 | 2.7 | 6.5 |
| 15–21 | 7.7 | 18.4 | 10.8 | 19.3 | 8.1 | 21.7 | 0 | 0 |
| 22–30 | 3.0 | 10.2 | 4.3 | 11.0 | 3.0 | 11.8 | 0 | 0 |
| 31–70 | 1.6 | 8.8 | 3.3 | 13.3 | 1.0 | 5.7 | 0 | 0 |
| 71 or Over | .1 | .5 | .1 | 1.1 | 0 | 0 | 0 | 0 |
| TOTAL | 100.0 | 100.0 | 100.0 | 100.0 | 100.0 | 100.0 | 100.0 | 100.0 |
| 5 or Under | 55.0 | 22.3 | 33.1 | 11.0 | 60.0 | 21.9 | 87.5 | 78.2 |
| 6–9 | 19.8 | 19.5 | 29.5 | 21.8 | 16.0 | 17.8 | 9.8 | 15.3 |
| 10 or Over | 25.2 | 58.2 | 37.4 | 67.2 | 24.0 | 60.3 | 2.7 | 6.5 |

* Comprehensive Plan sample.

422

TABLE 159.   Average Length of Stay by Type of Hospital
and Type of Admission

| | TYPE OF ADMISSION * | | |
| TYPE OF HOSPITAL | Medical | Surgical | Obstetrical |
| --- | --- | --- | --- |
| | NUMBER OF DAYS PER STAY | | |
| Voluntary | | | |
| Affiliated with Medical School | 13.4 | 8.8 | 5.1 |
| Approved for Training Residents | 10.6 | 6.8 | 4.3 |
| Other | 9.7 | 6.2 | 4.1 |
| Proprietary | 8.9 | 5.6 | 4.4 |

* Comprehensive Plan sample.

The lengthy average stays at medical-school-affiliated hospitals, as compared with other non-government hospitals, reflect a significantly smaller proportion of cases remaining 9 days or less and a larger proportion remaining 22 days or more.

This was generally true of both surgical and medical admissions, but particularly of medical. Thus, in the medical-school affiliates, 16 per cent of medical admissions remained in the hospital over three weeks, accounting for 40 per cent of the medical days credited to such hospitals, whereas only 4 per cent of proprietary medical admissions stayed more than 21 days, accounting for 14 per cent of all medical days in proprietary hospitals. Fewer than half (47 per cent) the medical cases in medical school affiliates were discharged within 9 days, and they accounted for only one fifth of the medical days for this category of hospital; in contrast, among other types of voluntary hospitals, as well as proprietary hospitals, 60 to 65 per cent of the medical cases incurred stays of under 10 days.

Surgical stays of under 10 days were typical of all types of hospitals, but to a lesser degree in medical school affiliates, where such cases accounted for only 26 per cent of aggregate surgical days as against 40 to 48 per cent in other hospital categories. The proportion of surgical cases remaining over three weeks was similar in all types of voluntary hospitals, ranging from 5 to 7 per cent, and negligible in proprietary hospitals—less than half of one per cent of their surgical cases (Table 160).

TABLE 160.  Per Cent of Surgical and Medical Admissions and Aggregate Days Accruing at Different Types of Hospitals for Stays of Specified Cumulated Intervals

| TYPE OF ADMISSION AND LENGTH OF STAY | PER CENT OF ADMISSIONS | | | | PER CENT OF AGGREGATE DAYS | | | |
| | TYPE OF HOSPITAL | | | | TYPE OF HOSPITAL | | | |
| | VOLUNTARY | | | PROPRIETARY | VOLUNTARY | | | PROPRIETARY |
| | Affiliated* | Approved† | Other | | Affiliated* | Approved† | Other | |
| *Surgical* | | | | | | | | |
| 3 Days or Under | 34.5 | 43.6 | 53.0 | 49.0 | 8.1 | 12.5 | 14.1 | 15.3 |
| 9 Days or Under | 61.8 | 73.9 | 80.5 | 79.6 | 26.2 | 39.7 | 40.2 | 47.5 |
| 14 Days or Under | 80.9 | 87.9 | 87.5 | 90.7 | 51.0 | 63.7 | 53.2 | 70.2 |
| 21 Days or Under | 93.6 | 95.2 | 93.0 | 99.6 | 75.2 | 82.2 | 68.9 | 97.5 |
| 22 Days or Over | 6.4 | 4.8 | 7.0 | .4 | 24.8 | 17.8 | 31.1 | 2.5 |
| *Medical* | | | | | | | | |
| 3 Days or Under | 11.1 | 14.3 | 17.9 | 17.9 | 1.6 | 2.9 | 3.7 | 4.8 |
| 9 Days or Under | 47.3 | 60.0 | 63.9 | 64.8 | 20.1 | 30.7 | 32.8 | 38.2 |
| 14 Days or Under | 67.5 | 78.4 | 82.5 | 86.9 | 38.2 | 51.2 | 55.6 | 67.7 |
| 21 Days or Under | 84.0 | 90.8 | 92.3 | 95.9 | 59.6 | 71.7 | 74.3 | 86.0 |
| 22 Days or Over | 16.0 | 9.2 | 7.7 | 4.1 | 40.4 | 28.3 | 25.7 | 14.0 |

* Affiliated with medical school.
† Approved for resident or intern training.

## Distribution Related to Diagnosis

The subject of diagnosis of hospital cases has previously been introduced in connection with presentations of population-based indices of frequency rates (see Table 147).

The remaining analyses are examples of the type which can be performed when the population at risk is not known—i.e. where hospital records are the only source of data.

### Distribution of Admissions and Days Among Diagnostic Categories

Over half the admissions (55 per cent) fell into four diagnostic categories, involving either the digestive tract, respiratory tract, circulatory system, or maternity care. Neoplasms and injuries were involved in another 16.5 per cent, and disorders of female organs in 5 per cent, of all admissions. No other single category accounted for as much as 4 per cent.

As between medical and surgical admissions, circulatory diseases were the single most important category for medical admissions and of relatively minor rank surgically; while neoplasms, the third-ranking cause of surgical admissions, were seldom listed as medical cases. In addition to circulatory disorders, admissions generally classified as medical included those involving infective, parasitic, allergic, blood, and nervous disorders. Admissions generally falling into the surgical category involved neoplasms, respiratory tract, eye, male and female genital organs or breast, and congenital malformations. Conditions affecting the digestive or urinary tracts, injuries, ear, skin and bone disorders each accounted for similar proportions of surgical and medical admissions but were more likely to be surgical than medical (Table 161).

### Diagnosis and Average Length of Stay

Average hospital stays ranged from 4.1 days for conditions of the respiratory tract to 12.0 days for diseases of the circulatory system. In practically all diagnostic categories, the average

TABLE 161. Distribution of Hospital Admissions and Days by Diagnostic Category, by Type of Admission

| | TYPE OF ADMISSION * | | | | | | | |
|---|---|---|---|---|---|---|---|---|
| | ALL | | MEDICAL | | SURGICAL | | OBSTETRICAL | |
| DIAGNOSTIC CATEGORY | Admissions | Days | Admissions | Days | Admissions | Days | Admissions | Days |
| | % | % | % | % | % | % | % | % |
| Infective and Parasitic Diseases | .8 | 1.1 | 2.3 | 2.3 | 0 | 0 | | |
| Neoplasms | 9.2 | 11.0 | 4.4 | 5.2 | 16.2 | 20.3 | | |
| Allergic, Endocrine System, Metabolic and Nutritional Diseases | 2.8 | 3.9 | 6.5 | 7.1 | 1.0 | 1.1 | | |
| Diseases of Blood and Blood-Forming Organs | .5 | .7 | 1.3 | 1.4 | .2 | .1 | | |
| Diseases of Nervous System | 1.9 | 2.3 | 4.0 | 4.0 | 1.1 | .9 | | |
| Diseases of the Eye | 2.0 | 1.5 | .5 | .4 | 3.8 | 3.2 | | |
| Diseases of the Ear | 1.1 | .8 | 1.2 | .9 | 1.4 | 1.0 | | |
| Diseases of the Circulatory System | 10.1 | 16.5 | 19.2 | 26.5 | 7.1 | 9.2 | | |
| Diseases of the Respiratory System | 13.1 | 7.3 | 11.8 | 10.7 | 18.8 | 5.2 | | |
| Diseases of the Digestive System | 14.8 | 18.6 | 18.1 | 15.5 | 17.7 | 26.5 | | |
| Diseases of the Urinary System | 3.7 | 3.9 | 5.4 | 4.6 | 3.7 | 4.0 | | |
| Diseases of the Male Genital Organs | 1.5 | 1.6 | .3 | .3 | 2.9 | 3.5 | | |
| Diseases of the Female Genital Organs and Breast | 5.2 | 4.5 | 1.6 | 1.2 | 9.8 | 9.3 | | |
| Deliveries and Complications of Pregnancy, Childbirth and Puerperium | 17.2 | 10.2 | 0 | 0 | 0 | 0 | 100.0 | 100.0 |
| Diseases of Skin and Subcutaneous Tissue | 1.9 | 1.4 | 2.8 | 1.9 | 2.0 | 1.3 | | |
| Diseases of Bones and Organs of Movement | 3.2 | 4.3 | 3.4 | 4.4 | 4.2 | 5.3 | | |
| Congenital Malformations | .8 | .8 | .3 | .3 | 1.3 | 1.5 | | |
| Certain Diseases of Early Infancy | .5 | .7 | 1.1 | 1.3 | .1 | .1 | | |
| Symptoms, Senility and Ill-Defined Conditions | 2.4 | 2.3 | 5.5 | 3.8 | .9 | 1.1 | | |
| Injuries and Adverse Effects of External Causes | 7.3 | 6.6 | 10.3 | 8.2 | 7.8 | 6.4 | | |
| TOTAL | 100.0 | 100.0 | 100.0 | 100.0 | 100.0 | 100.0 | 100.0 | 100.0 |

* Comprehensive Plan sample, excluding psychiatric admissions.

426

stays of surgically treated patients were much shorter than those of medical patients, the principal exception being disorders of the digestive system.

The average medical stay of 10.0 days was exceeded in seven categories—congenital malformations, neoplasms, blood diseases, bone diseases, allergies, diseases of early infancy, and circulatory diseases—each of which showed medical stays averaging between 11 and 13.8 days. Admissions with below-average medical stays were shown for most categories—skin and subcutaneous disorders, eye and ear disorders, disorders of male and female genital organs and breast, urinary and digestive conditions, injuries, respiratory diseases.

Surgical stays were longest for digestive conditions, circulatory disorders, bone disorders and neoplasms, shortest for respiratory, blood, skin, and ear conditions (Table 162).

### Distribution of Admissions and
### Days Within Each Diagnostic Category

The average length of stay shown in Table 162 for each diagnostic category fairly reflects major differences found. Variations may also be examined by noting for each diagnostic category the distribution of cases and aggregate days according to length of stay. The percentage of cases and days falling within specified length-of-stay intervals is shown in Table 163 for all cases and by type of case, in each category. Table 164, using the same data as Table 163, cumulates the distributions upward and downward to highlight similarities and differences found in the comparison of diagnostic categories.

In every diagnostic category, the majority of the admissions remained under 10 days but the range was from 54 per cent of circulatory conditions to 97 per cent of obstetrical cases. With few exceptions, however, more than half the aggregate days ascribed to each category were for admissions remaining 10 or more days. In all categories, relatively small proportions of admissions accounted for relatively large proportions of aggregate days. In categories typified by stays of 3 days or less —e.g. skin and respiratory conditions—only 25 to 30 per cent of

TABLE 162. Average Length of Stay, Surgical and Medical Admissions, by Major Diagnostic Categories

| | NUMBER OF DAYS PER STAY | | |
| DIAGNOSTIC CATEGORY | Hospital Admissions * | Surgical Admissions | Medical Admissions |
|---|---|---|---|
| Infective and Parasitic Diseases | 9.9 | — | 9.9 |
| Neoplasms | 8.8 | 8.2 | 11.8 |
| Allergic, Endocrine System, Metabolic and Nutritional Diseases | 10.4 | 7.5 | 11.0 |
| Diseases of Blood and Blood-Forming Organs | 9.4 | 2.0 | 10.8 |
| Diseases of the Nervous System | 8.8 | 5.4 | 10.0 |
| Diseases of the Eye | 5.6 | 5.4 | 6.9 |
| Diseases of the Ear | 5.6 | 4.5 | 7.5 |
| Diseases of the Circulatory System | 12.0 | 8.5 | 13.8 |
| Diseases of the Respiratory System | 4.1 | 1.7 | 9.0 |
| Diseases of the Digestive System | 9.3 | 9.8 | 8.5 |
| Diseases of the Urinary System | 7.8 | 7.1 | 8.5 |
| Diseases of the Male Genital Organs | 8.0 | 7.8 | 8.8 |
| Diseases of the Female Genital Organs and Breast | 6.3 | 6.2 | 7.6 |
| Deliveries and Complications of Pregnancy, Childbirth and Puerperium | 4.4 | — | — |
| Diseases of Skin and Subcutaneous Tissues | 5.4 | 3.9 | 6.8 |
| Diseases of Bones and Organs of Movement | 10.1 | 8.3 | 13.1 |
| Congenital Malformations | 7.7 | 6.9 | 11.2 |
| Certain Diseases of Early Infancy | 10.4 | 6.5 | 11.0 |
| Symptoms, Senility and Ill-Defined Conditions | 7.1 | 7.7 | 7.0 |
| Injuries and Adverse Effects of External Causes | 6.7 | 5.3 | 8.0 |
| TOTAL, Excluding Maternity | 8.0 | 6.5 | 10.0 |
| TOTAL, Including Maternity | 7.4 | — | — |

* Comprehensive Plan sample, excluding psychiatric admissions.

admissions remained as long as 6 days, but these cases accounted for 66 to 71 per cent of the aggregate days classified in these categories (Table 164 B). By the same token, 69 per cent of respiratory admissions remained under 4 days and accounted for only 22 per cent of aggregate days in this category, while 51 per cent of the admissions for skin disorders remained under 4 days and accounted for only 16 per cent of aggregate days charged to skin disorders (Table 164 A). In all categories, admissions remaining longer than 3 weeks were rare but the range was from 2.4 per cent of respiratory conditions to 11.6 per cent of circulatory conditions; in the latter instance, these admissions accounted for 34 per cent of aggregate days.

Blood diseases showed the largest proportion of cases remaining over 30 days—8.8 per cent; 37 per cent of aggregate days in this category resulted from such stays, as compared with 9 per cent for all categories combined.

TABLE 163. Distribution of Hospital
by Length of Stay
and by Type

A. ALL ADMISSIONS

| | PER CENT OF ADMISSIONS FOR EACH SPECIFIED | | | | | | | |
|---|---|---|---|---|---|---|---|---|
| | | | NUMBER OF DAYS HOSPITALIZED | | | | | |
| | TOTAL | | 1 | | 2 | | 3 | |
| DIAGNOSTIC CATEGORY | Adm. | Days | Adm. | Days | Adm. | Days | Adm. | Days |
| Infective and Parasitic Diseases | 100 | 100 | 0 | 0 | 5.4 | 1.1 | 8.1 | 2.5 |
| Neoplasms | 100 | 100 | 8.8 | 1.0 | 14.4 | 3.3 | 11.2 | 3.8 |
| Allergic, Endocrine System, Metabolic and Nutritional Diseases | 100 | 100 | 0 | 0 | 2.4 | .4 | 4.8 | 1.4 |
| Diseases of Blood and Blood-Forming Organs | 100 | 100 | 4.4 | .5 | 20.5 | 4.4 | 4.4 | 1.4 |
| Diseases of the Nervous System | 100 | 100 | 4.9 | .6 | 16.4 | 3.7 | 3.4 | 1.2 |
| Diseases of the Eye | 100 | 100 | 11.3 | 2.0 | 22.2 | 7.9 | 25.0 | 13.4 |
| Diseases of the Ear | 100 | 100 | 13.4 | 2.4 | 9.4 | 3.3 | 32.4 | 17.2 |
| Diseases of the Circulatory System | 100 | 100 | 1.9 | .1 | 3.5 | .6 | 6.1 | 1.5 |
| Diseases of the Respiratory System | 100 | 100 | 50.5 | 12.3 | 13.2 | 6.5 | 4.9 | 3.6 |
| Diseases of the Digestive System | 100 | 100 | 3.2 | .3 | 5.4 | 1.2 | 5.0 | 1.6 |
| Diseases of the Urinary System | 100 | 100 | 2.4 | .3 | 7.4 | 1.9 | 15.4 | 5.9 |
| Diseases of the Male Genital Organs | 100 | 100 | 21.4 | 2.7 | 7.2 | 1.7 | 7.2 | 2.7 |
| Diseases of the Female Genital Organs and Breast | 100 | 100 | 5.6 | .9 | 18.2 | 5.7 | 21.1 | 10.0 |
| Deliveries and Complications of Pregnancy, Childbirth and Puerperium | 100 | 100 | 2.4 | .6 | 6.5 | 3.0 | 12.8 | 8.7 |
| Diseases of Skin and Subcutaneous Tissues | 100 | 100 | 21.0 | 3.9 | 22.2 | 8.2 | 7.4 | 4.2 |
| Diseases of Bones and Organs of Movement | 100 | 100 | 4.0 | .5 | 19.8 | 5.6 | 15.9 | 5.7 |
| Congenital Malformations | 100 | 100 | 9.0 | 1.2 | 4.5 | 1.2 | 9.0 | 3.5 |
| Certain Diseases of Early Infancy | 100 | 100 | 0 | 0 | 0 | 0 | 4.8 | 1.4 |
| Symptoms, Senility and Ill-Defined Conditions | 100 | 100 | 2.8 | .4 | 11.1 | 3.2 | 12.5 | 5.3 |
| Injuries and Adverse Effects of External Causes | 100 | 100 | 16.3 | 2.4 | 14.7 | 4.4 | 12.9 | 5.8 |
| Undetermined Classifications | 100 | 100 | 15.5 | 1.8 | 19.4 | 4.6 | 5.6 | 2.0 |
| TOTAL, Including Obstetrics | 100 | 100 | 11.7 | 1.6 | 10.1 | 2.7 | 10.0 | 4.0 |
| TOTAL, Excluding Obstetrics | 100 | 100 | 13.6 | 1.7 | 10.9 | 2.7 | 9.4 | 3.5 |

* Comprehensive Plan sample.

# Admissions and Aggregate Days within Diagnostic Category of Admission

| | | | | | | | | | | | |
|---|---|---|---|---|---|---|---|---|---|---|---|
| NUMBER OF DAYS HOSPITALIZED | | | | | | | | | | | |
| 4–5 | | 6–9 | | 10–14 | | 15–21 | | 22–30 | | 31 *or more* | |
| Adm. | Days | Adm. | Days | Adm. | Days | Adm. | Days | Adm. | Days | Adm. | Days |
| 24.4 | 11.4 | 24.3 | 18.0 | 13.5 | 16.6 | 16.2 | 31.3 | 8.1 | 19.1 | 0 | 0 |
| 12.5 | 6.1 | 16.2 | 13.6 | 17.3 | 21.9 | 11.7 | 23.5 | 4.8 | 13.5 | 3.1 | 13.3 |
| 13.5 | 6.4 | 40.0 | 27.9 | 20.9 | 24.3 | 9.6 | 15.9 | 6.4 | 15.9 | 2.4 | 7.8 |
| 13.3 | 6.6 | 26.5 | 22.0 | 22.1 | 28.1 | 0 | 0 | 0 | 0 | 8.8 | 37.0 |
| 14.7 | 7.3 | 25.6 | 20.5 | 18.8 | 25.5 | 10.9 | 24.0 | 3.0 | 7.9 | 2.3 | 9.3 |
| 13.7 | 11.0 | 9.7 | 13.8 | 8.5 | 16.2 | 5.6 | 15.6 | 4.0 | 20.1 | 0 | 0 |
| 6.8 | 5.7 | 20.3 | 25.0 | 6.5 | 13.5 | 11.2 | 32.9 | 0 | 0 | 0 | 0 |
| 16.7 | 6.3 | 25.5 | 15.3 | 19.4 | 19.3 | 15.3 | 22.8 | 6.4 | 13.5 | 5.2 | 20.8 |
| 6.4 | 6.9 | 12.5 | 22.3 | 7.1 | 21.1 | 3.0 | 12.1 | 2.0 | 12.3 | .4 | 2.9 |
| 17.4 | 8.7 | 31.6 | 25.2 | 19.4 | 24.1 | 13.1 | 24.6 | 3.8 | 10.0 | 1.1 | 4.3 |
| 20.2 | 11.4 | 29.4 | 28.2 | 12.3 | 19.2 | 9.2 | 19.5 | 2.5 | 7.7 | 1.2 | 5.9 |
| 17.8 | 8.9 | 11.4 | 10.7 | 20.7 | 29.2 | 7.2 | 15.6 | 3.5 | 12.0 | 3.6 | 16.5 |
| 17.0 | 11.7 | 13.5 | 16.0 | 17.0 | 30.9 | 5.9 | 17.4 | 1.7 | 7.4 | 0 | 0 |
| 65.8 | 65.9 | 9.8 | 15.3 | 2.7 | 6.5 | 0 | 0 | 0 | 0 | 0 | 0 |
| 19.8 | 16.6 | 12.3 | 16.2 | 8.6 | 19.5 | 6.2 | 20.7 | 2.5 | 10.7 | 0 | 0 |
| 16.4 | 10.2 | 18.2 | 19.3 | 8.9 | 13.0 | 10.4 | 22.6 | 4.9 | 17.3 | 1.5 | 5.8 |
| 19.3 | 10.7 | 36.1 | 34.8 | 7.4 | 11.8 | 10.2 | 22.7 | 4.5 | 14.1 | 0 | 0 |
| 4.8 | 2.3 | 47.2 | 30.8 | 24.0 | 26.7 | 14.4 | 24.9 | 4.8 | 13.9 | 0 | 0 |
| 18.9 | 11.4 | 37.3 | 38.2 | 9.7 | 17.7 | 4.9 | 11.9 | 1.9 | 7.3 | .9 | 4.6 |
| 19.3 | 13.0 | 16.2 | 16.9 | 11.1 | 19.4 | 4.6 | 12.7 | 1.5 | 6.3 | 3.4 | 19.1 |
| 13.5 | 7.0 | 17.3 | 16.0 | 13.5 | 17.7 | 7.6 | 18.1 | 3.1 | 10.8 | 4.5 | 22.0 |
| 23.2 | 14.0 | 19.8 | 19.5 | 12.8 | 20.3 | 7.7 | 18.4 | 3.0 | 10.2 | 1.7 | 9.3 |
| 14.6 | 8.2 | 21.8 | 19.9 | 14.9 | 21.9 | 9.2 | 20.4 | 3.6 | 11.4 | 2.0 | 10.3 |

TABLE 163. *(Cont'd).* Distribution of Hospital
by Length of Stay
and by Type

B. SURGICAL ADMISSIONS

| | | | PER CENT OF ADMISSIONS FOR EACH SPECIFIED | | | | | |
|---|---|---|---|---|---|---|---|---|
| | | | NUMBER OF DAYS HOSPITALIZED | | | | | |
| | TOTAL | | 1 | | 2 | | 3 | |
| DIAGNOSTIC CATEGORY | Adm. | Days | Adm. | Days | Adm. | Days | Adm. | Days |
| Neoplasms | 100 | 100 | 9.0 | 1.1 | 15.7 | 3.8 | 11.2 | 4.1 |
| Allergic, Endocrine System, Metabolic and Nutritional Diseases | 100 | 100 | 0 | 0 | 0 | 0 | 0 | 0 |
| Diseases of Blood and Blood-Forming Organs | 100 | 100 | 0 | 0 | 100.0 | 100.0 | 0 | 0 |
| Diseases of the Nervous System | 100 | 100 | 14.3 | 2.5 | 57.2 | 20.8 | 0 | 0 |
| Diseases of the Eye | 100 | 100 | 12.5 | 2.3 | 21.9 | 8.0 | 25.0 | 13.7 |
| Diseases of the Ear | 100 | 100 | 7.7 | 1.8 | 15.4 | 6.9 | 46.1 | 31.0 |
| Diseases of the Circulatory System | 100 | 100 | 1.6 | .2 | 0 | 0 | 11.1 | 3.9 |
| Diseases of the Respiratory System | 100 | 100 | 73.0 | 40.4 | 16.4 | 18.2 | 4.8 | 7.9 |
| Diseases of the Digestive System | 100 | 100 | 2.4 | .2 | 4.2 | .9 | 5.4 | 1.6 |
| Diseases of the Urinary System | 100 | 100 | 2.5 | .3 | 12.8 | 3.6 | 23.1 | 9.7 |
| Diseases of the Male Genital Organs | 100 | 100 | 23.1 | 2.9 | 7.7 | 1.9 | 7.7 | 2.9 |
| Diseases of the Female Genital Organs and Breast | 100 | 100 | 5.7 | .9 | 19.8 | 6.4 | 22.6 | 11.0 |
| Diseases of Skin and Subcutaneous Tissues | 100 | 100 | 40.0 | 9.9 | 20.0 | 9.9 | 5.0 | 3.7 |
| Diseases of Bones and Organs of Movement | 100 | 100 | 4.9 | .6 | 17.1 | 4.1 | 19.5 | 7.0 |
| Congenital Malformations | 100 | 100 | 10.5 | 1.5 | 5.3 | 1.5 | 10.5 | 4.5 |
| Certain Diseases of Early Infancy | 100 | 100 | 0 | 0 | 0 | 0 | 0 | 0 |
| Symptoms, Senility and Ill-Defined Conditions | 100 | 100 | 0 | 0 | 25.0 | 6.5 | 8.3 | 3.3 |
| Injuries and Adverse Effects of External Causes | 100 | 100 | 24.4 | 4.5 | 18.3 | 6.8 | 15.8 | 8.9 |
| Undetermined Classifications | 100 | 100 | 13.6 | 1.9 | 22.7 | 6.3 | 4.6 | 1.9 |
| TOTAL | 100 | 100 | 20.7 | 3.2 | 14.2 | 4.3 | 11.7 | 5.3 |

* Comprehensive Plan sample.

# Admissions and Aggregate Days
## within Diagnostic Category
## of Admission

AND AGGREGATE DAYS INCURRED
LENGTH OF STAY *

| | | | | NUMBER OF DAYS HOSPITALIZED | | | | | | | |
|---|---|---|---|---|---|---|---|---|---|---|---|
| 4–5 | | 6–9 | | 10–14 | | 15–21 | | 22–30 | | 31 *or more* | |
| Adm. | Days | Adm. | Days | Adm. | Days | Adm. | Days | Adm. | Days | Adm. | Days |
| 12.4 | 6.6 | 14.6 | 13.1 | 19.1 | 26.2 | 11.8 | 25.4 | 5.1 | 15.3 | 1.1 | 4.4 |
| 0 | 0 | 90.0 | 81.3 | 10.0 | 18.7 | 0 | 0 | 0 | 0 | 0 | 0 |
| 0 | 0 | 0 | 0 | 0 | 0 | 0 | 0 | 0 | 0 | 0 | 0 |
| 0 | 0 | 7.1 | 7.8 | 7.1 | 13.0 | 7.2 | 27.3 | 7.1 | 28.6 | 0 | 0 |
| 12.5 | 10.3 | 9.4 | 13.7 | 9.4 | 18.3 | 6.2 | 17.7 | 3.1 | 16.0 | 0 | 0 |
| 7.7 | 8.6 | 15.4 | 22.4 | 0 | 0 | 7.7 | 29.3 | 0 | 0 | 0 | 0 |
| 28.6 | 15.1 | 34.9 | 27.8 | 11.1 | 14.9 | 7.9 | 15.1 | 1.6 | 4.3 | 3.2 | 18.7 |
| 2.1 | 5.6 | 2.1 | 9.1 | 0 | 0 | .5 | 5.0 | 1.1 | 13.8 | 0 | 0 |
| 16.2 | 7.6 | 30.5 | 23.1 | 19.1 | 22.7 | 16.8 | 29.7 | 4.8 | 11.8 | .6 | 2.4 |
| 23.1 | 14.4 | 7.7 | 7.2 | 15.4 | 26.3 | 12.8 | 28.8 | 2.6 | 9.7 | 0 | 0 |
| 19.2 | 9.7 | 7.7 | 7.2 | 19.2 | 27.6 | 7.7 | 16.9 | 3.8 | 13.0 | 3.9 | 17.9 |
| 17.0 | 12.0 | 10.4 | 12.7 | 17.0 | 31.5 | 5.6 | 17.0 | 1.9 | 8.5 | 0 | 0 |
| 20.0 | 23.5 | 0 | 0 | 10.0 | 29.5 | 5.0 | 23.5 | 0 | 0 | 0 | 0 |
| 14.6 | 7.9 | 14.6 | 13.5 | 9.8 | 12.3 | 12.2 | 25.8 | 4.9 | 17.6 | 2.4 | 11.2 |
| 15.8 | 9.7 | 42.1 | 44.0 | 5.3 | 9.7 | 5.2 | 11.2 | 5.3 | 17.9 | 0 | 0 |
| 0 | 0 | 100.0 | 100.0 | 0 | 0 | 0 | 0 | 0 | 0 | 0 | 0 |
| 8.3 | 4.3 | 33.3 | 32.6 | 8.4 | 15.2 | 16.7 | 38.1 | 0 | 0 | 0 | 0 |
| 17.1 | 13.6 | 9.7 | 12.3 | 6.1 | 14.1 | 3.7 | 12.3 | 2.4 | 12.7 | 2.5 | 14.8 |
| 13.6 | 8.2 | 22.7 | 23.3 | 13.6 | 20.7 | 4.6 | 11.9 | 0 | 0 | 4.6 | 25.8 |
| 13.4 | 9.1 | 16.0 | 17.8 | 11.9 | 21.1 | 8.1 | 21.7 | 3.0 | 11.8 | 1.0 | 5.7 |

TABLE 163 *(Concluded).*   Distribution of Hospital
by Length of Stay
and by Type

C. MEDICAL ADMISSIONS

|  | | | PER CENT OF ADMISSIONS FOR EACH SPECIFIED | | | | | |
|---|---|---|---|---|---|---|---|---|
|  | | | NUMBER OF DAYS HOSPITALIZED | | | | | |
|  | TOTAL | | 1 | | 2 | | 3 | |
| DIAGNOSTIC CATEGORY | Adm. | Days | Adm. | Days | Adm. | Days | Adm. | Days |
| Infective and Parasitic Diseases | 100 | 100 | 0 | 0 | 5.4 | 1.1 | 8.1 | 2.5 |
| Neoplasms | 100 | 100 | 8.1 | .7 | 8.1 | 1.4 | 11.3 | 2.9 |
| Allergic, Endocrine System, Metabolic and Nutritional Diseases | 100 | 100 | 0 | 0 | 2.9 | .5 | 5.8 | 1.6 |
| Diseases of Blood and Blood-Forming Organs | 100 | 100 | 5.3 | .5 | 5.3 | 1.0 | 5.3 | 1.5 |
| Diseases of the Nervous System | 100 | 100 | 1.5 | .2 | 1.5 | .3 | 4.7 | 1.4 |
| Diseases of the Eye | 100 | 100 | 0 | 0 | 25.0 | 7.3 | 25.0 | 10.9 |
| Diseases of the Ear | 100 | 100 | 22.2 | 3.0 | 0 | 0 | 11.1 | 4.4 |
| Diseases of the Circulatory System | 100 | 100 | 2.0 | .1 | 5.2 | .8 | 3.6 | .8 |
| Diseases of the Respiratory System | 100 | 100 | 2.6 | .3 | 6.2 | 1.4 | 5.2 | 1.7 |
| Diseases of the Digestive System | 100 | 100 | 4.2 | .5 | 6.9 | 1.6 | 4.5 | 1.6 |
| Diseases of the Urinary System | 100 | 100 | 2.4 | .3 | 2.4 | .6 | 8.2 | 2.9 |
| Diseases of the Male Genital Organs | 100 | 100 | 0 | 0 | 0 | 0 | 0 | 0 |
| Diseases of the Female Genital Organs and Breast | 100 | 100 | 4.3 | .6 | 4.3 | 1.2 | 8.7 | 3.4 |
| Diseases of Skin and Subcutaneous Tissues | 100 | 100 | 2.4 | .4 | 24.4 | 7.2 | 9.8 | 4.4 |
| Diseases of Bones and Organs of Movement | 100 | 100 | 3.8 | .3 | 1.9 | .3 | 3.8 | .9 |
| Congenital Malformations | 100 | 100 | 0 | 0 | 0 | 0 | 0 | 0 |
| Certain Diseases of Early Infancy | 100 | 100 | 0 | 0 | 0 | 0 | 5.5 | 1.5 |
| Symptoms, Senility and Ill-Defined Conditions | 100 | 100 | 3.4 | .5 | 7.9 | 2.3 | 13.5 | 5.8 |
| Injuries and Adverse Effects of External Causes | 100 | 100 | 8.0 | 1.0 | 11.1 | 2.8 | 9.9 | 3.7 |
| Undetermined Classifications | 100 | 100 | 17.8 | 1.8 | 15.6 | 3.2 | 6.7 | 2.0 |
| TOTAL | 100 | 100 | 4.0 | .4 | 6.4 | 1.3 | 6.4 | 1.9 |
|  | | | | | | | | |
| D. OBSTETRICAL ADMISSIONS | | | | | | | | |
|  | | | | | | | | |
| Deliveries and Complications of Pregnancy, Childbirth and Puerperium | 100 | 100 | 2.4 | .6 | 6.5 | 3.0 | 12.8 | 8.7 |

* Comprehensive Plan sample.

# Admissions and Aggregate Days
## within Diagnostic Category
## of Admission

AND AGGREGATE DAYS INCURRED
LENGTH OF STAY *

| | | | | NUMBER OF DAYS HOSPITALIZED | | | | | | | |
|---|---|---|---|---|---|---|---|---|---|---|---|
| 4–5 | | 6–9 | | 10–14 | | 15–21 | | 22–30 | | 31 *or more* | |
| *Adm.* | *Days* | *Adm.* | *Days* | *Adm.* | *Days* | *Adm.* | *Days* | *Adm.* | *Days* | *Adm.* | *Days* |
| 24.4 | 11.4 | 24.3 | 18.0 | 13.5 | 16.6 | 16.2 | 31.3 | 8.1 | 19.1 | 0 | 0 |
| 12.9 | 4.6 | 24.1 | 15.2 | 8.1 | 7.2 | 11.3 | 16.9 | 3.2 | 7.1 | 12.9 | 44.0 |
| | | | | | | | | | | | |
| 16.3 | 7.3 | 29.8 | 20.4 | 23.1 | 25.1 | 11.5 | 18.1 | 7.7 | 18.1 | 2.9 | 8.9 |
| | | | | | | | | | | | |
| 15.8 | 6.8 | 31.5 | 22.8 | 26.3 | 29.1 | 0 | 0 | 0 | 0 | 10.5 | 38.3 |
| 20.0 | 8.8 | 32.3 | 23.1 | 23.1 | 28.0 | 12.3 | 23.3 | 1.5 | 3.8 | 3.1 | 11.1 |
| 25.0 | 16.4 | 12.5 | 14.5 | 0 | 0 | 0 | 0 | 12.5 | 50.9 | 0 | 0 |
| 5.5 | 3.0 | 27.8 | 27.4 | 16.7 | 25.9 | 16.7 | 36.3 | 0 | 0 | 0 | 0 |
| 10.8 | 3.6 | 20.9 | 11.4 | 23.5 | 20.6 | 19.0 | 25.2 | 8.8 | 16.3 | 6.2 | 21.2 |
| 15.5 | 7.5 | 34.7 | 28.0 | 22.3 | 30.1 | 8.3 | 15.2 | 4.1 | 11.6 | 1.1 | 4.2 |
| 19.1 | 10.4 | 33.0 | 28.3 | 19.8 | 26.3 | 8.3 | 16.9 | 2.4 | 7.2 | 1.8 | 7.2 |
| 17.6 | 9.0 | 49.4 | 44.5 | 9.4 | 13.7 | 5.9 | 12.4 | 2.4 | 6.1 | 2.3 | 10.5 |
| 0 | 0 | 60.0 | 52.3 | 40.0 | 47.7 | 0 | 0 | 0 | 0 | 0 | 0 |
| | | | | | | | | | | | |
| 17.4 | 9.8 | 39.2 | 38.5 | 17.4 | 26.4 | 8.7 | 20.1 | 0 | 0 | 0 | 0 |
| 19.5 | 12.6 | 24.4 | 25.6 | 7.3 | 13.7 | 7.3 | 19.1 | 4.9 | 17.0 | 0 | 0 |
| 7.5 | 2.6 | 26.4 | 15.0 | 30.2 | 28.0 | 15.1 | 20.2 | 3.8 | 6.4 | 7.5 | 26.3 |
| 40.0 | 14.3 | 0 | 0 | 20.0 | 19.6 | 40.0 | 66.1 | 0 | 0 | 0 | 0 |
| 5.5 | 2.5 | 38.9 | 24.2 | 27.8 | 29.3 | 16.7 | 27.3 | 5.6 | 15.2 | 0 | 0 |
| | | | | | | | | | | | |
| 21.3 | 13.2 | 38.2 | 39.6 | 10.1 | 18.4 | 2.2 | 5.2 | 2.3 | 9.2 | 1.1 | 5.8 |
| | | | | | | | | | | | |
| 21.6 | 12.5 | 22.8 | 20.0 | 16.1 | 23.0 | 5.6 | 13.0 | .6 | 1.9 | 4.3 | 22.1 |
| 13.3 | 5.9 | 11.1 | 9.7 | 13.3 | 15.2 | 11.1 | 23.4 | 6.7 | 20.0 | 4.4 | 18.8 |
| | | | | | | | | | | | |
| 16.3 | 7.4 | 29.5 | 21.8 | 18.9 | 22.5 | 10.8 | 19.3 | 4.3 | 11.0 | 3.4 | 14.4 |
| | | | | | | | | | | | |
| | | | | | | | | | | | |
| 65.8 | 65.9 | 9.8 | 15.3 | 2.7 | 6.5 | 0 | 0 | 0 | 0 | 0 | 0 |

TABLE 164.   Cumulative Distribution of
by Length of Stay

**A. CUMULATED FROM SHORTEST STAYS**

| DIAGNOSTIC CATEGORY | PER CENT OF ADMISSIONS AND AGGREGATE | | | | | | | |
|---|---|---|---|---|---|---|---|---|
| | 1 DAY | | 1 OR 2 DAYS | | 1–3 DAYS | | 1–5 DAYS | |
| | Adm. | Days | Adm. | Days | Adm. | Days | Adm. | Days |
| Infective and Parasitic Diseases | 0 | 0 | 5.4 | 1.1 | 13.5 | 3.6 | 37.9 | 15.0 |
| Neoplasms | 8.8 | 1.0 | 23.2 | 4.3 | 34.4 | 8.1 | 46.9 | 14.2 |
| Allergic, Endocrine System, Metabolic and Nutritional Diseases | 0 | 0 | 2.4 | .4 | 7.2 | 1.8 | 20.7 | 8.2 |
| Diseases of Blood and Blood-Forming Organs | 4.4 | .5 | 24.9 | 4.9 | 29.3 | 6.3 | 42.6 | 12.9 |
| Diseases of the Nervous System | 4.9 | .6 | 21.3 | 4.3 | 24.7 | 5.5 | 39.4 | 12.8 |
| Diseases of the Eye | 11.3 | 2.0 | 33.5 | 9.9 | 58.5 | 23.3 | 72.2 | 34.3 |
| Diseases of the Ear | 13.4 | 2.4 | 22.8 | 5.7 | 55.2 | 22.9 | 62.0 | 28.6 |
| Diseases of the Circulatory System | 1.9 | .1 | 5.4 | .7 | 11.5 | 2.2 | 28.2 | 8.5 |
| Diseases of the Respiratory System | 50.5 | 12.3 | 63.7 | 18.8 | 68.6 | 22.4 | 75.0 | 29.3 |
| Diseases of the Digestive System | 3.2 | .3 | 8.6 | 1.5 | 13.6 | 3.1 | 31.0 | 11.8 |
| Diseases of the Urinary System | 2.4 | .3 | 9.8 | 2.2 | 25.2 | 8.1 | 45.4 | 19.5 |
| Diseases of the Male Genital Organs | 21.4 | 2.7 | 28.6 | 4.4 | 35.8 | 7.1 | 53.6 | 16.0 |
| Diseases of the Female Genital Organs and Breast | 5.6 | .9 | 23.8 | 6.6 | 44.9 | 16.6 | 61.9 | 28.3 |
| Deliveries and Complications of Pregnancy, Childbirth and Puerperium | 2.4 | .6 | 8.9 | 3.6 | 21.7 | 12.3 | 87.5 | 78.2 |
| Diseases of Skin and Subcutaneous Tissues | 21.0 | 3.9 | 43.2 | 12.1 | 50.6 | 16.3 | 70.4 | 32.9 |
| Diseases of Bones and Organs of Movement | 4.0 | .5 | 23.8 | 6.1 | 39.7 | 11.8 | 56.1 | 22.0 |
| Congenital Malformations | 9.0 | 1.2 | 13.5 | 2.4 | 22.5 | 5.9 | 41.8 | 16.6 |
| Certain Diseases of Early Infancy | 0 | 0 | 0 | 0 | 4.8 | 1.4 | 9.6 | 3.7 |
| Symptoms, Senility and Ill-Defined Conditions | 2.8 | .4 | 13.9 | 3.6 | 26.4 | 8.9 | 45.3 | 20.3 |
| Injuries and Adverse Effects of External Causes | 16.3 | 2.4 | 31.0 | 6.8 | 43.9 | 12.6 | 63.2 | 25.6 |
| Undetermined Classifications | 15.5 | 1.8 | 34.9 | 6.4 | 40.5 | 8.4 | 54.0 | 15.4 |
| TOTAL, Including Obstetrics | 11.7 | 1.6 | 21.8 | 4.3 | 31.8 | 8.3 | 55.0 | 22.3 |
| TOTAL, Excluding Obstetrics | 13.6 | 1.7 | 24.5 | 4.4 | 33.9 | 7.9 | 48.5 | 16.1 |

* Comprehensive Plan sample.

# Hospital Admissions and Aggregate Days within Diagnostic Category

## DAYS ACCUMULATED AT SPECIFIED INTERVALS *

| 1–9 DAYS | | 1–14 DAYS | | 1–21 DAYS | | 1–30 DAYS | | ALL | |
|---|---|---|---|---|---|---|---|---|---|
| Adm. | Days | Adm. | Days | Adm. | Days | Adm. | Days | Adm. | Days |
| 62.2 | 33.0 | 75.7 | 49.6 | 91.9 | 80.9 | 100.0 | 100.0 | | |
| 63.1 | 27.8 | 80.4 | 49.7 | 92.1 | 73.2 | 96.9 | 86.7 | 100.0 | 100.0 |
| 60.7 | 36.1 | 81.6 | 60.4 | 91.2 | 76.3 | 97.6 | 92.2 | 100.0 | 100.0 |
| 69.1 | 34.9 | 91.2 | 63.0 | 91.2 | 63.0 | 91.2 | 63.0 | 100.0 | 100.0 |
| 65.0 | 33.3 | 83.8 | 58.8 | 94.7 | 82.8 | 97.7 | 90.7 | 100.0 | 100.0 |
| 81.9 | 48.1 | 90.4 | 64.3 | 96.0 | 79.9 | 100.0 | 100.0 | | |
| 82.3 | 53.6 | 88.8 | 67.1 | 100.0 | 100.0 | | | | |
| 53.7 | 23.8 | 73.1 | 43.1 | 88.4 | 65.9 | 94.8 | 79.4 | 100.0 | 100.0 |
| 87.5 | 51.6 | 94.6 | 72.7 | 97.6 | 84.8 | 99.6 | 97.1 | 100.0 | 100.0 |
| 62.6 | 37.0 | 82.0 | 61.1 | 95.1 | 85.7 | 98.9 | 95.7 | 100.0 | 100.0 |
| 74.8 | 47.7 | 87.1 | 66.9 | 96.3 | 86.4 | 98.8 | 94.1 | 100.0 | 100.0 |
| 65.0 | 26.7 | 85.7 | 55.9 | 92.9 | 71.5 | 96.4 | 83.5 | 100.0 | 100.0 |
| 75.4 | 44.3 | | | | | | | | |
| | | 92.4 | 75.2 | 98.3 | 92.6 | 100.0 | 100.0 | | |
| 97.3 | 93.5 | 100.0 | 100.0 | | | | | | |
| 82.7 | 49.1 | 91.3 | 68.6 | 97.5 | 89.3 | 100.0 | 100.0 | | |
| 74.3 | 41.3 | 83.2 | 54.3 | 93.6 | 76.9 | 98.5 | 94.2 | 100.0 | 100.0 |
| 77.9 | 51.4 | 85.3 | 63.2 | 95.5 | 85.9 | 100.0 | 100.0 | | |
| 56.8 | 34.5 | 80.8 | 61.2 | 95.2 | 86.1 | 100.0 | 100.0 | | |
| 82.6 | 58.5 | 92.3 | 76.2 | 97.2 | 88.1 | 99.1 | 95.4 | 100.0 | 100.0 |
| 79.4 | 42.5 | 90.5 | 61.9 | 95.1 | 74.6 | 96.6 | 80.9 | 100.0 | 100.0 |
| 71.3 | 31.4 | 84.8 | 49.1 | 92.4 | 67.2 | 95.5 | 78.0 | 100.0 | 100.0 |
| 74.8 | 41.8 | 87.6 | 62.1 | 95.3 | 80.5 | 98.3 | 90.7 | 100.0 | 100.0 |
| 70.3 | 36.0 | 85.2 | 57.9 | 94.4 | 78.3 | 98.0 | 89.7 | 100.0 | 100.0 |

TABLE 164 *(Concluded).* Cumulative Distribution of
by Length of Stay

B. CUMULATED FROM LONGEST STAYS

| DIAGNOSTIC CATEGORY | PER CENT OF ADMISSIONS AND | | | | | |
|---|---|---|---|---|---|---|
| | 31 OR MORE DAYS | | 22 OR MORE DAYS | | 15 OR MORE DAYS | |
| | Adm. | Days | Adm. | Days | Adm. | Days |
| Infective and Parasitic Diseases | 0 | 0 | 8.1 | 19.1 | 24.3 | 50.4 |
| Neoplasms | 3.1 | 13.3 | 7.9 | 26.8 | 19.6 | 50.3 |
| Allergic, Endocrine System, Metabolic and Nutritional Diseases | 2.4 | 7.8 | 8.8 | 23.7 | 18.4 | 39.6 |
| Diseases of Blood and Blood-Forming Organs | 8.8 | 37.0 | 8.8 | 37.0 | 8.8 | 37.0 |
| Diseases of the Nervous System | 2.3 | 9.3 | 5.3 | 17.2 | 16.2 | 41.2 |
| Diseases of the Eye | 0 | 0 | 4.0 | 20.1 | 9.6 | 35.7 |
| Diseases of the Ear | 0 | 0 | 0 | 0 | 11.2 | 32.9 |
| Diseases of the Circulatory System | 5.2 | 20.6 | 11.6 | 34.1 | 26.9 | 56.9 |
| Diseases of the Respiratory System | .4 | 2.9 | 2.4 | 15.2 | 5.4 | 27.3 |
| Diseases of the Digestive System | 1.1 | 4.3 | 4.9 | 14.3 | 18.0 | 38.9 |
| Diseases of the Urinary System | 1.2 | 5.9 | 3.7 | 13.6 | 12.9 | 33.1 |
| Diseases of the Male Genital Organs | 3.6 | 16.5 | 7.1 | 28.5 | 14.3 | 44.1 |
| Diseases of the Female Genital Organs and Breast | 0 | 0 | 1.7 | 7.4 | 7.6 | 24.8 |
| Deliveries and Complications of Pregnancy, Childbirth and Puerperium | 0 | 0 | 0 | 0 | 0 | 0 |
| Diseases of Skin and Subcutaneous Tissues | 0 | 0 | 2.5 | 10.7 | 8.7 | 31.4 |
| Diseases of Bones and Organs of Movement | 1.5 | 5.8 | 6.4 | 23.1 | 16.8 | 45.7 |
| Congenital Malformations | 0 | 0 | 4.5 | 14.1 | 14.7 | 36.8 |
| Certain Diseases of Early Infancy | 0 | 0 | 4.8 | 13.9 | 19.2 | 38.8 |
| Symptoms, Senility and Ill-Defined Conditions | .9 | 4.6 | 2.8 | 11.9 | 7.7 | 23.8 |
| Injuries and Adverse Effects of External Causes | 3.4 | 19.1 | 4.9 | 25.4 | 9.5 | 38.1 |
| Undetermined Classifications | 4.5 | 22.0 | 7.6 | 32.8 | 15.2 | 50.9 |
| TOTAL, Including Obstetrics | 1.7 | 9.3 | 4.7 | 19.5 | 12.4 | 37.9 |
| TOTAL, Excluding Obstetrics | 2.0 | 10.3 | 5.6 | 21.7 | 14.8 | 42.1 |

* Comprehensive Plan sample.

**438**

# Hospital Admissions and Aggregate Days within Diagnostic Category

| DAYS ACCUMULATED AT SPECIFIED INTERVALS * | | | | | | | |
| 10 OR MORE DAYS | | 6 OR MORE DAYS | | 4 OR MORE DAYS | | 3 OR MORE DAYS | |
| Adm. | Days | Adm. | Days | Adm. | Days | Adm. | Days |
|---|---|---|---|---|---|---|---|
| 37.8 | 67.0 | 62.1 | 85.0 | 66.5 | 96.4 | 74.6 | 98.9 |
| 36.9 | 72.2 | 53.1 | 85.8 | 65.6 | 91.9 | 76.8 | 95.7 |
| 39.3 | 63.9 | 79.3 | 91.8 | 92.8 | 98.2 | 97.6 | 99.6 |
| 30.9 | 65.1 | 57.4 | 89.1 | 70.7 | 93.7 | 75.1 | 95.1 |
| 35.0 | 66.7 | 60.6 | 87.2 | 75.3 | 94.5 | 78.7 | 95.7 |
| 18.1 | 51.9 | 27.8 | 65.7 | 41.5 | 76.7 | 66.5 | 90.1 |
| 17.7 | 46.4 | 38.0 | 71.4 | 44.8 | 77.1 | 77.2 | 94.3 |
| 46.3 | 76.2 | 71.8 | 91.5 | 88.5 | 97.8 | 94.6 | 99.3 |
| 12.5 | 48.4 | 25.0 | 70.7 | 31.4 | 77.6 | 36.3 | 81.2 |
| 37.4 | 63.0 | 69.0 | 88.2 | 86.4 | 96.9 | 91.4 | 98.5 |
| 25.2 | 52.3 | 54.6 | 80.5 | 74.8 | 91.9 | 90.2 | 97.8 |
| 35.0 | 73.3 | 46.4 | 84.0 | 64.2 | 92.9 | 71.4 | 95.6 |
| 24.6 | 55.7 | 38.1 | 71.7 | 55.1 | 83.4 | 76.2 | 93.4 |
| 2.7 | 6.5 | 12.5 | 21.8 | 78.3 | 87.7 | 81.1 | 96.4 |
| 17.3 | 50.9 | 29.6 | 67.1 | 49.4 | 83.7 | 56.8 | 87.9 |
| 25.7 | 58.7 | 43.9 | 78.0 | 60.3 | 88.2 | 76.2 | 93.9 |
| 22.1 | 48.6 | 58.2 | 83.4 | 77.5 | 94.1 | 86.5 | 97.6 |
| 43.2 | 65.5 | 90.4 | 96.3 | 95.2 | 98.6 | 95.2 | 100.0 |
| 17.4 | 41.5 | 54.7 | 79.7 | 73.6 | 91.1 | 86.1 | 96.4 |
| 20.6 | 57.5 | 36.8 | 74.4 | 56.1 | 87.4 | 69.0 | 93.2 |
| 28.7 | 68.6 | 46.0 | 84.6 | 59.5 | 91.6 | 65.1 | 93.6 |
| 25.2 | 58.2 | 45.0 | 77.7 | 68.2 | 91.7 | 78.2 | 95.7 |
| 29.7 | 64.0 | 51.5 | 83.9 | 66.1 | 92.1 | 75.5 | 95.6 |

# INDEX